Landmark Papers in Psychiatry

Landmark Papers in ... series

Titles in the series

Landmark Papers in Psychiatry
Edited by Elizabeth Ryznar, Aderonke B. Pederson, Mark A. Reinecke, and John G. Csernansky

Landmark Papers in Otolaryngology
Edited by John S. Phillips and Sally Erskine

Landmark Papers in Pain
Edited by Paul Farquhar-Smith, Pierre Beaulieu, and Sian Jagger

Landmark Papers in Neurology
Edited by Martin R. Turner and Matthew C. Kiernan

Landmark Papers in Rheumatology
Edited by Richard A. Watts and David G. I. Scott

Landmark Papers in Neurosurgery, Second Edition
Edited by Reuben D. Johnson and Alexander L. Green

Landmark Papers in Anaesthesia
Edited by Nigel R. Webster and Helen F. Galley

Landmark Papers in Nephrology
Edited by John Feehally, Christopher McIntyre, and J. Stewart Cameron

Landmark Papers in Allergy
Edited by Aziz Sheikh, Thomas Platts-Mills, and Allison Worth, with Stephen Holgate

Landmark Papers in General Surgery
Edited by Graham MacKay, Richard Molloy, and Patrick O'Dwyer

Landmark Papers in Cardiovascular Medicine
Edited by Aung Myat and Tony Gershlick

Landmark Papers in Psychiatry

Seminal Papers with Expert Commentaries

Edited by

Elizabeth Ryznar

Resident in Psychiatry, McGaw Medical Center, Northwestern University's, Feinberg School of Medicine, Chicago, USA

Aderonke B. Pederson

Chief Resident in Psychiatry, McGaw Medical Center, Northwestern University's, Feinberg School of Medicine, Chicago, USA

Mark A. Reinecke

Professor of Psychiatry and Behavioral Sciences, Chief-Division of Psychology, Feinberg School of Medicine, Northwestern University, Chicago, USA

John G. Csernansky

Gilman Professor and Chair, Department of Psychiatry and Behavioral Sciences, Feinberg School of Medicine, Northwestern University, Chicago, USA

OXFORD
UNIVERSITY PRESS

OXFORD
UNIVERSITY PRESS

Great Clarendon Street, Oxford, OX2 6DP,
United Kingdom

Oxford University Press is a department of the University of Oxford.
It furthers the University's objective of excellence in research, scholarship,
and education by publishing worldwide. Oxford is a registered trade mark of
Oxford University Press in the UK and in certain other countries

First Edition published in 2020

Impression: 5

Published in the United States of America by Oxford University Press
198 Madison Avenue, New York, NY 10016, United States of America

British Library Cataloguing in Publication Data

Data available

Library of Congress Control Number: 2019950173

ISBN 978–0–19–883650–6

Printed in Great Britain by
Ashford Colour Press Ltd, Gosport, Hampshire

This book is dedicated to our students of psychiatry and psychology, whose intellectual curiosity continues to inspire.

Preface

Several decades ago, acclaimed developmental psychologist Jerome Bruner noted that books are like islands rising from the sea—they reflect an underlying geology and, ultimately, stem from long-developing tectonic movements and volcanic pressures. The same is true of research studies and conceptual innovations. The fields of psychiatry and clinical psychology have undergone momentous growth during recent years, and we have learned a great deal about vulnerability for psychopathology, resilience, prevention, and treatment. From neuroscience and genomics, to evidence-based practices, epigenetics, psychopharmacology, and a growing appreciation of broad social forces influencing human adaptation, advances in our field have been unprecedented during recent decades. These recent advances sit upon a bedrock of fundamental, seminal research and theory in psychiatry and mental health. That bedrock is the focus of this volume. Indeed, we believe that the ongoing advancement of psychiatry and clinical psychology requires a full appreciation of the major works in our field, their inspiration and methodology, and the insights garnered from them. Beyond this, it requires an understanding of their history, their philosophical foundations, and the contexts in which they emerged.

Such a volume is especially necessary given current trends. Information technology has significantly impacted how we conduct our research and understand our patients. We all regularly turn to our computers for a quick update on recent research or for reviews of clinical guidelines to aid us in caring for our patients. Computerized literature searches provide broad and immediate access to the most recent research in our field. Organized by number of citations and impact, search algorithms provide us with access to the most recent and important work in virtually any area of scholarship or clinical practice. Interestingly, by highlighting recent, high-impact work, our attention is directed away from older, more fundamental work. As a consequence, our likelihood of reading a paper, book, or chapter declines precipitously five years after it is published. Citations of research show a similar pattern. This temporal narrowness of focus comes at a cost. We have an all but exhaustive access to recent work, but are slowly and inexorably losing sight of our history, heritage, and the important work which forms the foundation of our current practices and scholarship. Our goal is to remedy this narrowing of focus.

This volume features over one hundred landmark works that have served as a foundation for the advances we have enjoyed in recent years. The book is divided into several thematic sections. The first section discusses major theoretical constructs, with chapters devoted to psychiatric diagnosis and epidemiology. Subsequent sections examine major facets of the theory and practice of psychiatry, such as pathogenesis, pharmacotherapy, psychotherapy, social interventions, and somatic treatments, with chapters devoted to specific disorders or modalities. A final section explores ethics, forensics, suicide, and research. This framework echoes the complexity of psychiatry, which cannot be reduced to a single set of diagnoses or subspecialty categories. Though we aimed to be comprehensive, we could not be exhaustive. We could not include all topics relevant to psychiatry, nor all seminal work within a specific topic. Nevertheless, the work discussed within forms a solid foundation for understanding the history of thought in psychiatry and psychology.

We are grateful for the efforts of so many who have worked to bring this project to fruition. Our contributors, through their understanding of the heritage and history of our profession, have illuminated not only seminal contributions to our understanding of human development, psychopathology, and treatment, but also recurrent themes, questions, issues, and challenges in our field. As we know, many essential questions are never fully resolved, they only reappear over time in a new guise. We left the choice of landmark works to the individual chapter contributors, given their expertise, and we acknowledge that the pool of foundational works extends beyond anything that can be included in any single volume.

We hope that you will find the chapters of this volume engaging, thought-provoking, and inspiring. The study of the human mind, its development, and its disease is challenging. As the chapters of this volume attest, its study cannot be limited to simple methodologies or strategies borrowed from other disciplines. As we stand on the lush islands of contemporary psychiatry and clinical psychology, it is worth noting that tectonic forces are continuing to move and grind beneath us. By appreciating our history and heritage, we will be better able to address the conceptual, empirical, and clinical challenges we encounter, and be, therefore, better able to serve our patients.

Elizabeth Ryznar, Aderonke B. Pederson,
Mark A. Reinecke, and John G. Csernansky

Contents

Abbreviations

ACT	acceptance and commitment therapy
ACT	assertive community treatment
ADHD	attention deficit hyperactivity disorder
AE	adverse event
AGP	Autism Genome Project
ANOVA	analysis of variance
APA	American Psychiatric Association
APD	antisocial personality disorder
APD	antipsychotic drug
ASC	Autism Sequencing Consortium
AT	automatic thought
ASD	autism spectrum disorder
BA	behavioural activation
BPD	borderline personality disorder
BPRS	Brief Psychiatric Rating Scale
BP	bipolar disorder
BPS	biopsychosocial
BS	between subject
CAD	computerized adaptive diagnostic
CAMS	Child/Adolescent Anxiety Multimodal Study
CAT	computerized adaptive testing
CATIE	clinical antipsychotic trials of intervention effectiveness
CBT	cognitive behavioural therapy
CDRS-R	Children's Depression Rating Scale-Revised
CGAS	Children's Global Assessment Scale
CGI	Clinical Global Impression
CI	confidence interval
CIDI	Composite International Diagnostic Interview
CMHA	community mental health agency
CNTRICS	Cognitive Neuroscience Treatment Research to Improve Cognition in Schizophrenia
CNV	copy number variant
Con A	concanavalin A
CORE	Consortium for Research on ECT
CPG	clinical practice guideline
CSF	cerebrospinal fluid
CT	computerized tomography
DA	dopamine
DALY	disability-adjusted life year
DB	double-blind
DBS	deep brain stimulation
DBT	dialectical behaviour therapy
DIS	Diagnostic Interview Schedule
DLPFC	dorsolateral prefrontal cortex
DOPA	dihydroxyphenylalanine
DREADDs	designer receptors exclusively activated by designer drugs
DSM	*Diagnostic and Statistical Manual of Mental Disorders*
DST	dexamethasone suppression test
DTI	diffusion tensor imaging
ECA	epidemiological catchment area
ECT	electroconvulsive therapy
EEG	electroencephalogram
EF	electric field
EHR	electronic health record
EPS	extrapyramidal side-effect
EPS	extrapyramidal syndrome
ES	effect size
FA	fractional anisotropy
GABA	gamma-aminobutyric acid
GAD	generalized anxiety disorder
GBD	global burden of disease
GHC	Group Health Cooperative
GWAS	genome-wide association study
HAM-D	Hamilton Rating Scale for Depression
HDRS	Hamilton Depression Rating Scale
HERV	human endogenous retroviral
HIAA	hydroxyindoleacetic acid
HMO	health maintenance organization
HPA	hypothalamic–pituitary–adrenal

HPLC	high-performance liquid chromatography
HPT	hypothalamic–pituitary–thyroid
HT	hydroxytryptophan
IASP	International Association for Suicide Prevention
ICD	International Statistical Classification of Diseases
ID	intellectual disability
LDA	longitudinal data analysis
IDS-SR	Inventory of Depressive Symptomatology–Self-Report
IED	intermittent explosive disorder
IMPS	Inpatient Multidimensional Psychiatric Scale
IPS	individual placement and support
IPT	interpersonal psychotherapy
IRT	item response theory
LC	locus coeruleus
LCMR	local glucose metabolic rate
LD	linkage disequilibrium
LIFUP	low-intensity focused ultrasound pulsation
LOCF	last observation carried forward
LSAS	Liebowitz Social Anxiety Scale
LSD	lysergic acid diethylamide
MAOI	monoamine oxidase inhibitor
MBCT	mindfulness-based cognitive therapy
MBSR	mindfulness-based stress reduction
m-CPP	meta-chlorophenylpiperazine
MD	mean diffusivity
MDD	major depressive disorder
MEG	magnetoencephalography
MHC	major histocompatibility complex
MIRT	multidimensional item response theory
MPH	methylphenidate hydrochloride
MRI	magnetic resonance imaging
MS	mood stabilizer
NA	negative affect
NAHR	non-allelic homologous recombination
NAMCS	National Ambulatory Medical Care Survey
NCS	National Comorbidity Survey
NCS-R	National Comorbidity Survey Replication
NDA	new drug application
NE	norepinephrine
NICE	National Institute for Health and Care Excellence
NIH	National Institutes of Health
NK	natural killer
NIMH	National Institute of Mental Health
NLR	neutrophil to lymphocyte ratio
NMDA	N-methyl-D-aspartate
NNH	number needed to harm
NNT	number needed to treat
NOS	not otherwise specified
NSDUH	National Survey on Drug Use and Health
NTS	nucleus tractus solitarius
NVIQ	non-verbal IQ
OCD	obsessive-compulsive disorder
PA	positive affect
PARS	Paediatric Anxiety Rating Scale
PCP	phencyclidine
PET	positron emission tomography
PGC	Psychiatric Genomics Consortium
PHA	phytohaemagluttinin
PHQ	Patient Health Questionnaire
PPI	protein–protein interaction
PR	psychosocial rehabilitation
PSE	present state exam
PWM	pokeweed mitogen
QIDS-SR	Quick Inventory of Depressive Symptomatology, Self-Report
QPR	question, persuade, and refer
RCT	randomized controlled trial
RDC	research diagnostic criteria
RDoC	research domain criteria
REM	rapid eye movement
rMT	resting motor threshold
RPCT	randomized placebo-controlled trial
RPS	risk profile score
RR	relative risk
RRM	random regression model
SAD	social anxiety disorder

SADS	Schedule for Affective Disorders and Schizophrenia
SCC	subcallosal cingulate cortex
SCID	Structured Clinical Interview for the DSM
SES	socioeconomic status
SEYLE	Saving and Empowering Young Lives in Europe
SGA	second-generation antipsychotic
SNP	single nucleotide polymorphism
SNV	single nucleotide variant
SPECT	single photon emission computed tomography
SRI	serotonin reuptake inhibitor
SSC	Simons Simplex Collection
SSCP	single-strand conformation polymorphism
SSRI	selective serotonin reuptake inhibitor
SSRS	Social Skills Rating System
START*D	Sequenced Treatment Alternatives to Relieve Depression
STEP-BD	Systematic Treatment Enhancement Program for Bipolar Disorder
tACS	transcranial alternating current stimulation
TADS	Treatment for Adolescents with Depression Study
TAU	treatment as usual
TCA	tricyclic antidepressant
TCL	training in community living
TDCRP	Treatment of Depression Collaboration Research Program
tACS	transcranial alternating current stimulation
tDCS	transcranial direct current stimulation
TES	transcranial electrical stimulation
TMS	transcranial magnetic stimulation
TORDIA	Treatment of Selective Serotonin Reuptake Inhibitor-Resistant Depression in Adolescents
TPH	tryptophan hydroxylase
TRD	treatment-resistant depression
TRS	treatment-resistant schizophrenia
VNS	vagus nerve stimulation
WHO	World Health Organization
WS	within subject
YLD	years lived with disability
YLL	years of life lost
YMRS	Young Mania Rating Scale

Contributors

Awais Aftab
Northcoast Behavioral Healthcare, Northfield, Ohio, USA; Department of Psychiatry, Case Western Reserve University, Cleveland, Ohio, USA

Nadia Al-Dajani
Department of Psychology, University of Toronto, Toronto, Ontario, Canada

Marina Bayeva
Department of Psychiatry, Northwestern University, Chicago, Illinois, USA

Emmalee Boyle
Boston University Medical Center, Department of Psychiatry, Boston, Massachusetts, USA

David V. Braitman
Department of Psychiatry, University of New Mexico, Albuquerque, New Mexico, USA

Juan R. Bustillo
Departments of Psychiatry and Neuroscience, University of New Mexico, Albuquerque, New Mexico, USA

Vladimir Carli
NationalCentre for Suicide Research and Prevention of Mental Ill-Health (NASP), Karolinska Institutet, Stockholm, Sweden

Kevin A. Caulfield
Brain Stimulation Laboratory, Medical University of South Carolina, Charleston, South Carolina, USA

Edwin H. Cook
Department of Psychiatry, University of Illinois at Chicago, Chicago, Illinois, USA

John G. Csernansky
Department of Psychiatry and Behavioral Sciences, Feinberg School of Medicine, Northwestern University, Chicago, Illinois, USA

Mark R. Dadds
Child Behaviour Research Clinic, University of Sydney, Sydney, New South Wales, Australia

Melissa DelBello
Dr. Stanley and Mickey Kaplan Professor and Chair, Department of Psychiatry and Behavioral Neuroscience, University of Cincinnati College of Medicine, Cincinnati, Ohio USA

Lynn E. DeLisi
Professor of Psychiatry, Harvard Medical School, Brockton, Massachusetts, USA

Stephen H. Dinwiddie
Department of Psychiatry and Behavorial Neurosciences, Feinberg School of Medicine, Northwestern University, Chicago, Illinois, USA

Keith S. Dobson
Department of Psychology, University of Calgary, Calgary, Alberta, Canada

Shaun M. Eack
School of Social Work, University of Pittsburgh, Pittsburgh, Pennsylvania, USA

Valsamma Eapen
School of Psychiatry and Ingham Institute, University of New South Wales, Sydney, New South Wales, Australia

Jenni E. Farrow
Department of Psychiatry and Behavioral Neuroscience, University of Cincinnati College of Medicine, Cincinnati, Ohio, USA

Amanda Ferguson
Department of Psychology, University of Toronto, Toronto, Ontario, Canada

Mark S. George
Brain Stimulation Laboratory, Medical University of South Carolina, Charleston, South Carolina, USA

Robert D. Gibbons
Departments of Medicine and Public Health Sciences, The University of Chicago Biological Sciences, Chicago, Illinois, USA

Paul E. Holtzheimer
Geisel School of Medicine at Dartmouth, Dartmouth Hitchcock Medical Center, Lebanon, New Hampshire, USA

Yixin Jiang
School of Psychology, University of Sydney, Sydney, New South Wales, Australia

Neil Jordan
Department of Psychiatry and Behavorial Sciences, Feinberg School of Medicine, Northwestern University, Chicago, Illinois, USA; Center of Innovation for Complex Chronic Healthcare, Edward Hines Jr VA Hospital, Hines, Illinois, USA

Rodrigo Machado-Vieira
Department of Psychiatry and Behavorial Sciences, University of Texas Health Science Center, Houston, Texas, USA

Helen Mayberg
Center for Advanced Circuit Therapeutics, Icahn School of Medicine at Mount Sinai, New York, USA

Kevin S. McCarthy
Chestnut Hill College, Philadelphia, Pennsylvania, USA

Herbert Y. Meltzer
Department of Psychiatry and Behavorial Sciences, Feinberg School of Medicine, Northwestern University, Chicago, Illinois, USA

Keith G. Rasmussen
Department of Psychiatry and Psychology, Mayo Clinic, Rochester, Minnesota, USA

Francisco Romo-Nava
Associate Chief Research Officer, Lindner Center of HOPE, Department of Psychiatry and Behavioral Neuroscience, University of Cincinnati College of Medicine, Cincinnati, Ohio, USA

Wulf Rössler
Department of Psychiatry and Psychotherapy, Charité - Universitätsmedizin Berlin, Berlin, Germany

Elizabeth Ryznar
Resident in Psychiatry, McGaw Medical Center, Northwestern University, Chicago, Illinois, USA

John Z. Sadler
Department of Psychiatry, The University of Texas Southwestern Medical Center, Dallas, Texas, USA

Marsal Sanches
Department of Psychiatry and Behavorial Sciences, University of Texas Health Science Center, Houston, Texas, USA

Stephen Scott
Institute of Psychiatry, Psychology and Neuroscience, King's College London, London, UK

Zindel V. Segal
Department of Psychology, University of Toronto, Toronto, Ontario, Canada

Jair C. Soares
Department of Psychiatry and Behavorial Sciences, University of Texas Health Science Center, Houston, Texas, USA

Marcus Sokolowski
National Centre for Suicide Research and Prevention of Mental Ill-Health (NASP), Karolinska Institutet, Stockholm, Sweden

Dan J. Stein
Department of Psychiatry and Neuroscience Institute, University of Cape Town and South African Medical Research Council Unit on Risk & Resilience in Mental Disorders, Cape Town, South Africa

Richard F. Summers
Perelman School of Medicine, University of Pennsylvania, Philadelphia, Pennsylvania, USA

Ozan Toy
Department of Psychiatry, Boston University Medical Center, Boston, Massachusetts, USA

Mariam Ujeyl
Department of Psychiatry and Psychotherapy, Charité-Universitätsmedizin Berlin, Berlin, Germany

Amanda A. Uliaszek
Department of Psychology, University of Toronto, Toronto, Ontario, Canada

Danuta Wasserman
National Centre for Suicide Research and Prevention of Mental Ill-Health (NASP), Karolinska Institutet, Stockholm, Sweden

Harvey Whiteford
School of Public Health, University of Queensland, Brisbane, Australia; Institute of Health Metrics and Evaluation, University of Washington, Seattle, Washington, USA

Rachel E. Zettl
Resident of Psychiatry, The University of Texas Southwestern Medical Center, Dallas, Texas, USA

Section I

Foundational topics

Chapter 1

Diagnosis and conceptualization of mental illness

Awais Aftab and John G. Csernansky

Introduction

This chapter charts the evolution of the conceptualization of mental disorders. We have selected seven landmark papers that have informed our current nosology; these texts also reflect the history of paradigm shifts within psychiatry. We begin with the eighth edition of Emil Kraepelin's famous textbook *Psychiatrie,* in which we find a mature version of his foundational distinction between *dementia praecox* and manic-depressive insanity; Kraepelin is widely acknowledged as having proposed the first systematized nosology in psychiatry based on a detailed understanding of clinical picture and longitudinal course. In the late nineteenth and early twentieth century, the principal means of conveying new ideas in psychiatry was through textbooks rather than articles, and the selection of a volume of Kraepelin's textbook in lieu of a paper represents that historical reality. We then jump to Robert Kendell and colleagues' classic 1971 paper from the US–UK diagnostic project, which reported drastic differences in the clinical application of diagnostic descriptions between American and British psychiatrists, particularly regarding schizophrenia. The poor reliability among experts on the two sides of the Atlantic raised serious concerns about the integrity of the diagnostic process and served as a powerful wake-up call for the field. In response to this crisis, operational criteria were developed in an attempt to improve both reliability and validity.

Building on Eli Robins and Samuel Guze's criteria for diagnostic validity, the paper by John Feighner and colleagues in 1972 represented the first systematic application of operational criteria for clinical diagnosis in psychiatry. Feighner's approach was eventually taken up and expanded by Robert Spitzer and colleagues to form the Research Diagnostic Criteria. The Research Diagnostic Criteria in turn became the backbone for the revolutionary third edition of the *Diagnostic and Statistical Manual of Mental Disorders* (DSM) in 1980, which adopted operationalized diagnostic criteria for the first time, in contrast to the first and second editions, which had relied on vague descriptions of disorders often based on psychodynamically driven aetiological theories.

Operationalized criteria relied heavily on the 'medical model' and dovetailed well with the growing 'biological psychiatry' movement. This movement gained steam following the discovery of effective psychotropics in the 1950s, and subsequent decades saw a growing rift between 'biological psychiatry' and 'psychodynamic psychiatry'. George Engel addressed the ongoing tension between psychological/psychodynamic theory and the medical model by proposing a biopsychosocial model, which provided a practical, but perhaps temporary, solution aimed at uniting the diverse camps within psychiatry. The discussion on the biopsychosocial model is represented here by Engel's 1977 paper in *Science*. Jerome Wakefield's highly influential philosophical account of mental disorder as harmful dysfunction is addressed next. This account, albeit not without philosophical limitations, helped reframe the conceptual debate by reintroducing concepts of disease mechanisms and their relationship to the appearance of psychiatric disorders.

Finally, the last pair of articles highlight the endophenotype concept, proposed by Irving Gottesman, and the Research Domain Criteria (RDoC), proposed by Tom Insel, which seek to unite clinical diagnosis with an understanding of aetiologic and pathogenetic mechanisms. These articles also reflect an ongoing paradigm shift in psychiatry, the fruits of which are yet to be seen. The RDoC framework, if successful in linking underlying neurobiological mechanisms to clinical syndromes, could fundamentally alter the way we think about psychiatric diagnosis and classification.

Kraepelin and the foundations of modern clinical nosology

Main citation

Kraepelin, E. (1913). *Psychiatrie*, Vol. III (8th edn). Leipzig: Barth.

English translations of relevant chapters from main citation

Kraepelin, E. (1913). 'Dementia praecox and paraphrenia', trans. R. M. Barclay (1919). Edinburgh: E. & S. Livingstone.

Kraepelin, E. (1913). 'Manic-depressive insanity and paranoia', trans. R. M. Barclay (1921). Edinburgh: E. & S. Livingstone.

Background

The German psychiatrist Emil Kraepelin (1856–1926) is a towering figure in the history of psychiatry. His classification of mental disorders provides a foundation for modern psychiatric nosology, and post-psychoanalytic twentieth-century psychiatrists were proud to be a part of the self-identified 'neo-Kraepelinian revolution' (Compton & Guze, 1995). Kraepelin presented his grand psychiatric framework in a series of editions of textbooks. These textbooks began to attract widespread attention with the fourth edition in 1893. The eighth and final edition was published in five volumes between 1909 and 1915. Edward Shorter states that editions of Kraepelin's textbooks were 'anticipated with the same rapt attention that awaits new editions of the DSM today' (Shorter, 2015).

Kraepelin is most well-known for his dichotomy of endogenous psychoses; that is, the separation of '*dementia praecox*' (schizophrenia) from manic-depressive insanity (psychotic mood disorders), first proposed in the sixth edition of 1899. He justified this classification using commonalities and differences in clinical picture, course, and outcomes. Prior to Kraepelin, chronic illnesses with delusions, hallucinations, thought disorder, inappropriate affect, and social isolation did not exist as a unified category and were not differentiated from affective disorders. Benedict Morel had coined the term '*dementia praecox*' in French ('demence precoce') in 1852 to describe young patients with premature dementia. German psychiatrists Ewald Hecker and Karl Ludwig Kahlbaum had used the terms 'hebephrenia' and 'paraphrenia hebetica' respectively for a disease of younger patients manifesting florid psychosis and a deteriorating course. Kraeplin borrowed from Kahlbaum and developed these ideas further (Adityanjee et al., 1999; Zivanovic & Nedic, 2012). Prior to Kraepelin, German psychiatry had not systematically classified mental disorders by using course and outcomes as critical defining features (Engstrom & Kendler, 2015).

The term '*dementia praecox*' first appears in the fourth edition of Kraepelin's textbook (1893) under the group heading of 'psychic degenerative processes'. It became an independent disease in the fifth edition. The sixth edition marked his greatest nosological contribution with two distinct, broad categories of disorder—*dementia praecox* and manic-depressive insanity. He included Kahlbaum's catatonia, Hecker's hebephrenia, and paranoia in his description of *dementia praecox*, and in the seventh edition, these appear as the hebephrenic, catatonic, and paranoid subtypes of *dementia praecox*. In the eighth edition, Kraepelin recognized that some cases of *dementia praecox* may have a late onset and that a few cases may recover.

Methods

Kraepelin was an astute and experienced psychiatric clinician. He aimed to accurately describe and classify psychiatric symptoms, in contrast to other psychiatric researchers of his era who were preoccupied with neuroanatomical and neuropathological research and paid little attention to nuances of clinical presentation and course.

Kraepelin's work was based on detailed clinical observation and case notes of thousands of patients; it is estimated that he cared for over 8,000 patients in Munich and Heidelberg (Zivanovic & Nedic, 2012). Kraeplin believed in the necessity of systematic and objective observation of his patients. To accomplish that, he utilized 'diagnostic cards', which were developed for the purpose of record-keeping in psychiatric institutions. He kept records of, among other things, age, age of onset, family history, medical history, treatment and duration of treatment, clinical features, and course of symptoms (Zivanovic & Nedic, 2012).

Kraepelin utilized a validation schema that foreshadowed the one proposed by Robins and Guze later in the twentieth century; he emphasized clinical presentation, features of course and outcomes, and family aggregation of disease as factors distinguishing different conditions. He also found premorbid personality and temperament to be useful for classification purposes.

Results

At the heart of Kraepelin's classification system is the division between *dementia praecox* and manic-depressive insanity. In his own words: '*Dementia praecox* consists of a series of states, the common characteristic of which is a peculiar destruction of the internal connections of the psychic personality. The effects of this injury predominate in the emotional and volitional spheres of mental life' (Kraepelin/Barclay, 1913/1919, p. 3). 'Manic-depressive insanity ... includes on the one hand the whole domain of so called *periodic and circular insanity*, on the other hand *simple mania*, the greater part of the morbid states termed *melancholia* and also a not inconsiderable number of cases of *amentia*. Lastly, we include here certain slight and slightest colourings of *mood*, some of them periodic, some of them continuously morbid, which on the one hand are to be regarded as the rudiment of more severe disorders, on the other hand pass over without sharp boundary into the domain of *personal predisposition*' (Kraepelin/Barclay, 1913/1921, p. 1).

Kraepelin was convinced that each condition represented a distinct morbid process, despite variation in clinical presentations of *dementia praecox* and manic-depressive insanity. He elaborated on various differences in past history, symptoms/signs, and course of illness to arrive at his differential diagnosis. *Dementia praecox* was in the majority of cases a chronic condition with poor prognosis, resulting in a state of 'dementia', while manic-depressive insanity was more cyclical and had a relatively good prognosis. Episodes of manic-depressive insanity could be prolonged, but recovery was expected. The recovery between episodes was not always complete; recurrent attacks could lead to some residual impairment. Kraepelin was sceptical of the search for the pathognomonic symptom, and he always stressed the importance of considering the total clinical picture (Kendler, 1986).

Kraepelin did not view *dementia praecox* as always chronic nor manic-depressive insanity as always remitting with complete recovery in between episodes. He was aware that we cannot distinguish satisfactorily between these two illnesses based on clinical picture and course alone. However, he continued to assert that fundamentally different basic pathological processes underpinned these two conditions.

Conclusions and critique

Kraeplin's methodology and classification have proven to be of lasting significance (Compton & Guze, 1995; Zivanovic & Nedic, 2012; Kendler, 1986). His landmark contributions lie in utilizing disease course and outcomes as principles for classification and in distinguishing *dementia praecox* as a distinct entity from psychotic mood disorders.

Kraepelin's concept of *dementia praecox* is well preserved in modern psychiatry in the construct of schizophrenia; his unitary notion of affective disorders, in comparison, has not been adopted by contemporary classifications. It is a common misconception that manic-depressive insanity corresponds to modern bipolar disorder. In fact, it includes the entire affective spectrum. Manic-depressive insanity, as conceptualized by Kraepelin, comprises the entire range of disorders with singular or recurrent episodes of both polarities. His views align with more modern dimensional concepts of mood disorders (Ghaemi, 2013).

The recognition that many patients experience a 'schizoaffective disorder' with features of both illnesses has, from the very beginning, raised the question of whether schizophrenia can be clinically categorized as a distinct entity from mood disorders. Recent genetic studies have also cast doubt on the notion that schizophrenia and bipolar disorder have distinct genetic underpinnings (Miller & Rockstroh, 2013). Whether future aetiology-based classifications will preserve the Kraepelinian distinction is an open question.

Kraepelin's emphasis on course and outcome as critical defining features of psychiatric illnesses was revived in American psychiatry, in the second half of the twentieth century, by Robins and Guze (see the section 'The development of operationalized criteria'). By and large, current diagnostic thinking, as exemplified by the DSM, remains neo-Kraepelinian in spirit.

Crisis of reliability: the US–UK diagnostic project

Main citation

Kendell, R. E., Cooper, J. E., Gourlay, A. J., Copeland, J. R., Sharpe, L., & Gurland, B. J. (1971). Diagnostic criteria of American and British psychiatrists. *Archives of General Psychiatry*, 25, 123–130.

Background

Multiple studies from the first half of the twentieth century suggested problematically poor interrater reliability for psychiatric diagnoses. For instance, in one study, three clinicians agreed on a psychiatric diagnosis only 20% of the time when seeing the same patient (Ash, 1949). The 1960s and early 1970s further highlighted this crisis of reliability with the discovery of stark differences in diagnostic practices between psychiatrists from the UK and the US. Studies of hospital records had revealed that the diagnosis of schizophrenia in the inpatient setting was consistently more prevalent in America, while in Britain, the diagnosis of manic-depressive illness was more frequently used (Gurland et al., 1970). In one study, American psychiatrists diagnosed depressive neurosis more readily as compared to British psychiatrists' preference for manic-depressive illness (Sandifer et al., 1968). In another study, American psychiatrists provided a range of diagnoses of schizophrenia, neurosis, and personality disorder after viewing a single diagnostic interview, while 60% of British psychiatrists diagnosed personality disorder and none diagnosed schizophrenia on watching the same interview (Katz et al., 1969).

These findings prompted the creation of the Cross-National Project for the Study of the Diagnosis of Mental Disorders in the United States and the United Kingdom, which began as a series of studies in 1965. The project used semi-structured interviews, ratings of videotapes, and systematic examinations of case records, and was carried out by multidisciplinary teams based in New York and London (Gurland et al., 1970; US–UK

Cross-National Project, 1974). The Kendell and colleagues' paper is perhaps the most well-known of these, given the striking findings it reported from a well-designed experiment, and will be discussed here in detail.

Methods

The study was conducted using videotapes of unstructured diagnostic interviews with eight patients, 20 to 50 minutes in duration. Given the audience, five of these patients were British and three were American. The investigators selected cases that included both classic presentations and presentations that would evoke dissent. Around 240 British psychiatrists and 450 American psychiatrists participated in rating the videos; the American sample was drawn predominantly from the New York Psychiatric Institute and other New York metropolitan area hospitals. A minimum of four years' experience of psychiatry was required (average length of experience was 12–15 years). All clinical information was to be gleaned from the videos only; however, certain slang phrases and allusions were explained.

Participating psychiatrists were asked to provide three sets of ratings:

1) Lorr's Inpatient Multi-dimensional Psychiatric Scale (IMPS), which consists of ratings in non-technical language covering a variety of abnormal behaviours;
2) Checklist of 116 technical terms to describe observed psychopathology (such as retardation, blocking, and flattening of affect);
3) Primary diagnosis (to be picked only from ICD-8 diagnoses), with provisions for a subsidiary diagnosis and an alternative diagnosis if needed. In addition, participants could also provide a 'personal diagnosis' unrestricted by ICD-8 terminology. A five-point confidence scale was attached to the main diagnosis, since the investigators thought that many psychiatrists might not be sufficiently confident about a diagnosis based on the limited information provided in the video.

Results

Three out of these eight patients exhibited typical symptoms of classical diagnostic stereotypes (paranoid schizophrenia with the possibility of an alcoholic psychosis, depressive illness, and schizophrenic illness), and there was substantial agreement between the ratings of American and British psychiatrists for these videos. Three other patients showed a mixture of psychotic and affective symptoms. The proportion of British psychiatrists making a diagnosis of affective psychosis was higher compared to American psychiatrists. Despite this relative difference, the majority of psychiatrists on both sides arrived at the same diagnosis.

The most serious disagreement occurred with two cases, where the majority of American psychiatrists diagnosed some form of schizophrenia, while the majority of British psychiatrists diagnosed personality disorder or neurotic illness. Many American psychiatrists utilized the diagnosis of 'pseudoneurotic schizophrenia' (a now obsolete diagnostic category in which prominent symptoms of anxiety, obsessions, compulsions, and phobias were believed to mask a latent psychotic disorder), while this diagnosis was rarely utilized by British raters.

The study also revealed that American and British psychiatrists not only differed in the diagnosis given, but also in their detection of observed symptomatology. In the case of patient F, for example, 67% of American psychiatrists rated the patient as having delusions, 63% as having passivity feelings, and 58% as showing thought disorder. This was in contrast to British psychiatrists, whose ratings were 12%, 8%, and 5%, respectively. Even when using IMPS ratings (which are straightforward, non-technical descriptions), American psychiatrists were more likely to perceive symptomatology as having stronger schizophrenic connotations.

There were other differences as well: for instance, the British observed hysteria more commonly than Americans, and the Americans diagnosed involutional melancholia in middle-aged women, where British psychiatrists diagnosed manic depression. However, the differences in schizophrenia diagnosis were the starkest finding: many of the patients diagnosed with schizophrenia in New York would have been diagnosed with manic-depressive illness in London (Gurland et al., 1970; US–UK Cross-National Project, 1974).

Conclusions and critique

The study demonstrated very clearly that the concept of schizophrenia in the US, at the very least among psychiatrists on the east coast, was broader than the British concept of schizophrenia. In the discussion of the paper, the authors noted that the diagnosis of schizophrenia 'is now made so freely on the east coast of the United States that it is losing much of its original meaning and is approaching the point at which it becomes a synonym for functional mental illness' (Kendell et al., 1971). Seven of the eight patients in the study had been diagnosed as schizophrenic by over two thirds of American psychiatrists.

As stated previously, the Kendell paper was part of the larger US–UK Project, which found that inconsistent diagnostic methods for routine hospital admissions in the two countries led to large discrepancies in diagnosis. These findings highlighted the crucial need for diagnostic reliability and prompted the development of operationalized diagnostic criteria. The problem of reliability also had implications for the validity of psychiatric diagnosis, since a lack of reliability precluded a lack of validity.

Another highly publicized, and much more theatrical, study from the early 1970s was the Rosenhan Experiment ('On being sane in insane places') (Rosenhan, 1973). The study was conducted by David Rosenhan, a psychologist at Stanford, and highlighted problems with the overall reliability of identifying individuals with mental illness. The experiment involved sending eight healthy volunteers to different hospitals across the US with feigned auditory hallucinations (voices saying the words 'empty', 'hollow', and 'thud') and no other psychiatric symptoms and no prior psychiatric history. All the 'patients' were admitted to psychiatric units. After admission, these patients acted as their normal selves and reported no further auditory hallucinations. Despite normal behaviour on the unit, hospital staff viewed their behaviour as reflective of a mental illness. All were given antipsychotic medications (which the 'pseudopatients' did not swallow). Seven were diagnosed with schizophrenia and one with manic-depressive psychosis. The duration of admission ranged from seven to fifty-two days. The biggest critique of this study is that it lacked realism—psychiatrists, and physicians in general, do not begin with the assumption that a patient is feigning symptoms.[1] Nevertheless, the study highlighted the problem of reliability of the overarching category of 'mental disorder', and further spurred the psychiatric community to place psychiatric diagnoses on a more solid footing.

The development of operationalized criteria

Main citation

Feighner, J. P., Robins, E., Guze, S. B., Woodruff Jr, R. A., Winokur, G., & Munoz, R. (1972). Diagnostic criteria for use in psychiatric research. *Archives of General Psychiatry*, 26, 57–63.

Related references

Robins, E. & Guze, S. B. (1970). Establishment of diagnostic validity in psychiatric illness: its application to schizophrenia. *American Journal of Psychiatry*, 126, 983–987.

Spitzer, R. L., Endicott, J., & Robins, E. (1978). Research Diagnostic Criteria: rationale and reliability. *Archives of General Psychiatry*, 35, 773–782.

Background

In the mid-twentieth century, American psychiatry displayed little interest in psychiatric diagnosis. The dominant framework of psychoanalysis emphasized individual differences rather than commonalities in presentation, with little use for the types of broad diagnostic labels used by other medical specialties. In the 1950s, when nearly every psychiatry department in the US was dominated by psychoanalytic theory and practice, the Department of Psychiatry at Washington University in St Louis, Missouri, was a prominent exception (Kendler et al., 2010). Edwin Gildea, then Department Chair, believed in open-minded inquiry with respect to biological theories. With this support, a small group of psychiatrists in the department led by Eli Robins and Samuel Guze set out on the ambitious project of providing psychiatry with operationalized diagnostic criteria that were valid and reliable. Robins and Guze viewed psychiatry from the lens of the medical model, where diagnosis plays a central role. They outlined a five-phase diagnostic validation model for psychiatric diagnosis (Robins & Guze, 1970). Their way of thinking, with its emphasis on the clinical picture and longitudinal course, was clearly neo-Kraepelinian in spirit.

Robins and Guze continued to promote this line of inquiry in their department with colleagues and trainees. In 1967, John Feighner, then a psychiatry resident, created a discussion group with Eli Robins as senior mentor, along with Samuel Guze, George Winokur,

[1] Recent investigation by Susannah Cahalan, as described in her book 'The Great Pretender', suggests that Rosenhan may have exaggerated his findings and excluded data to support his thesis.

Robert Woodruff, and Rod Muñoz as active participants. They initially intended to write a literature review of key contributions to psychiatric diagnosis but ultimately claimed the more ambitious task of developing a set of operationalized diagnostic criteria for multiple mental disorders. These criteria were published in 1972 and are generally referred to as the 'Feighner criteria'. The criteria filled a much-needed void (DSM-I and DSM-II only contained brief and vague descriptions of mental disorders and were of little help in making the process of diagnosis reliable) and were quickly and widely adopted by clinicians and researchers, making this article one of the most cited publications in psychiatry.

Methods

As mentioned previously, Robins and Guze had earlier devised a strategy for validating a psychiatric diagnosis, based on the following five phases (Robins & Guze, 1970):

1. Clinical description: the constellation of signs and symptoms associated with the condition, including items such as race, gender, age of onset, and precipitating factors.
2. Laboratory studies: chemical, physiological, radiological, anatomical findings, as well as findings from psychological testing.
3. Delimitation from other disorders: exclusion criteria to exclude other disorders with similar clinical features.
4. Follow-up studies: looking at diagnostic stability, longitudinal course, and treatment response. Marked difference in outcomes, such as between complete recovery and chronic illness, suggests that the group is not homogeneous and challenges the validity of the original diagnosis.
5. Family history: increased prevalence of same disorder among close relatives of original patients.

The Feighner criteria followed this framework and drew data from a thorough literature review, clinical experience, and group discussion. The meetings continued for approximately nine months, and Feighner gathered the materials for the literature review and developed working outlines of the diagnostic criteria. The other authors would meet, review Feighner's proposed criteria, revise them in light of their own knowledge, research, and clinical experience, and finalize them based on consensus.

Results

The project resulted in operationalized diagnostic criteria for 15 psychiatric conditions: primary affective disorders (depression and mania) and secondary affective disorder (depression only), schizophrenia, anxiety neurosis, obsessive-compulsive neurosis, phobic neurosis, hysteria, antisocial personality disorder, alcoholism, drug dependence, mental retardation, organic brain syndrome, homosexuality, transsexualism, and anorexia nervosa. The criteria also allowed clinicians to note that a patient had 'undiagnosed psychiatric illness' when his/her symptoms did not fit any other specific disorder

(Feighner et al., 1972). For example, the Feighner criteria for depression (Feighner et al., 1972) required:

- a dysphoric mood (including feeling 'depressed, sad, blue, despondent, hopeless, "down in the dumps", irritable, fearful, worried, or discouraged').
- at least four additional symptoms for 'probable' depression and at least five additional symptoms for 'definite' depression; these symptoms can be 'poor appetite or weight loss', 'sleep difficulty', 'loss of energy', 'agitation or retardation,' 'loss of interest in usual activities, or decrease in sex drive,' 'feelings of self-reproach or guilt,' 'complaints of or actually diminished ability to think or concentrate,' 'recurrent thoughts of death or suicide'.
- a time duration of at least one month with 'no preexisting psychiatric conditions'. The criteria specifically excluded 'schizophrenia, anxiety neurosis, phobic neurosis, obsessive compulsive neurosis, hysteria, alcoholism, drug dependency, antisocial personality, homosexuality and other sexual deviations, mental retardation, or organic brain syndrome'. They also further specified that 'patients with life-threatening or incapacitating medical illness preceding and paralleling the depression do not receive the diagnosis of primary depression'.

Contemporary readers will notice the striking resemblance with the symptom profile for current DSM criteria for major depression, though the time duration has been shortened and the exclusion criterion has been lifted.

The reliability and validity of the criteria were established in an 18-month follow-up study of 314 psychiatric emergency-room patients and a seven-year follow-up study of 87 psychiatric inpatients at Washington University in St Louis. Reliability, as measured by interrater agreement about diagnosis, was 86–95% in the emergency room and 92% for inpatients. Validity, defined as the agreement between initial and follow-up diagnoses, was 93% and 92% respectively (Feighner et al., 1972).

Conclusions and critique

The influence and legacy of the Feighner criteria are manifold (Kendler et al., 2010). First and foremost, the Feighner criteria represented the first systematic application of operationalized criteria for psychiatric diagnosis into psychiatric practice. Moreover, Feighner demonstrated that the approach could identify a broad array of disorders. Second, the success of the Feighner criteria forced American psychiatry to pay attention to the course and outcome of a clinical syndrome as critical defining features. This line of thinking had been a prominent feature of European descriptive psychiatry, exemplified by the work of Kraepelin, but had been lost to American psychiatry. Third, the Feighner criteria were a major milestone in a broader research programme aimed at developing empirically validated psychiatric diagnoses. It is important to keep in mind that the Feighner criteria were based on research findings whenever available, but that the available research data at that time was highly limited.

Another important way in which the Feigner criteria shaped history is by serving as a forerunner to the development of DSM-III, via the Research Diagnostic Criteria (RDC) (Spitzer et al., 1978). Robert Spitzer at Columbia, along with psychologist Jean Endicott, had been working on improving psychiatric diagnosis for many years. Their initial efforts came in the form of a computer algorithm called DIAGNO, which provided diagnoses based on raw clinical data entered by clinicians. DIAGNO was not easily adopted into research or clinical practice. After the publication of the Feighner criteria, Spitzer and Endicott collaborated with Eli Robins, one of the original authors of the Feighner criteria, to create an updated version (known as RDC) that laid out operationalized criteria for 25 major diagnostic categories (Spitzer et al., 1978).

While the Feighner group was primarily interested in improving the validity of psychiatric diagnosis, the Spitzer group was primarily interested in establishing reliability. The Spitzer group believed that variability in the criteria used for diagnosis was the biggest contributor to poor reliability among clinicians, and stressed the use of specific inclusion and exclusion criteria for each disorder as crucial to this endeavour. The Spitzer group were among the first to use the kappa coefficient statistic to measure diagnostic reliability while correcting for chance agreement (Spitzer et al., 1978) (see Chapter 23 for a discussion of kappa).

Spitzer and Endicott believed that there were three major lessons from the Feighner group that influenced the development of RDC and subsequently of DSM-III: the use of operationalized criteria; paying attention to course of illness and prognosis in addition to the acute clinical picture; and, wherever possible, basing diagnostic criteria on research data rather than just clinical experience and consensus (Kendler et al., 2010).

The RDC were developed to enable researchers to apply a consistent set of criteria for the description or selection of subjects with psychiatric disorders, and the final version was published in 1978 (Spitzer et al., 1978). The reliability of the RDC was shown to be considerably better than psychiatric diagnoses otherwise determined. The success of the RDC paved the way for the inclusion of specified diagnostic criteria for more than 200 mental disorders in DSM-III. Spitzer later wrote that the inclusion of diagnostic criteria in DSM-III was only possible because RDC 'tested the water, and clinicians and researchers saw the advantage of replacing vague descriptions of psychiatric disorders with precise definitions using specified criteria' (Spitzer, 1999).

The biopsychosocial revolution

Main citation

Engel, G. (1977). The need for a new medical model: a challenge for biomedicine. *Science*, 196, 129–136.

Related reference

Engel, G. (1980). The clinical application of the biopsychosocial model. *American Journal of Psychiatry*, 137, 535–544.

Background

The biopsychosocial (BPS) model, proposed by George Engel, is now so commonplace in contemporary psychiatry as to be accepted as axiomatic. It is a difficult to imagine a time when this was not the case. The BPS model represents both a philosophy of clinical care and a practical clinical guide. Biologically oriented research in the 1960s and 1970s led to a sharp increase in support for the medical model, which viewed disorders in more biological terms, and perhaps with the implicit inference that clinicians need not be concerned with psychosocial issues. This exacerbated tensions between psychoanalytically minded and biologically minded psychiatrists.

Methods

Engel constructed the BPS model utilizing a basic framework provided by general systems theory. According to systems theory, nature is organized in the form of a hierarchically arranged continuum of systems (or levels of explanations), with more complex, larger units superordinate to the less complex, smaller units. Each system—such as cell, organ, person, or family—is at a particular level of complexity, with its own distinctive qualities and relationships, requiring explanatory frameworks that are unique to that level. Each system is not merely an assemblage of its constituent parts, but also exists in relationship to other systems. Building on this theoretical foundation, Engel offered a framework that accounted for all systems relevant to the biological, psychological, and social domains involved in mental illness.

Results

Engel's purpose in writing these two classic papers was twofold: firstly, to show the deficiencies of biomedical reductionism, and secondly, to propose the BPS model as the preferred alternative. The biomedical model, as Engel viewed it, assumed 'disease to be fully accounted for by deviations from the norm of measurable biological (somatic) variables' (Engel, 1977). In other words, the biomedical model could conceptualize disorders as entities independent of social behaviour.

Engel argued that biological abnormalities, at best, constitute a necessary but not sufficient condition for illness and, in particular, for the human experience of the disease. To take into account the human experience of disease—whether and when patients come to view themselves or be viewed by others as sick, how illness is reported, and how it impacts human lives—is impossible without considering psychological, social, and cultural factors (Engel, 1977, 1980).

Establishing a relationship between a clinical presentation and an underlying biological aetiology requires a scientific understanding of behaviour and psychosocial aspects, because that is how patients report their symptoms. Patients seek help from the clinician because either they do not know what is wrong or, if they do, they feel incapable of helping themselves. Engel argued that the 'psychobiological unity of man' requires that clinicians accept the responsibility to evaluate and manage whatever problems the patient presents, regardless of whether they can be reduced to biological disruptions in the body.

Engel recognized the unique position of psychiatry within the medical profession as the only clinical discipline still concerned primarily with the study of the human condition. He considered it a lasting contribution of Sigmund Freud and Adolf Meyer that they had provided frames of reference which led to the inclusion of psychological processes in the concept of disease.

Engel maintained that the clinician must accurately determine the patient's experience of illness, formulate possible explanations for the clinical presentation, utilize further interviewing or laboratory studies to verify and reject hypotheses, and then determine a treatment plan in which the patient's cooperation is ensured. All these practical steps require a thorough understanding of psychological and social factors influencing the patient: 'To provide a basis for understanding the determinants of disease and arriving at rational treatments and patterns of health care, a medical model must also take into account the patient, the social context in which he lives, and the complementary system devised by society to deal with the disruptive effects of illness, that is, the physician role and the health care system. This requires a biopsychosocial model' (Engel, 1977).

Conclusions and critique

Engel conceptualized the biopsychosocial model as 'a blueprint for research, a framework for teaching, and a design for action in the real world of health care' (Engel, 1977). Philosophically, it is a way of understanding how suffering and illness are affected by multiple levels of organization, from the social to the molecular. At a practical level, it is a way of understanding the patient's subjective experience as an essential contributor to accurate diagnosis, health outcomes, and humane care (Borrell-Carrio et al., 2004).

The BPS model has been of tremendous influence in psychiatry and psychology, and within a short period of time it achieved the status of psychiatric orthodoxy. It has at least partially resolved the debates between the psychodynamic and biological camps within psychiatry by offering a model acceptable to all parties. There is no doubt that the BPS model is an advance over earlier models. However, critics argue that in contemporary practice the biopsychosocial model has evolved into a confusing set of assumptions about the content of psychiatric conditions, leading the clinicians into a state of lazy eclecticism (Ghaemi, 2009). As interpreted by most mental health professionals today, this model does little but assert that all illnesses have components that are, unsurprisingly, biological, psychological, and social (Ghaemi, 2009).

Paul McHugh and Phillip Slavney argue that the biopsychosocial model is excessively broad and provides no real guidance to clinicians or researchers. They compare the model to a list of ingredients, as opposed to a recipe. In their view, the BPS model only lists relevant aspects of psychiatry. It is silent as to how to understand those aspects under different conditions and in different circumstances (McHugh & Slavney, 1998).

Biopsychosocial thinking has evolved into a mature philosophy of psychiatric pluralism in recent years. The conceptual framework of pluralism in psychiatry originates from the work of early twentieth-century psychiatrist and philosopher Karl Jaspers, and has been elaborated by contemporary thinkers such as McHugh, S. Nassir Ghaemi, and Kenneth Kendler. The basic viewpoint of pluralism is that multiple independent methods and levels of explanations are necessary to understand and treat mental illness. Pluralism explicitly recognizes the strengths and limits of each method or explanation, and recommends using whichever is best suited for the specific circumstances based on empirical evidence (Ghaemi, 2009). Kendler advocates for an 'integrative pluralism' in which active efforts are made to incorporate divergent levels of analysis. For complex disorders, single-level analyses usually lead to partial answers; integrative pluralism seeks to establish small 'local' integrations across levels of analysis (Kendler, 2005). Pluralism is the natural successor to the BPS model and may very well supplant it in the future.

Mental disorder as harmful dysfunction

Main citation

Wakefield, J. C. (1992). The concept of mental disorder: on the boundary between biological facts and social values. *American Psychologist*, 47, 373–388.

Related reference

Wakefield, J. C. (1992). Disorder as harmful dysfunction: a conceptual critique of DSM-IIIR's definition of mental disorder. *Psychological Review*, 99, 232–247.

Background

The concept of mental illness has been the subject of heated debate for several decades, particularly as psychiatry has been routinely charged with addressing normal suffering or problems of living. Philosophically, disease concepts can involve normative, value-based judgements or scientific, fact-based judgements. Value-based judgements include matters such as social deviance, moral disapproval, and considerations of harm, while fact-based judgements include notions of statistical deviation, biological disadvantage with regards to fertility or mortality, and presence of biological pathology. This basic division is at the heart of the dispute, with the debate often being framed in terms of whether the identification of an individual as disordered is sociopolitical or biomedical. Philosophers such as Michel Foucault, and psychiatrists such as Thomas Szasz and R. D. Laing were of the position that psychiatric diagnoses were masked sociopolitical judgements (a position embraced by the antipsychiatry movement), while commentators such as John G. Scadding, Robert Kendell, and Christopher Boorse were in the biomedical camp.

Thomas Szasz created intense controversy in the field with his 1960 article and book *The Myth of Mental Illness*, in which he began by defining disease as demonstrable anatomical or physiological lesions. This definition implies that the only sort of disease that can exist is physical, since disease cannot be non-physical. In other words, the 'mind' cannot be diseased in the literal, physical sense since it is non-physical. His conclusion was that mental disorders can therefore only be diseases in a metaphorical sense. If psychiatric symptoms are due to a neurological defect, then these conditions are brain diseases, and if psychiatric symptoms are not due to a brain disease, then they are only non-pathological problems in living. In either case, Szasz argues, the concept of mental illness is unnecessary and misleading (Szasz, 1960).

Jerome Wakefield defines disorder (including mental disorder) as 'harmful dysfunction' and maintains that the concept of disorder must include a factual component so that disorders can be distinguished from disvalued conditions. At the same time, observable facts alone are not enough, and disorder also requires harm, which involves values. By this hybrid account, Wakefield suggests a unifying and appealing ground that has understandably been of great influence.

Wakefield agrees with Szasz that disorder requires physical abnormality but does not accept Szasz's argument or conclusion. Wakefield sees the notion of 'lesion' as too narrow and inapplicable to many conditions in medicine. Furthermore, Wakefield does not conceptualize mental disorders as disorders of the non-physical 'mind', but rather as disorders of 'mental functions' in the brain. Thus, the same concept of disorder can apply to physical as well as mental disorders.

Methods

Wakefield conducts a conceptual analysis of the concept of disorder. He recognizes that we value many conditions negatively, but that our notion of disorder is not reduced to the notion of merely a disvalued condition. Our notion of disorder also seems to make inherent reference to abnormality or malfunction in some biomedical processes. Based on his analysis, Wakefield proposes a hybrid definition requiring both a fact-based criterion and a value-based criterion.

Results

Wakefield argues that the notion of function and dysfunction are central to the fact component of disorder. Dysfunction implies that there is a failure of some mechanism in the organism to perform its function. This failure is not failure to function in a socially preferred manner, but rather failure to function in the manner for which it is naturally designed. Functions can have tremendous explanatory value. Wakefield argues that 'natural mechanisms, like artifacts, can be partially explained by referring to their effects, and natural functions, like artifact functions, are those effects that enter into such explanations' (Wakefield, 1992, p. 382).

Wakefield goes on to argue that functional explanations have utility even when the actual nature of the mechanism that is dysfunctional is poorly understood. He then connects his notion of natural function with evolutionary perspective. Evolutionary theory provides an explanation of how a mechanism's effects can explain the mechanism's presence, since those mechanisms whose effects contributed to the reproductive success of the organisms of a species increased in frequency in the population ('natural selection'). For Wakefield, 'dysfunction' is the breakdown of a mechanism that was naturally selected in the process of evolution. Dysfunction, in this respect, is different from an evolutionary maladaptation, since in the case of a maladaptation the naturally selected mechanism remains intact but is no longer well-suited for the organism's current environment. At the same time, the value criterion of the definition prevents it from collapsing into an evolutionary account. 'The mental health theoretician is interested in the functions that people care about and need within the current social environment, not those that are interesting merely on evolutionary theoretical grounds' (Wakefield, 1992, p. 384).

DSM takes the approach that what makes a disorder 'mental' is the behavioural nature of the symptoms rather than the kind of dysfunction. But Wakefield argues that for a disorder to be mental, the presence of dysfunction must involve mental mechanisms.

On the surface there is a great similarity between the DSM definition of dysfunction (at the time of Wakefield's proposal, it was DSM-III-R) and Wakefield's definition of harmful dysfunction. However, while DSM-III-R identified dysfunction and harm as two necessary conditions for mental disorder, it did not explicitly describe or define dysfunction, thus providing little meaningful guidance. Utilizing the writings of Spitzer and Endicott, Wakefield shows that DSM-III operationalizes the concept of harmful dysfunction as 'unexpectable distress or disability', which fails to capture the notion of dysfunction as Wakefield envisions it (Wakefield, 1992).

Conclusions and critique

Wakefield defines disorder as a harmful failure of a natural function, with 'natural function' referring to functioning as designed in evolution. Wakefield's account has been popular in psychiatry, and in many ways the interpretation of the DSM definition has shifted over time to be more aligned with Wakefield's definition. Robert Spitzer called it 'a considerable advance over the DSM definition of mental disorder' (Spitzer, 1999) and suggested that it should formally be adopted by DSM-5. Allen Frances, chairman of the DSM-IV taskforce, has praised it: Wakefield 'has come up with a definition that works extremely well on paper. His harmful dysfunction and evolutionary perspective provide the best possible abstract definition of mental disorder' (Frances, 2013).

Wakefield's account runs into problems in its application to psychiatry for two primary reasons. Firstly, too little is known about the cerebral mechanisms underlying basic psychological functions, and their evolution, to determine with any degree of certainty if a dysfunction of evolutionary design is present. Therefore, the presence of dysfunction in most cases is highly inferential. Secondly, there are many ways for things to 'go wrong' in the psychological realm. While one possibility is failure of a mechanism to perform a function as designed in evolution, there are a number of other possibilities that do not count as dysfunction as Wakefield sees it. The practical implication is that Wakefield's account turns into (in Derek Bolton's words) 'a hypothesis that would typically be, for most psychiatric conditions, uncertain, speculative, provisional, for some quite likely false—and in probably all cases controversial' (Bolton, 2008, p. xxv).

Despite these limitations, Wakefield's conceptual analysis of mental disorder and proposed definition have played a tremendous role in redefining the debate, and even philosophical commentators who disagree with his account find it to be the leading objectivist account of mental disorder: 'Wakefield's analysis has much to be said for it, and it may well be the best or the only way of providing an objective, scientific basis for the notion of disorder' (Bolton, 2008, p. xxiv).

The endophenotype concept in psychiatry

Main citation

Gottesman, I. I. & Gould, T. D. (2003). The endophenotype concept in psychiatry: etymology and strategic intentions. *American Journal of Psychiatry*, 160, 636–645.

Background

Psychiatric disorders have complex genetic underpinnings, and syndromal diagnosis—exemplified by DSM classification—has proven to be non-optimal for genetic research. In the context of genetic theories of schizophrenia in the 1970s, Irving Gottesman and James Shields described 'endophenotypes' as internal phenotypes discoverable by a biochemical test or microscopic examination (Gottesman & Shields, 1973); they adapted the term from Bernard John and Kenneth R. Lewis, who had used it to explain concepts in evolution and insect biology. Endophenotypes are measurable entities at an intermediate level, connecting a disease syndrome with the underlying genotype. An endophenotype may be neurophysiological, biochemical, endocrinological, neuroanatomical, cognitive, or neuropsychological. Even though the endophenotype concept had been introduced in the 1970s, it did not have much widespread impact in psychiatry until publication of the 2003 review paper, which reintroduced this notion to psychiatry, generating excitement and a large body of research (Gottesman & Gould, 2003). Gregory Miller and Brigitte Rockstroh have called 2003–2013 'the decade of the endophenotype' (Miller & Rockstroh, 2013).

Since behavioural syndromes are complex entities with complex genetic underpinnings, endophenotypes are expected to represent relatively less complex phenomena, and the number of genes required to produce variations in endophenotypic traits are expected to be fewer than those involved in producing psychiatric syndromes. Thus, many hoped that we would have better success in linking endophenotypes with genes, and linking endophenotypes with syndromes, rather than linking genes with syndromes directly. In medicine, endophenotype-based methods have been successful in identifying genes related to long QT syndrome, idiopathic hemochromatosis, juvenile myoclonic epilepsy, and familial adenomatous polyposis coli (Gottesman & Gould, 2003).

Methods

The authors reviewed the literature and reintroduced the concept of endophenotypes in the context of intense research into psychiatric biomarkers.

Results

'Endophenotype' is similar to the concept of 'biomarker', but a biomarker differs primarily from an endophenotype in that it has no genetic underpinnings. Gottesman and Gould suggested the following criteria for identifying endophenotypes:

1. The endophenotype is associated with illness in the population.
2. The endophenotype is heritable.
3. The endophenotype is primarily state-independent (manifests in an individual whether or not illness is active).
4. Within families, endophenotype and illness co-segregate.
5. The endophenotype found in affected family members is found in non-affected family members at a higher rate than in the general population.

The article subsequently discusses sensory motor gazing, eye-tracking dysfunction, and working memory as potential candidates for endophenotypes in schizophrenia as salient examples.

Conclusions and critique

The endophenotype concept was innovative and revitalized research efforts at a time when traditional avenues of research were struggling to tackle the complexity of genetic contributions. Years of research in endophenotypes has led to multiple successes but also humility, as the aetiology and pathogenesis of most psychiatric disorders have remained elusive. Many potential endophenotypes have been identified (for instance, executive function and sensory gating in schizophrenia), but there has not been much success yet in finding the genes involved or relevant gene–environment interactions (Miller & Rockstroh, 2013). The assumption that endophenotypes in psychiatry would have less complex genetic underpinnings than syndromes has not yet been demonstrated.

Over time, the endophenotype concept led to the realization that existing syndromic, categorical disorders may hinder research; the National Institute of Mental Health (NIMH) thought along similar lines as it developed its RDoC framework. Moreover, most researchers would now agree that it is naive to assume that endophenotypes would align along conventional diagnostic lines. Endophenotype research supports a transdiagnostic perspective on mental disorder, and it can be reasonably argued that the RDoC initiative represents a natural extension and elaboration of the endophenotype tradition (Miller & Rockstroh, 2013).

Research Domain Criteria and the future of psychiatric classification

Main citations

Insel, T., et al. (2010). Research domain criteria (RDoC): toward a new classification framework for research on mental disorders. *American Journal of Psychiatry*, 167, 748–751.

Sanislow, C. A., et al. (2010). Developing constructs for psychopathology research: research domain criteria. *Journal of Abnormal Psychology*, 119, 631–639.

Background

A large body of research has shown that consensus-based diagnostic categories that utilize clinical descriptions of psychiatric syndromes do not align with findings from clinical neuroscience and genetics research. Research findings do not validate the boundaries of DSM constructs in a way we would expect if these constructs represented distinct disease processes. In addition, clinical syndromes do not have high predictive validity with regards to treatment response. All this suggests that DSM categories are unlikely to capture fundamental mechanisms of dysfunction and aetiology.

In this context, the NIMH launched the Research Domain Criteria (RDoC) project to generate a framework for neuroscientific research on the pathophysiology of mental disorders. It is hoped that the RDoC project will create a future classification that better reflects underlying neurobiological mechanisms. The two selected citations are representative articles that introduced this project to the psychiatric community (Insel et al., 2010; Sanislow et al., 2010).

Methods

The RDoC framework was adapted from a method that had been successfully deployed for studying cognition in schizophrenia—the Cognitive Neuroscience Treatment Research to Improve Cognition in Schizophrenia (CNTRICS) project. The RDoC approach rests on three fundamental assumptions:

1) Mental disorders are brain disorders; that is, they are complex, multi-level disorders of brain circuitry.
2) Dysfunction in neural circuits can be identified with clinical neuroscience tools, such as electrophysiology, functional neuroimaging, and new methods for quantifying connections *in vivo*.
3) Genetics and clinical neuroscience will yield biosignatures or biomarkers that can refine clinical diagnosis and management.

Results

RDoC can be conceived of as a matrix in which the columns of the matrix represent different levels of analysis, starting with genetic, molecular, and cellular levels; proceeding to the circuit level; and on to the level of the individual, family environment, and social context. Though the matrix accommodates all levels of biological, psychological, and social analysis in its framework, the primary focus of RDoC is on neural circuitry. Levels of analysis progress in one of two directions—upwards from measures of circuitry function to variation in clinical function, or downwards to the genetic and molecular/cellular factors. This framework acknowledges that causal influences are multidirectional across levels (e.g. across genes, molecules, cellular systems, neural circuits, and behaviour) and is consistent with the idea of 'explanatory pluralism' with modest hopes of 'patchy reductionism' (Kendler, 2005).

The rows of the matrix represent various constructs grouped hierarchically into broad domains of function (e.g. negative emotionality, cognition). There are five candidate domains in the current conceptualization, which were decided upon by collaborative effort of leading scientists involved in the development of RDoC; and more domains may potentially be added in the future (Insel et al., 2010; Sanislow et al., 2010):

- Negative affect (negative valence systems): includes constructs that are primarily responsible for responses to aversive situations or context, such as fear, distress, and aggression.
- Positive affect (positive valence systems): includes constructs that aggregate for positive emotionality such as reward seeking and learning and habit formation.
- Cognition: includes constructs dealing with attention, perception, working memory/executive function, long-term memory, and cognitive control.
- Systems for social processes: includes constructs that mediate responses in interpersonal settings, such as affiliation and attachment and social communication.
- Arousal/regulatory systems: includes constructs that are responsible for generating activation of neural systems as appropriate for various contexts and providing appropriate homeostatic regulation of such systems as energy balance and sleep.

As an example, Table 1.1 shows the RDoC matrix for positive valence systems at the time of writing this chapter (these domains and constructs are subject to periodic updates by the NIMH) (National Institute of Mental Health, n.d.).

RDoC is by design transdiagnostic; that is, it emphasizes cross-cutting mechanisms for constructs like fear or working memory that can be applied across an array of related diagnoses and de-emphasizes conventionally defined mental disorder categories. RDoC research studies are intended to be conducted in clinical samples, but these samples may include one or more DSM disorders (or they may span across clinical syndromes and subclinical phenomena) based on a hypothesized shared mechanism of interest, such as fear response across anxiety disorders.

Conclusions and critique

Critics have argued that the RDoC's emphasis on brain circuitry as the preferred level of explanation will not be applicable to many psychiatric disorders, that the neuroscience models it relies on are insufficiently developed at present, that it leans towards biological reductionism, and that it gives limited consideration to psychosocial factors in psychopathology and treatment (Paris & Kirmayer, 2016). These are not fatal criticisms, however, as the RDoC can be expanded to incorporate research insights from the domains of psychology, phenomenology, and social sciences.

The NIMH hopes that research conducted within the RDoC framework will lead to new molecular and neurobiological parameters that will predict prognosis and treatment

Table 1.1 Research Domain Criteria matrix for positive valence systems

Construct/Subconstruct		Genes	Molecules	Cells	Circuits	Physiology	Behaviour	Self-Report	Paradigms
Approach motivation	Reward valuation								
	Effort valuation/ Willingness to work								
	Expectancy/Reward prediction error								
	Action selection/ Preference-based decision making								
Initial responsiveness to reward attainment									
Sustained/Longer-term responsiveness to reward attainment									
Reward learning									
Habit									

Adapted from National Institute of Mental Health. RDoC Matrix response more successfully than conventional syndromes. Thus, the utility of the RDoC becomes an empirical matter. If research conducted under the RDoC framework leads to the identification of a genetic polymorphism that identifies responders or non-responders to an intervention, or if a copy number variant identifies a subtype with high remission rates, or if a neuroimaging marker in mood disorders predicts lithium response, such findings will have high impact on future psychiatric classification and practice (Insel et al., 2010; Sanislow et al., 2010).

Conclusion

While psychiatry has made great advances in the diagnosis and conceptualization of mental illness, significant problems and unanswered questions remain and will continue to preoccupy the field in the future. Kraepelin's hope that a classification based on course of illness would ultimately lead to a classification based on brain pathology has not yet been realized. Operationalized criteria have improved the reliability of diagnosis (though there is still room for improvement, as demonstrated by the DSM-5 field trials (Regier et al., 2013)), but not yet the validity of diagnosis. Robins and Guze provided a basis for examining the construct validity of a syndromic diagnosis, but validity based on aetiological considerations remains elusive. The biopsychosocial model provided a unified framework for a divided psychiatry, but it has declined into a lazy eclecticism in practice, necessitating its evolution into a more sophisticated explanatory pluralism. The RDoC framework represents a potential paradigm shift in psychiatric nosology, with hopes of creating a classification fundamentally based on an understanding of disease mechanisms rather than descriptive phenomenology.

Our understanding of the complexity of brain and psychiatric conditions will increase exponentially in the coming decades, and it will be a surprise to none if future conceptualizations of psychiatric conditions are as incommensurable with contemporary views as the notion of 'mental disorder' is with 'madness'.

References

Adityanjee, Aderibigbe, Y. A., Theodoridis, D., & Vieweg, V. R. (1999). Dementia praecox to schizophrenia: the first 100 years. *Psychiatry and Clinical Neurosciences*, **53**, 437–448.

Ash, P. (1949). The reliability of psychiatric diagnoses. *Journal of Abnormal Psychology*, **44**, 272–276.

Bolton, D. (2008). *What is Mental Disorder? An Essay in Philosophy, Science, and Values*. Oxford: Oxford University Press.

Borrell-Carrio, F., Suchman, A. L., & Epstein, R. M. (2004). The biopsychosocial model 25 years later: principles, practice, and scientific inquiry. *Annals of Family Medicine*, **2**, 576–582.

Compton, W. M. & Guze, S. B. (1995). The neo-Kraepelinian revolution in psychiatric diagnosis. *European Archives of Psychiatry and Clinical Neuroscience*, **245**, 196–201.

Engel, G. L. (1977). The need for a new medical model: a challenge for biomedicine. *Science*, **196**, 129–136.

Engel, G. L. (1980). The clinical application of the biopsychosocial model. *American Journal of Psychiatry*, **137**, 535–544.

Engstrom, E. J. & **Kendler, K. S.** (2015). Emil Kraepelin: icon and reality. *American Journal of Psychiatry*, **172,** 1190–1196.

Feighner, J. P., Robins, E., Guze, S. B., Woodruff Jr, R. A., Winokur, G., & **Munoz, R.** (1972). Diagnostic criteria for use in psychiatric research. *Archives of General Psychiatry*, **26,** 57–63.

Frances, A. (2013). DSM in philosophyland: curiouser and curiouser. In: *Making the DSM-5: Concepts and Controversies*, ed. J. Paris & J. Phillips. New York: Springer; pp. 95–103.

Ghaemi, S. N. (2009). The rise and fall of the biopsychosocial model. *British Journal of Psychiatry*, **195,** 3–4.

Ghaemi, S. N. (2013). Bipolar spectrum: a review of the concept and a vision for the future. *Psychiatry Investigations*, **10,** 218–224.

Gottesman, I. I. & **Gould, T. D.** (2003). The endophenotype concept in psychiatry: etymology and strategic intentions. *American Journal of Psychiatry*, **160,** 636–645.

Gottesman, I. I. & **Shields, J.** (1973). Genetic theorizing and schizophrenia. *British Journal of Psychiatry* **122** 15–30.

Gurland, B. J., Fleiss, J. L., Cooper, J. E., Sharpe, L., Kendell, R. E., & **Roberts, P.** (1970). Cross-national study of diagnosis of mental disorders: hospital diagnoses and hospital patients in New York and London. *Comprehensive Psychiatry*, **11,** 18–25.

Insel, T., et al. (2010). Research domain criteria (RDoC): toward a new classification framework for research on mental disorders. *American Journal of Psychiatry*, **167,** 748–751.

Katz, M. M., Cole, J. O., & **Lowery, H. A.** (1969). Studies of the diagnostic process: the influence of symptom perception, past experience, and ethnic background on diagnostic decisions. *American Journal of Psychiatry*, **125,** 937–947.

Kendell, R. E., Cooper, J. E., Gourlay, A. J., Copeland, J. R., Sharpe, L., & **Gurland, B. J.** (1971). Diagnostic criteria of American and British psychiatrists. *Archives of General Psychiatry*, **25,** 123–130.

Kendler, K. S. (1986). Kraepelin and the differential diagnosis of dementia praecox and manic-depressive insanity. *Comprehensive Psychiatry*, **27,** 549–558.

Kendler, K. S. (2005). Toward a philosophical structure for psychiatry. *American Journal of Psychiatry* **162,** 433–440.

Kendler, K. S., Munoz, R. A., & **Murphy, G.** (2010). The development of the Feighner criteria: a historical perspective. *American Journal of Psychiatry*, **167,** 134–142.

Kraepelin, E. (1913). Dementia praecox and paraphrenia (trans. R. M. Barclay) (1919). Edinburgh: E. & S. Livingstone.

Kraepelin, E. (1913). Manic-depressive insanity and paranoia (trans. R. M. Barclay) (1921). Edinburgh: E. & S. Livingstone.

McHugh, P. R. & **Slavney, P. R.** (1998). *The Perspectives of Psychiatry*, 2nd edn Baltimore: Johns Hopkins University Press.

Miller, G.A. & **Rockstroh, B.** (2013). Endophenotypes in psychopathology research: where do we stand? *Annual Review of Clinical Psychology*, **9,** 177–213.

National Institute of Mental Health. (n.d.) *RDoC Matrix*. Available at: https://www.nimh.nih.gov/research-priorities/rdoc/constructs/rdoc-matrix.shtml (accessed 6 April 2018).

Paris, J. & **Kirmayer, L. J.** (2016). The National Institute of Mental Health Research Domain Criteria: a bridge too far. *Journal of Nervous and Mental Disease*, **204,** 26–32.

Regier, D.A., et al. (2013). DSM-5 field trials in the United States and Canada. Part II: test-retest reliability of selected categorical diagnoses. *American Journal of Psychiatry*, **170,** 59–70.

Robins, E. & **Guze, S. B.** (1970). Establishment of diagnostic validity in psychiatric illness: its application to schizophrenia. *American Journal of Psychiatry*, **126,** 983–987.

Rosenhan, D. L. (1973). On being sane in insane places. *Science*, **179**, 250–258.

Sandifer, M. G., Hordern, A., Timbury, G. C., & Green, L. M. (1968). Psychiatric diagnosis: a comparative study in North Carolina, London and Glasgow. *British Journal of Psychiatry*, **114**, 1–9.

Sanislow, C.A., et al. (2010). Developing constructs for psychopathology research: research domain criteria. *Journal of Abnormal Psychology*, **119**, 631–639.

Shorter, E. (2015). The history of nosology and the rise of the Diagnostic and Statistical Manual of Mental Disorders. *Dialogues in Clinical Neuroscience*, **17**, 59–67.

Spitzer, R. L. (1999). Harmful dysfunction and the DSM definition of mental disorder. *Journal of Abnormal Psychology*, **108**, 430–432.

Spitzer, R. L., Endicott, J., & Robins, E. (1978). Research diagnostic criteria: rationale and reliability. *Archives of General Psychiatry*, **35**, 773–782.

Szasz, T. S. (1960). The myth of mental illness. *American Psychologist*, **15**, 113.

US–UK Cross-National Project (1974). The diagnosis and psychopathology of schizophrenia in New York and London. *Schizophrenia Bulletin*, Winter(11), 80–102.

Wakefield, J. C. (1992). The concept of mental disorder. On the boundary between biological facts and social values. *American Psychology*, 47, 373–388.

Zivanovic, O. & Nedic, A. (2012). Kraepelin's concept of manic-depressive insanity: one hundred years later. *Journal of Affective Disorders*, **137**, 15–24.

Chapter 2

Epidemiology

Elizabeth Ryznar and Harvey Whiteford

Introduction

Psychiatric epidemiology is the study of the distribution and determinants of mental disorders in populations, as well as its application in the prevention and treatment of mental disorders. The perspective that clinicians have about a specific disorder comes solely from those who access treatment; however, in almost all countries this only represents a minority of those with the disorder. The individuals who access treatment do not represent all clinical dimensions that exist in the disorder; therefore, it is necessary to study mental disorders at the population level.

Modern psychiatric epidemiology has historical roots in the sociological and ecological studies of the late nineteenth and early twentieth centuries. Frenchman Emile Durkheim concluded that suicide rates were higher among Protestant societies compared to Catholic societies, and were higher in men than women (Durkheim, 1897 [1951]). Robert Faris and Warren Dunham demonstrated the increased risk of schizophrenia in neighbourhoods with a high degree of social disorganization in Chicago (Faris & Dunham, 1939).

After World War II, investigators began to survey participants in the community about their psychological status. One such example is the Midtown Manhattan Study (Srole et al., 1962), which found that 23% of respondents had a substantial mental impairment, while only 19% of respondents lacked significant symptoms and could be considered to have good mental health (Srole et al., 1962). However, a major limitation of these studies was their reliance on scales that gauged either non-specific psychological distress or symptoms for a probable mental disorder but without a diagnosis using specific criteria. Moreover, some surveys used measures of impairment rather than diagnostic criteria, which presented difficulties with reliability and validity[1] (Lapouse & Monk, 1958; Rutter, 1989). These limitations reflected the controversies surrounding the nature of mental health and illness and the lack of a common language to describe mental disorders, which slowed progress in psychiatric epidemiology relative to other areas of epidemiology.

[1] Similarly, the early epidemiological studies in child psychiatry did not produce formal diagnoses. The Buffalo Study (Lapouse & Monk, 1958) examined a non-representative sample of children and found a high frequency of emotional and behavioural problems, many of which decreased with age. Michael Rutter conducted the first large-scale epidemiological investigation in child psychiatry, the Isle of Wight Study (Rutter, 1989), using multiple data sources to survey the entire population and collecting clinical symptoms, but again mental disorders were not formally diagnosed.

To improve the reliability of psychiatric diagnoses, John Wing and his colleagues in London developed the Present State Exam (PSE) (Wing et al., 1974), a semi-structured interview using symptom ratings to assess current diagnosis. The PSE was used in the World Health Organization (WHO) International Pilot Study of Schizophrenia (Sartorius et al., 1974), which established that international comparative psychiatric epidemiology was feasible. Furthermore, with the development of the Diagnostic Interview Schedule (DIS) and publication of the third edition of the *Diagnostic and Statistical Manual of Mental Disorders* (DSM-III) came a consistent set of criteria to measure the presence of mental disorders, and hence prevalence, heralding the beginning of modern psychiatric epidemiology (Dohrenwend & Dohrenwend, 1982).

This chapter highlights key developments in psychiatric epidemiology. The first two papers represent landmark publications that provided quantitative approaches to measuring the prevalence of mental disorders in general populations. The Epidemiological Catchment Area (ECA) Study provided the first comprehensive picture of the current and lifetime prevalence of DSM-III mental disorders in the USA (Robins et al., 1984). The National Comorbidity Survey (NCS) was the first study to estimate current and lifetime prevalence of DSM-III-R mental disorders in a nationally representative American sample (Kessler et al., 1994). These studies established the methods of modern psychiatric epidemiology now employed in many countries, including the use of reliable, lay-administered, structured, diagnostic assessment tools to ascertain standardized diagnostic criteria; the comparison of clinical interviews with lay interviews to evaluate diagnostic validity; and the application of sampling strategies to identify nationally representative samples.

The third paper (Murray & Lopez, 1997d), from the first Global Burden of Disease (GBD) Study, demonstrated how mental illness in the community can be measured using the disability-adjusted life year (DALY), a metric allowing the morbidity and mortality from all diseases and injuries to be compared; it also showed mental disorders to be the leading cause of disability globally. Finally, the fourth study demonstrated how epidemiology can elucidate the causes of mental disorder. A series of studies by American and Danish collaborators established the role of genetic inheritance in schizophrenia, by separating the effect of the family environment using adoption studies (Kety et al., 1971).

One chapter cannot capture all facets of psychiatric epidemiology, and some areas are not covered. Prospective studies are important in epidemiology, as they minimize retrospective recall bias and allow for the separation of risk factors from subsequent factors that occur with or arise from the disorder. One example is the Dunedin Multidisciplinary Health and Development Study in New Zealand, an ongoing cohort study of health and behaviour in 1,037 participants born between 1 April 1972 and 30 March 1973, with retention rates of over 90%. Whilst the study itself represents a landmark, the individual contributions from it have been more incremental and do not lend themselves to the 'landmark paper' format. Additionally, this chapter does not specifically focus on advances in epidemiological research methodology, though this is addressed when discussing the aforementioned papers (and see also Chapter 23), nor on specific populations, such as children or ethnic subpopulations.

Assessing presence of mental disorders in the general population

Main citation

Robins, L. N., et al. (1984). Lifetime prevalence of specific psychiatric disorders in three sites. *Archives of General Psychiatry*, 41, 949–958.

Background

In 1977, then American President Jimmy Carter commissioned a report on the 'mental health needs of the Nation' (Carter, 1977). During its preparation, many psychiatrists recognized that extant epidemiological knowledge could not adequately assess this request (Dohrenwend & Dohrenwend, 1982; Regier et al., 1978; Robins 1978; Weissman & Klerman, 1978): the earliest prevalence studies examined treated populations (i.e. asylums), which were not representative of the general community; meanwhile, community studies from the 1950s and 1960s were non-diagnostic and not particularly replicable. Thus, a new approach was needed.

The ECA Study is considered the first modern psychiatric epidemiological study, presenting lifetime diagnostic prevalence of the major mental disorders for the general population, rather than describing individuals with symptoms or impairments. It harnessed several decades of work rigorously defining mental illness and identifying diagnostic criteria that culminated in DSM-III (see Chapter 1). While the ECA Study was ultimately comprised of multiple phases at five sites, the study investigators presented preliminary findings after completing the first wave of interviews at three sites. A set of five papers was published in 1984—two focusing on objectives and design (Eaton et al., 1984; Regier et al., 1984), one on lifetime prevalence (Robins et al., 1984), one on six-month prevalence (Myers et al., 1984), and one on six-month health service utilization (Shapiro et al., 1984). The lifetime prevalence paper is the most cited and influential of these papers and is discussed here.

Methods

The design was a multisite cross-sectional survey of adults, 18 years and older, in three communities in the USA: New Haven, Baltimore, and St Louis. Each site selected over 3,000 residents, representative of individuals residing in households. Trained lay interviewers administered the DIS, which probed for the presence and severity of current or past psychiatric symptoms. A computerized algorithm determined the diagnoses for each respondent, with respondents' data weighted to account for sampling variation. The response rate was high (75–80%). The paper presented lifetime prevalence in each site for 15 mental disorders including schizophrenia spectrum disorders, affective disorders, anxiety and somatoform disorders, anorexia, antisocial personality disorder, severe cognitive impairment, and substance use disorders.

Results

Approximately one third of the population (29% in New Haven, 31% in St Louis, 38% in Baltimore) had experienced a mental disorder in their lifetime, with the most common being alcohol abuse and dependence (11.5–15.7%), phobias (7.8–23.3%), major depression (3.7–6.7%), and drug abuse and dependence (5.5–5.8%). Antisocial personality disorder and alcohol abuse and dependence were more common in men, whereas depressive disorders and phobias were more common in women. Young adults (aged 25 to 44 years) had the highest prevalence rates for most disorders. Apart from phobias (which were higher in Baltimore), variation in prevalence across the three sites was not significant. There were few racial or ethnic differences (comparing black and non-black people), and where differences were found, they were insignificant compared to age and sex differences, and not consistent across sites.

Conclusions and critique

This study is a landmark for several reasons. First, it established a new era of psychiatric epidemiology that used case definitions for specific diagnoses, thus aligning psychiatric epidemiology with the broader field of population epidemiology. Second, it introduced the method of using trained, non-clinician interviewers to administer a structured interview with a pre-designed algorithm for generating the diagnosis, thus creating the potential for a more cost-effective and standardized collection of population prevalence data across multiple sites. Third, it was the largest epidemiological study up until that time, with each site sampling over 3,000 people; in comparison, the largest studies prior to the ECA Study had assessed 1,010 people (Stirling County in Canada) and 1,660 people (Midtown Manhattan Study in the USA) (Regier et al., 1984). Fourth, the information on service use (and the linkage of epidemiologic and health service use data) revealed that, while a considerable proportion of people in the community met diagnostic criteria for psychiatric illness, only a small subset of these individuals sought treatment from primary care or mental health services (Shapiro et al., 1984).

Despite these advances, the ECA Study had its limitations. The number of diagnoses assessed was restricted and low prevalence disorders were not well represented in household surveys. Later ECA publications reported on data from institutions such as psychiatric hospitals, prisons, and nursing homes in their sampling frameworks to help overcome this limitation. Although the authors of the DIS presented data showing that DSM-III diagnoses given by lay interviewers were in general agreement with those obtained at an independent assessment by a psychiatrist or with chart diagnoses (Robins et al., 1981), comparisons of disorders in remission or borderline conditions produced less satisfactory results. The use of trained lay interviewers remained controversial (Anthony et al., 1985), but became an accepted option in subsequent research.

Developing nationally representative mental health surveys

Main citation

Kessler, R. C., et al. (1994). Lifetime and 12-month prevalence of DSM-III-R psychiatric disorders in the United States. Results from the National Comorbidity Survey. *Archives of General Psychiatry*, 51, 8–19.

Background

The ECA Study established the feasibility of conducting lay-administered structured diagnostic interviews in a community. This foundation allowed researchers to work toward designing and undertaking a nationally representative study. The result was the American NCS, which set the gold standard for community survey methodological design in psychiatric epidemiology.

The NCS relied on the Composite International Diagnostic Interview (CIDI), which evolved from the ECA Study's DIS methodology. Designed by the WHO and the Alcohol, Drug, and Mental Health Administration of the USA, the CIDI was compatible with multiple diagnostic criteria (DSM-III-R and the International Statistical Classification of Diseases (ICD)) and across multiple cultures (with versions available in different languages) (Kessler, 2000). The CIDI was released in 1990, in time for NCS interviews, which occurred in 1990–1992. Presented here is the most cited and influential of the NCS papers, describing lifetime and 12-month prevalence rates of psychiatric disorders in the USA.

Methods

The design was a nationally representative cross-sectional community sample of people aged 15 to 54 (the younger age was meant to capture early onset of disease to minimize recall bias). There were 8,098 respondents, with an overall response rate of 82.6%. Specially trained non-clinician interviewers administered a modified version of the CIDI to generate DSM-III-R diagnoses. These diagnoses included affective disorders, anxiety disorders, substance use disorders, antisocial personality disorder, and non-affective psychosis. Reliability and validity of the CIDI for acute psychotic disorder was low, thus the NCS incorporated clinician re-interviews for respondents with psychotic symptoms using the Structured Clinical Interview for the DSM-III-R. Data was adjusted for the higher non-response rate of people with current and lifetime psychiatric disorders, for probabilities of being selected as a respondent, and for multiple demographic factors in accordance with a separate national health survey.

Results

Nearly half of the respondents (48%) had experienced a mental disorder during their lifetime, and over a quarter (29.5%) met criteria within the previous 12 months. The most prevalent disorder groups were substance use disorders and anxiety disorders, affecting a quarter of the respondents over their lifetimes (26.6% and 24.9%, respectively) and a smaller percentage within the past 12 months (11.3% and 17.2%, respectively). At an individual diagnostic level, the most prevalent disorders were major depressive episode, alcohol dependence, social phobia, and simple phobia.

Comorbidity between mental disorders was common: 26% of lifetime disorders occurred in people with two lifetime disorders, and 54% of lifetime disorders occurred in people with three or more disorders. Put differently, the majority of lifetime disorders in this population were comprised of comorbid disorders (among the whole sample, 14% of respondents had three or more lifetime disorders, 13% had two lifetime disorders, and 21% had one lifetime disorder).

Health service utilization was low: only 42% of people with a lifetime diagnosis ever received care; the percentages were lower for treatment specifically with a psychiatrist or psychologist (26.2%) or in a substance abuse facility (8.4%).

Several statistically significant demographic factors were found to be associated with a lifetime diagnosis. Sex-specific differences resembled those reported in the ECA Study. Respondents aged 25–34 years had higher odds relative to other groups. Black respondents had lower odds of some disorders compared to white respondents; Hispanic respondents had no differences. Lower income and educational level generally correlated with higher odds, though the degree varied by diagnostic category. Geographic region, but not level of urbanization, showed some differences.

Conclusions and critique

The NCS found a higher than expected prevalence of mental illness in a nationally representative sample of the USA, with half of the population experiencing a mental illness over the course of their lifetime, and a quarter experiencing a mental illness within the past 12 months. Mental disorder comorbidity was concentrated in a much smaller group. Most people with mental illness had not received treatment.

There were three main advances from the NCS and CIDI. First, diagnoses were made using DSM-III-R and ICD-10 criteria. Second, the NCS was designed to also assess risk factors and included questions about family psychiatric history, childhood adversity, social networks and support, and stressful life events. Third, the NCS was drawn from a national sampling frame that allowed an examination of regional variations in prevalence, risk factors, and treatment coverage.

There were two main limitations in the NCS. First, the use of trained but lay interviewers, without supplementary information on the respondent, reduced diagnostic precision. Second, the NCS was a cross-sectional survey that relied on retrospective reports by the respondent to assess lifetime prevalence, which introduced recall bias, despite efforts in the design of the interviews (e.g. commitment and memory probes) to minimize this.

As part of the original NCS there were many publications exploring risk factors, comorbidity patterns, and service utilization patterns for specific disorders. A replication study was undertaken in the USA in 2001–2002, adapting the CIDI to produce prevalence using DSM-IV criteria (Kessler et al., 2005). Out of this work emerged the World Mental Health Survey Initiative, which has since undertaken CIDI-based surveys in nearly 30 countries from around the world (Harvard Medical School, 2016).

Identifying mental disorders as the leading cause of disability globally

Main citation

Murray, C. J. & Lopez, A. D. (1997). Regional patterns of disability-free life expectancy and disability-adjusted life expectancy: Global Burden of Disease Study. *Lancet*, 349, 1347–1352.

Background

Historically, priority settings in global health were largely determined by mortality rates, and so mental disorders remained a low global health priority. In 1993, the World Bank released a World Development Report that focused on health (World Bank, 1993). This report used a new time-based metric, the DALY, which combined the years of life lost from premature mortality (YLL) and years lived with disability (YLD). This metric allowed the comparison of health loss from different diseases and injuries using one measure. Thus, disorders that were not considered a cause of death, but which caused substantial morbidity, became recognized as important causes of health loss. The Report was followed by the first GBD Study, which presented mortality and disability rates for 1990 as well as projected rates through 2020. This was published as a book (Murray & Lopez, 1996) and then as four papers in *The Lancet* (Murray & Lopez 1997a, 1997b, 1997c, 1997d). The paper on the burden from disability (Murray & Lopez, 1997d) is presented here.

Methods

Systematic reviews of published and unpublished studies generated data on the incidence, prevalence, duration, and mortality of each disorder (and its disabling sequalae). These were then made internally consistent for each region, by age group, using a specially developed software modelling tool, DisMod.

One DALY equals one healthy year of life lost (YLL + YLD). DALY estimates were made for 107 diseases and injuries for the year 1990 with projections to 2020. YLL were calculated from the number of deaths at each age multiplied by a global standard life expectancy for the age at which the death occurred. YLD for each disorder for each time period was calculated by the number of incident cases in that period multiplied by the average duration of the disorder and a disability weight that reflected the severity of the disorder on a scale from 0 (perfect health) to 1 (death). Projections of the change in mortality and disability for each disorder to 2020 were made using trends in population growth and ageing and the decline in age-specific mortality from communicable, maternal, perinatal, and nutritional disorders.

Results

This study highlighted major differences in the leading causes of premature mortality as measured by YLL, compared to the leading causes of disability, as measured by YLD. The burden from mental illnesses was found to have been seriously underestimated by traditional approaches that only accounted for deaths and not disability (Murray & Lopez, 1996, p. 284). Although mental illnesses (including substance abuse) were found to be responsible for little more than 1% of deaths, they accounted for over 10% of disease burden worldwide. In 1990, there were no mental disorders in the top ten causes of mortality, but five of the ten leading causes of disability were mental disorders (major depression, alcohol use disorder, bipolar disorder, schizophrenia, and OCD), with depression the number one cause of disability globally.

The other major finding from the overall study (Murray & Lopez, 1996) was the declining contribution to global disease burden from communicable, maternal, perinatal, and nutritional disorders, and the increasing contribution from non-communicable disorders and injuries. The decline in child mortality allowed more of the population to survive into the age groups where mental disorders and other non-communicable disorders predominate. The proportionate share of the global burden of disease due to neuropsychiatric disorders (mental and neurological disorders) was projected to rise from 10.5% in 1990 to 14.7% in 2020.

Conclusions and critique

This original study, and all subsequent annual GBD studies (most recently for 328 disorders and injuries in 195 countries), have consistently demonstrated that mental disorders rank as prominent causes of burden (DALYs) and are the leading cause of disability (YLD) globally (Vos et al., 2017). This has raised the profile of mental health on the global stage and influenced how governments and international agencies prioritize mental health in many parts of the world.

The DALYs for mental disorders are predominately due to the YLD component, which reflects the high prevalence and persistence of these disorders, as well as their high level of impairment (acute psychosis has the highest disability weight of all disorders in GBD) (Whiteford et al., 2013). The premature mortality of people with mental disorders is not included in the YLL component because GBD assigns one cause of death and this follows the ICD classification (where suicide is assigned to injuries). Mental disorders are rarely identified as the primary cause of death. GBD estimates could be improved if the increased risk of death in individuals with a mental disorder was captured as part of the comparative risk assessment protocol component of the GBD.

Separating family environment and genetics in schizophrenia

Main citation

Kety, S. S., Rosenthal, D., Wender, P. H., & Schulsinger, F. (1971). Mental illness in the biological and adoptive families of adopted schizophrenics. *American Journal of Psychiatry*, 128, 302–306.

Background

It had long been known that mental disorders tended to run in families but beliefs about why, greatly influenced by the writings of dominant figures such as Sigmund Freud and Emil Kraepelin, led to profoundly different views on the origin and pathophysiology of mental illness. The controversy raged for over a century, with one school arguing that mental illness was a result of dysfunctional relationships in the family, especially between parent and child, and the other proposing a hereditary cause. Early research tried to address this controversy in schizophrenia by showing that the disorder had higher concordance rates in monozygotic twins than in dizygotic twins (Kallmann, 1946; Slater, 1953). While this was compatible with genetic factors, there were alternative explanations for these concordance rates as the environmental factors and relationships within the family, even for twins, were not the same (Gottesman & Shields, 1976). The probability of a genetic component was strengthened by the findings from a study showing a higher prevalence of schizophrenia and other disorders in the children of mothers hospitalized with chronic schizophrenia who were reared in foster homes, compared to a control group (Heston, 1966). The rate of schizophrenia in the adopted and biological parents of adopted individuals with schizophrenia, carried out over 25 years by American and Danish collaborators, produced the most definitive evidence for the importance of genetic factors in the aetiology of schizophrenia. The findings were first published as a book chapter (Kety et al., 1968; see also discussion in Chapter 4) and then as an article in the *American Journal of Psychiatry* (Kety et al., 1971).

Methods

Kety et al. (1971) used the comprehensive population and health registries in Denmark to identify adoptees and their adoptive and biological parents, and to obtain hospitalization records and diagnoses of each individual. Out of 5,483 children adopted to non-biological families in Copenhagen between 1924 and 1948, 507 were admitted to a psychiatric hospital for any reason. Abstracts of these 507 cases were prepared and presented to the authors, who identified 33 "index cases" of schizophrenia based on consensus review. Thirty-three controls were chosen from the sample of adoptees who had not been admitted to a psychiatric hospital; they were matched on sex, age, time spent with biological family, preadoption history, and adoptive family's socioeconomic class. A registry search was then undertaken to identify the biological and adoptive family members (parents, siblings, and half-siblings) of the index and control cases, yielding 463 total relatives. Hospital, police, and military records for these relatives were then reviewed to identify any possible psychiatric disorders. Those records were abstracted and presented to authors, who again identified diagnoses by consensus review. They considered several 'schizophrenia spectrum' diagnoses: definite schizophrenia, possible schizophrenia, and 'inadequate personality' (a category similar to 'borderline schizophrenia'). The prevalence of schizophrenia spectrum disorders among biological and adoptive family members of index cases versus controls were compared.

Results

Of the 463 relatives, 67 were considered to have some form of mental illness. Consensus review of those relatives revealed 21 relatives with schizophrenia spectrum disorders. Among biological relatives, 13/150 relatives of index cases had a schizophrenia spectrum disorder (8.7%) compared to 3/156 relatives of control cases (1.9%). This difference was statistically significant ($p = 0.0072$). Among adoptive relatives, 2/74 relatives of index cases had a schizophrenia spectrum disorder (2.7%) compared to 3/83 relatives of control cases (3.6%). This difference was not statistically significant. This pattern was even stronger among adoptees who were separated from their biological families within one month of birth: 9/93 biological relatives of index cases had a schizophrenia spectrum disorder (9.6%) compared with 0/92 biological relatives of control cases ($p = 0.0018$); 2/45 adoptive relatives of index cases had a schizophrenia spectrum disorder (4.4%) compared with 1/51 adoptive relatives of control cases (1.9%). There did not seem to be a correlation between the type of schizophrenia (acute, chronic, or borderline) in the index cases and the type and severity of schizophrenia spectrum disorders in their biological family members, which to the authors suggested polygenic inheritance.

Conclusions and critique

This study, and subsequent studies by the same research collaboration, confirmed that children born to a mother with schizophrenia, but reared in an adoptive family, develop schizophrenia at a similar rate as those reared by the biological mother. They also found that biological relatives of an adopted person with schizophrenia have significantly elevated rates of schizophrenia, whereas the adoptive families of that person do not have elevated rates of schizophrenia.

Though revolutionary at the time, this landmark paper has several limitations. A limitation shared with all registry studies is the sole reliance on governmental and hospital records. Additional limitations include a small sample size and inability of their study design to examine the environment of the index cases and controls. Subsequent research by the group addressed these limitations. They employed an innovative 'cross-fostering' design to examine psychotic illnesses in adoptees reared by non-biological parents with schizophrenia. Adoptees from biological families in which there was no schizophrenia raised by adoptive parents *with* schizophrenia were no more likely to develop schizophrenia than adopted children from biological families without schizophrenia raised by adoptive parents without schizophrenia (Wender et al., 1974).

Thus, genetic factors were shown to be important in the development of schizophrenia, opening the door to an explosion of genetic research in many mental disorders. Since 2009, genome-wide analyses have searched for the individual genetic regions (loci) associated with schizophrenia, with 108 loci now identified as contributing to schizophrenia susceptibility (Schizophrenia Working Group of the Psychiatric Genomics, 2014) (see Chapters 4 and 7). However, it will be important to uncover the gene–environment interplay that determines how expression of genetic vulnerability leads to the development of psychopathology (van Os et al., 2010).

Conclusion

The landmark papers describe breakthroughs in how we count mental disorders in the general population, how we measure their impact on an individual in comparison to other health conditions, and how we understand causes of mental disorders.

The breakthroughs in these papers depended heavily on cross-sectional assessments of the population. To address additional questions in psychiatric epidemiology, other study designs are necessary. Ongoing work from prospective cohort studies examines developmental trajectories, psychosocial risk factors, and early manifestations of emerging mental disorder. Combining epidemiological evidence with that from genetics and neuroscience increases the opportunities for understanding the aetiology of mental illness and, with that, the possibility for primary prevention.

While the prospect of uncovering more about the cause of mental illness is exciting, epidemiology has immediate practical relevance for health policy. It provides information about those at risk in the population, those who have a mental disorder, and the impact on their lives. It provides information on accessibility of treatment and the barriers to or facilitators of receiving effective interventions. Additionally, it can track changes in all these areas over time. As such, epidemiology is a basic tool for public health planning (McGrath et al., 2018).

References

Anthony, J. C., et al. (1985). Comparison of the lay Diagnostic Interview Schedule and a standardized psychiatric diagnosis. Experience in eastern Baltimore. *Archives of General Psychiatry*, **42**(7), 667–675.

Carter, J. (1977). *President's Commission on Mental Health*. Available at: http://www.presidency.ucsb.edu/ws/?pid=6643 (accessed 17 March 2018).

Dohrenwend, B. P. & Dohrenwend, B. S. (1982). Perspectives on the past and future of psychiatric epidemiology. The 1981 Rema Lapouse Lecture. *American Journal of Public Health*, **72**(11), 1271–1279.

Durkheim, É. (1897 [1951]). *Suicide: A Study in Sociology*. New York: Free Press.

Eaton, W. W., et al. (1984). The design of the Epidemiologic Catchment Area surveys. The control and measurement of error. *Archives of General Psychiatry*, **41**(10), 942–948.

Faris, R. E. L. & Dunham, W. H. (1939). *Mental Disorders in Urban Areas: An Ecological Study of Schizophrenia and Other Psychoses.* Chicago, Illinois: The University of Chicago Press.

Gottesman, I. I. & Shields, J. (1976). A critical review of recent adoption, twin, and family studies of schizophrenia: behavioral genetics perspectives. *Schizophrenia Bulletin*, **2**(3), 360–401.

Harvard Medical School (2016). *The World Mental Health Survey Initiative.* Available at: https://www.hcp.med.harvard.edu/wmh/ (accessed 17 March 2018).

Heston, L. L. (1966). Psychiatric disorders in foster home reared children of schizophrenic mothers. *British Journal of Psychiatry*, **112**(489), 819–825.

Kallmann, F. J. (1946). The genetic theory of schizophrenia: an analysis of 691 schizophrenic twin index families. *American Journal of Psychiatry*, **103**(3), 309–322.

Kessler, R. C. (2000). Psychiatric epidemiology: selected recent advances and future directions. *Bulletin of the World Health Organization*, **78**(4), 464–474.

Kessler, R. C., et al. (2005). Lifetime prevalence and age-of-onset distributions of DSM-IV disorders in the National Comorbidity Survey replication. *Archives of General Psychiatry*, **62**(6), 593–602.

Kessler, R. C., et al. (1994). Lifetime and 12-month prevalence of DSM-III-R psychiatric disorders in the United States. Results from the National Comorbidity Survey. *Archives of General Psychiatry*, **51**(1), 8–19.

Kety, S. S., Rosenthal, D., Wender, P. H., & Schulsinger, F. (1968). The types and prevalence of mental illness in the biological and adoptive families of adopted schizophrenics. In: *The Transmission of Schizophrenia*, ed. D. Rosenthal & S. S. Kety. Oxford: Pergamon Press.

Kety, S. S., Rosenthal, D., Wender, P. H., & Schulsinger, F. (1971). Mental illness in the biological and adoptive families of adopted schizophrenics. *American Journal of Psychiatry*, **128**(3), 302–306.

Lapouse, R. & Monk, M. A. (1958). An epidemiologic study of behavior characteristics in children. *American Journal of Public Health and the Nation's Health*, **48**(9), 1134–1144.

McGrath, J. J., Mortensen, P. B., & Whiteford, H. A. (2018). Pragmatic psychiatric epidemiology–if you can't count it, it won't count. *Journal of the American Medical Association: Psychiatry*, **75**(2), 111–112.

Murray, C. J. L. & Lopez, A. D. (1996). *The Global Burden of Disease: A Comprehensive Assessment of Mortality and Disability from Diseases, Injuries, and Risk Factors in 1990 and Projected to 2020.* Cambridge, MA: Harvard School of Public Health on behalf of the World Health Organization and the World Bank.

Murray, C. J. L. & Lopez, A. D. (1997a). Alternative projections of mortality and disability by cause 1990–2020: Global Burden of Disease Study. *Lancet*, **349**(9064), 1498–1504.

Murray, C. J. L. & Lopez, A. D. (1997b). Global mortality, disability, and the contribution of risk factors: Global Burden of Disease Study. *Lancet*, **349**(9063), 1436–1442.

Murray, C. J. L. & Lopez, A. D. (1997c). Mortality by cause for eight regions of the world: Global Burden of Disease Study. *Lancet*, **349**(9061), 1269–1276.

Murray, C. J. L. & Lopez, A. D. (1997d). Regional patterns of disability-free life expectancy and disability-adjusted life expectancy: Global Burden of Disease Study. *Lancet*, **349**(9062), 1347–1352.

Myers, J. K., et al. (1984). Six-month prevalence of psychiatric disorders in three communities 1980 to 1982. *Archives of General Psychiatry*, **41**(10), 959–967.

Regier, D. A., Goldberg, I. D., & Taube, C. A. (1978). The de facto US mental health services system: a public health perspective. *Archives of General Psychiatry*, **35**(6), 685–693.

Regier, D. A., et al. (1984). The NIMH Epidemiologic Catchment Area program. Historical context, major objectives, and study population characteristics. *Archives of General Psychiatry*, **41**(10), 934–941.

Robins, L. N. (1978). Psychiatric epidemiology. *Archives of General Psychiatry*, **35**(6), 697–702.

Robins, L. N., Helzer, J. E., Croughan, J., & Ratcliff, K. S. (1981). National Institute of Mental Health Diagnostic Interview Schedule. Its history, characteristics, and validity. *Archives of General Psychiatry*, **38**(4), 381–389.

Robins, L. N., et al. (1984). Lifetime prevalence of specific psychiatric disorders in three sites. *Archives of General Psychiatry*, **41**(10), 949–958.

Rutter, M. (1989). Isle of Wight revisited: twenty-five years of child psychiatric epidemiology. *Journal of the American Academy of Child and Adolescent Psychiatry*, **28**(5), 633–653.

Sartorius, N., Shapiro, R., & Jablensky, A. (1974). The International Pilot Study of Schizophrenia. *Schizophrenia Bulletin*, **1**(11), 21–34.

Schizophrenia Working Group of the Psychiatric Genomics, Consortium (2014). Biological insights from 108 schizophrenia-associated genetic loci. *Nature*, **511**(7510), 421–427.

Shapiro, S., et al. (1984). Utilization of health and mental health services. Three Epidemiologic Catchment Area sites. *Archives of General Psychiatry*, **41**(10), 971–978.

Slater, E. & Shields, J. (1953). *Psychotic and Neurotic Illness in Twins.* Medical Research Council Special Report Series No. 278. London: Her Majesty's Stationery Office.

Srole, L., Langner, T. S., Michael, S. T., Opler, M. K., & Rennie, T. A. C. (1962). *Mental Health in the Metropolis: The Midtown Manhattan Study.* New York: McGraw-Hill.

van Os, J., Kenis, G., & Rutten, B. P. F. (2010). The environment and schizophrenia. *Nature*, **468**(7321), 203–212.

Vos, T. & GBD 2016 Disease and Injury Incidence and Prevalence Collaborators (2017). Global, regional, and national incidence, prevalence, and years lived with disability for 328 diseases and injuries for 195 countries, 1990–2016: a systematic analysis for the Global Burden of Disease Study 2016. *Lancet*, **390**(10100), 1211–1259.

Weissman, M. M. & Klerman, G. L. (1978). Epidemiology of mental disorders: emerging trends in the United States. *Archives of General Psychiatry*, **35**(6), 705–712.

Wender, P. H., Rosenthal, D., Kety, S. S., Schulsinger, F., & Welner, J. (1974). Crossfostering. A research strategy for clarifying the role of genetic and experiential factors in the etiology of schizophrenia. *Archives of General Psychiatry*, **30**(1), 121–128.

Whiteford, H. A., et al. (2013). Global burden of disease attributable to mental and substance use disorders: findings from the Global Burden of Disease Study 2010. *Lancet*, **382**(9904), 1575–1586.

Wing, J. K., Cooper, J. E., & Sartorius, N. (1974). *Measurement and Classification of Psychiatric Symptoms: An Instruction Manual for the PSE and Catego Program.* London/New York: Cambridge University Press.

World Bank (1993). *World Development Report 1993: Investing in Health.* New York: Oxford University Press.

Section II

Pathogenesis

Chapter 3

The neurochemical basis of psychiatric disorders

Elizabeth Ryznar and Herbert Y. Meltzer

Introduction

Neurochemical theories of mental illness were offered in ancient times, but the first evidence-based theories emerged in the 1950s, stimulated by the discovery of effective medications for schizophrenia (chlorpromazine, reserpine), major depression (tricyclic amine reuptake inhibitors and monoamine oxidase inhibitors), and bipolar disorder or manic-depressive illness (lithium carbonate). These serendipitously discovered medications revolutionized the treatment of patients with these disorders and stimulated the development of sophisticated methods to test drug efficacy, develop animal models, and establish outpatient treatment networks. Thanks to these outpatient centres, which administered medications and provided additional support services, patients were able to lead better lives outside of the huge asylums that had developed in the nineteenth and early twentieth centuries. Moreover, for the first time, a wide range of neuroscientists (including medicinal chemists, neuroanatomists, pharmacologists, physiologists, microscopists, and ethnopsychopharmacologists based not only in academic centres but also in the developing modern pharmaceutical industry, which had its origins in pharmacies or chemical companies) had valid starting points for exploring the wonders of the human brain and the basis for its dysfunction, which afflicted people of all ages and ethnicities, male and female. In a relatively short period of time after their introduction in the 1950s, first-generation antidepressants and antipsychotics inspired novel pathophysiological theories of the underlying disease process, which were then used to develop and test putative next-generation antidepressant and antipsychotic drugs (APDs).

This chapter illustrates how some of the most heuristic neurochemical theories of schizophrenia and depression arose. Although there are many papers that illustrate this fascinating slice of research, we have chosen four papers that demonstrate in a historical context how hypotheses are developed and tested. We begin with the monoamine theory of depression,[1] which proposes that the illness labelled as major depression by current criteria (dysphoria, sadness, hopelessness, motor retardation, flat affect, suicidal ideation,

[1] 'Monoamine' refers to the chemical structure of small molecules like serotonin, norepinephrine, epinephrine, and dopamine; the last three share a 'catechol' group and are often called catecholamines.

weight loss, loss of interest in sexual activity) is caused by a deficiency of the monoamine neurotransmitter, norepinephrine (NE), and could respond to a restoration of the function and availability of this neurotransmitter. The second theory we have chosen to discuss was pioneered by Dutch psychiatrist Herman van Praag and others, who articulated the 'serotonin hypothesis' of depression. Together these two hypotheses dominated biological psychiatry and drug discovery relative to depression, until recent developments in understanding the role of gamma-aminobutyric acid (GABA) and glutamate in neurotransmission, including their effects on NE and serotonin (5-hydroxytryptophan, or 5-HT).

We next discuss two seminal papers that are relevant to understanding the pathophysiology of schizophrenia. We have chosen a paper by Herbert Meltzer and colleagues which advanced the theory that effects on 5-HT_{2A} receptors may contribute to the 'atypical' properties of clozapine, an antipsychotic drug that was first noted to have low extrapyramidal symptoms compared to other first-generation antipsychotics and was later shown to be more efficacious in treatment-resistant psychosis. As this novel hypothesis was percolating, the prior theory that psychosis was due to excessive dopamine D_2 receptor stimulation in the limbic brain was widely accepted as the definitive theory of psychosis, which was then considered synonymous with schizophrenia itself (a view which has been challenged by the theory that it is the dorsal striatum which is responsible for psychosis). The final article discusses the role of the excitatory neurotransmitter glutamate in the pathogenesis of schizophrenia and broadens the concept of schizophrenia to include negative symptoms and cognitive impairment. In discussing each of these papers, this chapter also highlights other key studies that informed or followed these landmark contributions to our understanding of the aetiology and treatment of these two key disorders and their treatment.

We have also endeavoured to point out that the development of these theories and novel treatments for schizophrenia and major depression also led to many breakthroughs in understanding the neurobiology of the brain (for a more detailed account, see Robinson (2001) or Valenstein (2005)). Ever since Spanish histologist Santiago Ramón y Cajal theorized, in the late 1880s, that neurons were distinct cells separated by a gap, physiologists sought to understand how neurons communicated with each other across this gap (termed 'synapse' by English neurophysiologist Charles Scott Sherrington in 1897).[2] While prevailing scientific opinion favoured electricity as the method of synaptic communication, some researchers speculated that small molecules like curare, muscarine, and adrenal extracts might be the basis for synaptic communication. In 1921, German researcher Otto Loewi provided the first direct evidence of chemical synaptic transmission, demonstrating that a chemical substance excreted from the vagus nerve slowed the heart rate (this '*Vagusstoff*' was soon proven to be acetylcholine). It took another decade for the scientific community to fully accept chemical transmission as the mode of synaptic communication in the peripheral nervous system. However, the notion that synaptic chemical transmission occurred in the central nervous system remained speculative and highly controversial,

[2] Remarkably, because of the light microscope's resolution limits, the synapse was never directly visualized until the 1950s, thanks to the electron microscope.

even as researchers demonstrated the presence of acetylcholine, serotonin, norepinephrine, and epinephrine in brain tissues during the 1930s and the following two decades.

Psychotropic medications proved to be invaluable tools for establishing the role of neurotransmitters and neuromodulators in neuronal communication in the brain. Decoding how psychotropic medications worked within synapses was honoured by the award of two Nobel Prizes. Julius Axelrod used first-generation antidepressant drugs to clarify our understanding of the importance of reuptake of norepinephrine as an essential feature of neurotransmission, while Arvid Carlsson, studying the action of amphetamine and chlorpromazine, identified dopamine as a neurotransmitter (specifically that amphetamine enhances the availability of dopamine and norepinephrine, and that chlorpromazine blocks the action of dopamine at specific dopamine receptors).

The 'catecholamine hypothesis' of depression

Main citation

Schildkraut, J. J. (1965). The catecholamine hypothesis of affective disorders: a review of supporting evidence. *American Journal of Psychiatry*, 122, 509–522.

Background

Three drugs were crucial to understanding the neurochemical basis of major depression, which Winston Churchill famously referred to as his 'black dog': reserpine, iproniazid, and imipramine. All were first used for treatments of other medical disorders, but astute clinicians noted important effects on mood: reserpine caused depression, while iproniazid and imipramine alleviated depression. Reserpine, first isolated in 1952 from a plant used in Indian medicine as a calming agent, was found to be an effective sedative and antihypertensive agent. Though it received limited use for these two indications, its ability to cause a high incidence of clinically relevant depressive symptoms that resembled those of endogenous depression became evident, stimulating speculation on the mechanism of this unwanted side-effect. Iproniazid, a widely used antitubercular agent developed in 1951, was found to produce 'mild euphoria' as a side-effect (Selikoff et al., 1952). This stimulated open and then controlled studies, primitive by today's standards, in depressed patients, which demonstrated its beneficial effects, leading it to be labelled a 'psychic energizer' (Loomer et al., 1957). Finally, imipramine was initially developed in Sweden as a putative antipsychotic, derived from the tricyclic antipsychotic phenothiazines, of which chlorpromazine was the prototype. Imipramine was not as effective as a treatment for schizophrenia. However, psychiatrist Roland Kuhn tested it in three patients with major depression in the mid-1950s and found it to be effective after several weeks of treatment (as described in Miller (2014) and also in Chapter 8). Subsequent clinical trials confirmed his observations, and imipramine and its analogues became the mainstay for decades for treating depression, despite their slow onset of action and their side-effects.

Because of these effects on mood, researchers sought to understand the mechanisms of action of the three agents. One group at the National Institutes of Health (NIH), led by Bernard Brodie, noted the structural similarity of reserpine to serotonin. They used their novel method of measuring brain serotonin levels via spectrophotofluorimetry to assess the effect of systemic reserpine on serotonin levels in rabbit brain homogenates, demonstrating a severe dose-dependent depletion (Brodie et al., 1955; Pletscher et al., 1956). Of note, this was the first demonstration of chemical synaptic transmission in the central nervous system.[3] Soon after, they showed that reserpine also depleted norepinephrine (Brodie et al., 1957). That group then discovered that iproniazid, already known to inhibit monoamine oxidase, increased serotonin and norepinephrine levels in rat brain homogenates (Brodie et al., 1959). Meanwhile, Julius Axelrod, also at the NIH, used radiolabelled ^{3H}NE to show that reserpine caused the release of norepinephrine from vesicles within presynaptic neurons and imipramine prevented the reuptake of norepinephrine into presynaptic neurons where it could be repackaged for release (Axelrod et al., 1962).

All of this convergent clinical and preclinical evidence led to speculation that depression could result from alterations in brain biogenic amines. In 1965, Joseph Schildkraut synthesized the existing literature to advocate for the 'catecholamine hypothesis', which states that 'some, if not all, depressions are associated with an absolute or relative deficiency of catecholamines, particularly norepinephrine, at functionally important [nor] adrenergic receptor sites in the brain' (Schildkraut, 1965). Other reviewers came to the same conclusion (Coppen, 1967; Bunney & Davis, 1965), though Schildkraut's paper became the most cited.

Methods

A critical review and synthesis of preclinical and clinical studies.

Results

Schildkraut begins by summarizing the neuroanatomical distribution of monoamines. He then cites the controversy over whether biogenic amines, such as NE, are neurotransmitters or neuromodulators whose primary effects are through other neurotransmitters. The article then discusses the metabolism of catecholamines, and specifically the use of their metabolites to measure turnover (like, for example, vanillylmandelic acid for norepinephrine).

Next, Schildkraut reviews the links between antidepressant medications and monoamines. He cites the fact that effective antidepressants like iproniazid increase NE and 5-HT levels in the brain. He also notes that amphetamine, known to enhance synaptic levels of NE, alleviates depression, while amphetamine withdrawal, which may reflect a relative decrease in NE levels, leads to depressive symptoms. Finally, he describes then-recent evidence demonstrating that imipramine blocks norepinephrine reuptake into the presynaptic terminal and increases the duration of synaptic stimulation of noradrenergic receptors, thus further supporting the 'catecholamine hypothesis'.

3 In his Nobel Prize lecture, Arvid Carlsson, who briefly worked in Brodie's lab before pursuing his own catecholamine research, described the impact of this finding: 'For the first time, a bridge seemed to have been built between the biochemistry of the brain and some important brain functions' (lecture given on 8 December 2000; transcript available at https://www.nobelprize.org/prizes/medicine/2000/carlsson/lecture/).

Schildkraut then describes the link between reserpine and catecholamines. He highlights the temporal association between reserpine-induced behavioural changes and measurable decreases in synaptic levels of NE. Moreover, he notes that administration of dihydroxyphenylalanine (DOPA), the precursor of DA and NE, rescues reserpine-induced decreases in locomotor activity and other symptoms of depression. This linkage of reserpine-induced depression and the antidepressant action of MAO-Is and imipramine provides a coherent model for causation and treatment of depression based upon the availability of brain NE.

Schildkraut also summarizes the evidence that urine levels of norepinephrine, and especially its metabolites, support the catecholamine hypothesis, with the qualification that the urine levels may not reflect what is occurring in the brain.

Conclusions and critique

This review article elegantly summarized the evidence available at the time for the role of NE in depression, and was very influential in transforming views of depression as an illness that reflected biological vulnerability, which could be triggered by stress and other causes (e.g. agents which depleted the availability of neurotransmitters). It was modest in its claims, leaving room for other causes of depression. It recognized that while drugs may produce similar effects, they may do so via different pathways. It also acknowledged a need for much more direct examination of the role of NE in the brains of depressed patients, both living and deceased. Numerous brain banks were started in this era which proved to be of enormous value in enabling investigators to study the pathophysiology of depression and suicide. Schildkraut predicted there would be evidence for other neurotransmitters and neuromodulators as causes of depression. Post-mortem studies (and eventually brain imaging studies) that capture basal levels in a case-control design, or within-subject studies of change in mood state and drug effects, were on the horizon in this era. Ultimately, they provided confirmatory evidence for diminished noradrenergic activity in depressed patients (Klimek et al., 1997; Horton, 1992). In subsequent decades, the importance of genetic and epigenetic factors to regulate noradrenergic activity would be discovered and used to refine and circumscribe the catecholamine hypothesis (Zhu et al., 2019).

The 'serotonin hypothesis' of depression

Main citation

van Praag, H. M., Korf, J., & Puite, J. (1970). 5-hydroxyindoleacetic acid levels in the cerebrospinal fluid of depressive patients treated with probenecid. *Nature*, 225, 1259–1260.

Background

While Schildkraut and many others focused on the role of NE, glucocorticoids, and to a lesser extent, dopamine (DA), in the aetiology of depression, others, especially Herman van Praag in the Netherlands, and Alec Coppen and Merton Sandler in England, emphasized the importance of decreased levels of 5-HT as a cause of specific types of depressive illness. The evidence that was available at the time was quite analogous to that available for the role of NE in depression, including the depletion of 5-HT by reserpine in the brains of laboratory animals. The previously mentioned Brodie lab at NIMH vigorously debated whether depletion of 5-HT or NE was important to the loss of motor activity following reserpine. Additional evidence for the role of serotonin came from the observation that replenishment of 5-HT with tryptophan, a serotonin precursor, alleviated depression in some people, especially when given with a monoamine oxidase inhibitor. Furthermore, people who completed suicide had lower cerebrospinal fluid (CSF) levels of serotonin and its major metabolite, 5-hydroxyindoleacetic acid (5-HIAA). Low levels of 5-HIAA in plasma and CSF of depressed patients were reported from many laboratories.

Amidst this mounting evidence for serotonin's role in depression, Herman van Praag and colleagues devised an elegant experiment to test the 'serotonin hypothesis of depression' (van Praag et al., 1970). They proposed that increases in CSF 5-HIAA concentrations following administration of probenecid, a drug that blocks transport of 5-HIAA from the brain to the bloodstream, could serve as a real-time measure of the brain's rate of serotonin synthesis, and thus demonstrate whether a 'serotonin deficiency' was present in some depressed patients. van Praag was an early champion of subtyping on phenomenological and presumptive causal bases. He believed that 'reactive' depression (what we might now consider stress-induced depression) was a separate subtype compared to 'vital' or endogenous depression, a variant of the illness which emerges from internal changes in brain chemistry that are independent of stresses or other environmental causes.

Methods

van Praag conducted biological examinations in a research unit in which he measured CSF levels of 5-HIAA in 14 patients with 'endogenous' depression and 11 age- and sex-matched controls; all participants had not received medications for at least one week. Baseline CSF 5-HIAA concentrations were obtained on the first day via lumbar puncture. All participants then received multiple doses of probenecid on the second and third days, and a final dose on the fourth day, followed by a repeat lumbar puncture to measure the accumulation of 5-HIAA.

Results

Baseline CSF 5-HIAA levels were lower at baseline in depressed patients compared to controls (see Table 3.1). After probenecid treatment, CSF concentrations of 5-HIAA

Table 3.1 Concentrations of 5-HIAA in the cerebrospinal fluid (μg/mL)

	Baseline	After probenecid	Change
Depressed patients	0.017 +/− 0.017	0.039 +/− 0.025	0.022 +/− 0.020
Controls	0.040 +/− 0.024	0.074 +/− 0.026	0.035 +/− 0.018

Adapted with permission from Van Praag, H. M. and Puite, J. 5-Hydroxyindoleacetic Acid Levels in the Cerebrospinal Fluid of Depressive Patients treated with Probenecid. *Nature, 225*:1259–1260. Copyright © 1970, Springer Nature. https://doi.org/10.1038/2251259b0.

increased in both groups, but less so in the patients with depression (see Table 3.1). The authors noted that seven patients with depression had a mean change of less than 0.020 ug/ml, compared to only one patient in the control group; this difference was statistically significant ($p < 0.05$).

Conclusions and critique

The authors developed a method to measure the overall rate of synthesis and metabolism of serotonin in the brain of depressed patients and controls, and thus, of providing a test of the serotonin hypothesis of depression. They found an overall decrease in serotonin release and metabolism, in line with their hypothesis.

Limitations of the study are that CSF levels of 5-HIAA provided only a limited picture of 5-HT neuronal activity. Regional differences were not assessed; these are no doubt present and important in understanding the brain areas involved in causing depression. The sample size was small and did not account for differences between vital and reactive depression. The drug washout time was short by any standard. Nevertheless, this study provided important evidence from depressed patients consistent with the idea of diminished synthesis and release of 5-HT in the brain.

This paper helped inspire the development of selective serotonin reuptake inhibitors (SSRIs). The first of these drugs to be introduced was zimelidine, developed by Arvid Carlsson and Astra-Zeneca in Sweden. It was prematurely withdrawn in 1983 due to a single fatal case of Guillain Barre syndrome, enabling fluoxetine (Prozac) to become the dominant drug of this class. Fluoxetine revolutionized treatment of depression because of its improved safety profile relative to the tricyclics and monoamine oxidase inhibitors, which can be fatal in overdose.

The role of serotonin in depression is now known to be more nuanced than simple deficiency. Modern research emphasizes the balance of serotoninergic activity overall, as well as the differing roles of various serotonin receptors. SSRIs require three weeks before they are effective, correlated with the time period needed to desensitize presynaptic 5-HT_{1A} receptors, which normally serve to inhibit the synthesis and release of 5-HT. Desensitization of the autoreceptor must occur before release of 5-HT and stimulation of post-synaptic 5-HT_{1A} receptors. Furthermore, 5-HT_7 and 5-HT_{1A} receptors have been shown to be important targets for treating depression. 5-HT_{1A} agonism and 5-HT_7 antagonism are key aspects of the pharmacology of atypical antipsychotic drugs, which are known to work as effective antidepressants. For example, it has been demonstrated that amisulpride's antidepressant action is based on its 5-HT_7 antagonism.

Current interest in ketamine, rapastinel, and scopolamine as rapidly acting antidepressant drugs has shifted the focus of depression research and treatment to glutamate, GABA, and acetylcholine. There are no strong links between these agents and primary abnormalities in NE and 5-HT, but it is important to note that ketamine and rapastinel are used to augment the efficacy of the antidepressant drugs that arose out of the monoamine theories of depression.

The dopamine and serotonin hypotheses of schizophrenia

Main citation

Meltzer, H. Y., Matsubara, S., & Lee, J. C. (1989). Classification of typical and atypical antipsychotic drugs on the basis of dopamine D-1, D-2 and serotonin$_2$ pK_i values. *The Journal of Pharmacology and Experimental Therapies*, 251, 238–246.

Background

The accidental ingestion of lysergic acid diethylamide (LSD) by Albert Hofmann, the Swiss medical chemist who synthesized it while studying the role of ergot alkaloids, quickly became invaluable to studying the causes and treatment of psychosis because it reliably produced vivid visual hallucinations and disturbances in attention and thought processes. The structural similarity of LSD to 5-HT led to hypotheses promoting endogenous 5-HT-based compounds with psychotomimetic properties as a cause of psychosis (Woolley & Shaw, 1954; Gaddum, 1954). However, the inability of various laboratories, particularly that of Arnold Friedhoff at New York University, to demonstrate the production of psychotomimetic indoles such as N,N-dimethyltryptamine in patients with schizophrenia led to the rejection of this hypothesis. Nevertheless, this line of research produced much valuable information about the role of 5-HT receptors in psychosis. Ultimately, 14 5-HT receptors were cloned and of these, the 5-HT$_{2A}$ receptor was shown to be the one most responsible for the ability of LSD and psychotomimetic indoles, such as psilocybin, to cause psychotic experiences and thought disorganization. Today, the value of these compounds as enabling psychotherapy is more significant than their ability to cause psychosis, but as will be discussed, the role of 5-HT$_{2A}$ receptors in the action of atypical APDs is of very great interest.

Indeed, for decades and lasting until the present time, many believed that only dopamine D$_2$ receptor blockade was effective to treat psychosis. More of the early history of the development of the DA hypothesis is reviewed by Alan Baumeister and Jennifer Francis (2002). They highlighted the studies of Jacques van Rossum, who showed that DA rather than NE was relevant to amphetamine-induced psychosis, and that overstimulation of DA receptors led to an exacerbation of psychosis. Arvid Carlsson and colleagues convincingly demonstrated that depletion of DA rather than 5-HT was related to the antipsychotic-like effects of reserpine in rabbits, using locomotor stimulation as a proxy for psychosis, and that the antipsychotic and parkinsonian effects of chlorpromazine and other first-generation APDs were related to blockade of DA receptors. This led to the identification of the five types of DA receptors with all signs pointing towards D$_2$ receptor, coupled to adenylyl cyclase, as the main one involved in schizophrenia and other forms of psychosis, including L-DOPA-induced psychosis in patients with Parkinson's disease. We now know that all five DA receptors are involved in schizophrenia and are targets for treating the illness. D$_1$ receptor stimulation is finally coming to the fore as a target for treating negative symptoms of schizophrenia: that is, withdrawal, lack of motivation, flat affect, and anergia (Arnsten et al., 2017).

Efforts to find drugs that increase synthesis and release of DA in regions of the brain persist until the present time. At first the ventral striatum, also known as the nucleus accumbens, was considered the source of the hyperdopaminergic activity leading to positive symptoms. Recent PET studies have pointed towards the dorsal striatum, but this issue is far from settled (Kegeles et al., 2010). The impetus for increased dopaminergic activity, in either or both regions, has not been determined. It is well established that blockade of D_2 receptors in the dorsal striatum is the cause of parkinsonism, tardive dyskinesia, and the sometimes fatal neuroleptic malignant syndrome. Recently, tardive dyskinesia has been shown to be involved in the cognitive impairment of schizophrenia.

A key breakthrough in our understanding of schizophrenia was the discovery of clozapine, a dibenzodiazepene, by Swiss chemists seeking to find an antipsychotic which did not produce extrapyramidal side-effects (EPSs). Although a low-potency agent (requiring doses averaging 400–500 mg/day, compared to 2–5 mg of haloperidol), it produced minimal EPSs in man and laboratory animals. However, 1% of patients who take clozapine will develop agranulocytosis and must be taken off the medication to avoid developing infections. About 1 in 1,000 or fewer will die if infection sets in despite stopping the medication. For this reason, weekly and then monthly white blood cell (WBC) monitoring is required for up to several years in most countries, and indefinitely in the USA (based on irrational risk–benefit considerations by the Food and Drug Administration). Meltzer and colleagues demonstrated that clozapine is effective in treating the more than half of patients with schizophrenia who do not respond to D_2 receptor antagonists such as haloperidol (i.e. patients with treatment-resistant schizophrenia (TRS)) (Kane et al., 1988) (see Chapter 7).

The need for safer drugs which are as, or more, effective in TRS is obvious. Whether low EPS risk and efficacy for TRS were due to the same aspects of clozapine's complex pharmacology was not known. Clozapine has affinities for a large number of 5-HT, DA, acetylcholine, NE, histamine receptors, and numerous other actions leading to many hypotheses as to which actions are most relevant to its unique profile. Early leading candidates were antimuscarinic blockade and D_1 antagonism. There was also some evidence pointing towards 5-HT_{2A} antagonism. To test which, if any, were correct, Meltzer and colleagues took the approach of comparing APDs which did and did not produce EPS at equivalent doses on these three measures (Meltzer et al., 1989). The *in vivo* effects of these compounds in humans were not always available, but there were effects for all of them in laboratory animals. In no cases was there a discrepancy between the EPS data for laboratory animals and man.

Methods

Meltzer and colleagues compared the affinities of 37 compounds for D_2, 5-HT_{2A}, and D_1 receptors by measuring binding to brain membranes containing these receptors. The study included an initial reference group to identify the measure that best discriminated which compounds were like haloperidol (so-called typical APDs) and which were like clozapine (atypical APDs). The drugs used in the reference group were *a priori* defined as typical or atypical APDs based on their effects on humans and animals (typical drugs had notable extrapyramidal side-effects and/or high serum prolactin elevations).

Results

In the reference group, mean pK_i values differed among typical and atypical antipsychotics, though the difference was only significant for the D_2 receptor; pK_i ratios were statistically significantly different for the $5HT_{2A}/D_2$ ratio and showed no overlap between the typical and atypical groups.

The $5HT_{2A}/D_2$ ratio was then used to perform a cluster analysis of the 37 drugs. The cluster analysis yielded two groups. The first cluster included 19 out of the 20 drugs identified as typical based on clinical and preclinical data. The second cluster included 15 out of the 17 drugs identified as atypical based on clinical and preclinical data. Only three drugs clustered differently from their preclinical or clinical data (amoxapine clustered as atypical, and HP-370 and zotepine clustered as typical). Thus, 92% of all drugs were 'correctly' classified.

Conclusions and critique

This study demonstrated that subgroups of APDs could be distinguished by their pharmacodynamic profiles: atypical antipsychotics had relatively lower D_2 binding affinity compared to their higher $5HT_{2A}$ binding affinity. Ultimately, the $5HT_{2A}/D_2$ biochemical 'profile' became a 'blueprint' for a new generation of atypical APDs (e.g. risperidone, olanzapine, quetiapine, ziprasidone, lurasidone, iloperidone), which became the preferred treatment for schizophrenia and other disorders, such as bipolar disorder, in which antipsychotic agents were indicated. This work also inspired the development of pimavanserin, a relatively pure $5HT_{2A}$ antagonist recently approved for the treatment of psychosis in patients with Parkinson's disease.

This study also re-established 5-HT as having a key role in the pathophysiology of schizophrenia and its treatment, and revealed that the key to developing a more effective psychotropic drug was not high receptor specificity. Rather, it may be that efficacy may be more related to patterns of drug–receptor interactions. Investigation of drugs that have multiple effects on different brain receptor targets continues today.

The glutamate hypothesis of schizophrenia

Main citation

Javitt, D. C. & Zukin, S. R. (1991). Recent advances in the phencyclidine model of schizophrenia. *American Journal of Psychiatry*, 148, 1301–1308.

Background

Insufficient control of psychosis, despite adequate trials of first-generation APDs, is found in about 30% of patients with schizophenia, including 10% of first-episode patients (Meltzer, 1997). As the disease progresses, up to 30% become refractory in terms of psychosis. These findings question the validity of hypotheses that focus on dopamine, serotonin, or their interaction as the key pathophysiological target. As described previously, the dopamine hypothesis grew in part from the 'amphetamine model' of schizophrenia, which primarily addressed the positive symptoms of the disorder. However, there was a different drug that more faithfully replicated a more complete clinical picture of schizophrenia: phencyclidine (PCP).

PCP was synthesized in the 1950s as an anaesthetic and referred to as Sernyl or 1-(1-phenylcyclohexyl) piperidine monohydrochloride. Soon after its introduction, psychiatrists noted that Sernyl induced certain disruptive cognitive and perceptual experiences in healthy volunteers: 'alternations in ego boundaries' and reality testing, a sense of isolation, hostility, and thought disorganization. Reflecting on their experiences with patients that had schizophrenia, they considered these experiences more representative of the broad syndrome and more relevant than the production of hallucinations evoked by LSD (Luby et al., 1959). Furthermore, administration of Sernyl, but not LSD, destabilized patients with schizophrenia (Luby et al., 1959). These findings suggested that PCP provided a higher-fidelity model of schizophrenia (Luby et al., 1962, 1959).

It took another two or three decades to determine PCP's mechanism of action. In 1979, researchers identified a unique 'PCP receptor', and in the 1980s they localized this site to the N-methyl-D-aspartate (NMDA) receptor complex, though PCP has actions on other receptors as well. In their landmark 1991 review, Daniel Javitt and Stephen Zukin reaffirmed the utility of PCP as a model for schizophrenia and argued that PCP exerts it schizophrenia-like effects at plasma concentrations necessary to block NMDA receptors (Javitt & Zukin, 1991). They were therefore the first to explicitly implicate NMDA receptor dysfunction in the pathophysiology of schizophrenia.

Methods

This is a review of the literature.

Results

Javitt and Zukin first review clinical studies of PCP, which was introduced as a general anaesthetic in the 1950s. It differed from other anaesthetics by causing a dissociated mental state rather than a loss of consciousness. Subanaesthetic doses produced disturbances in thinking and impulse control, that sometimes caused violent and bizarre behaviour. Subanaesthetic doses of PCP (0.05–0.1 mg/kg intravenously) given to healthy volunteers produced symptoms similar to the negative symptoms of schizophrenia, including withdrawal and poverty of speech and thought. PCP administered to patients with schizophrenia caused an exacerbation of their primary symptoms, even if they had been previously stabilized. In contrast, patients with schizophrenia that has been well controlled did not experience psychotic symptoms when given amphetamine, which 'suggests that the neural substrates affected by PCP are vulnerable in subjects with the schizophrenic trait, while the neural substrates affected by amphetamine are vulnerable only in subjects in the acutely decompensated state' (Javitt & Zukin, 1991, p. 1302).

The authors then discuss PCP's site of action. They note the serum levels needed to cause various effects (psychosis at levels less than 100 ng/mL; gross impairment of consciousness at levels over 100 ng/mL; and coma, seizures, and respiratory arrest at over 250 ng/mL). They reason that the site at which psychosis is initiated must be the one of greatest importance for schizophrenia. This is the NMDA receptor binding site. They provide a variety of animal and biochemical data to support the NMDA receptor as the site of psychomimetic action. For example, they posit that this site must also bind other drugs that produce similar effects (like ketamine), and they reference studies showing that doses at which these drugs produce PCP-like effects correlate with their potency in binding the 'PCP receptor'.

They conclude that 'the ability of PCP to induce schizophreniform psychosis by inhibiting NMDA receptor-mediated neurotransmission suggests that endogenous dysfunction or dysregulation of NMDA receptor-mediated transmission might occur in schizophrenia and contribute to symptom generation. PCP-induced psychosis thus provides a neurochemical hypothesis of schizophrenia distinct from the dopamine hypothesis' (Javitt & Zukin, 1991, p. 1305). They suggest that schizophrenia is a heterogeneous syndrome with different disease processes. Linking their hypothesis with the most classic formulations of schizophrenia as a syndrome, they point out that amphetamine-induced psychosis coincides with the Schneiderian model of schizophrenia, in which positive symptoms make the diagnosis, whereas PCP-induced psychosis matches with Eugen Bleuler's description of the '4 As' of schizophrenia (association of thought, affect, autism, and ambivalence). They also state that NMDA receptor dysfunction better explains the combination of positive symptoms and cognitive symptoms, which reflect, respectively, DA hyperactivity and DA hypoactivity.

Conclusions and critique

The authors concluded that PCP offers a higher-fidelity model of schizophrenia, given its ability to induce cognitive dysfunction and negative symptoms, as well as psychosis, in healthy individuals and to exacerbate these forms of psychopathology in patients with schizophrenia. Based on PCP's action as a non-competitive inhibitor of the NMDA receptor, they posited that alterations in NMDA receptor-mediated neurotransmission could explain the pathogenesis of schizophrenia. This theory implicated the excitatory neurotransmitter glutamate in a neurodevelopmental context, which could be revealed at adolescence or later on in adulthood. It also implicated the inhibitory amino acid neurotransmitter, GABA, and the balance between glutamate and GABA. Finally, this paper was important in broadening the focus of understanding and treating schizophrenia beyond delusions and hallucinations, which was the legacy of the emphasis on dopamine, amphetamine psychosis, and D_2 receptor blockers. Much research now takes into account cognitive and psychosocial impairments.

Ketamine (another NMDA receptor antagonist, albeit much weaker than PCP) also produces a spectrum of psychopathology including psychosis and cognitive impairment. John Krystal and colleagues (1994) demonstrated the development of positive and negative symptoms in healthy individuals who received ketamine. They also noted an antidepressant action of ketamine as discussed previously. Adrienne Lahti and colleagues (1995) showed that patients with schizophrenia who were stable on conventional antipsychotic treatment experienced a resurgence of their specific symptoms when receiving ketamine. Preclinical studies from the Millan and Meltzer labs showed that the behavioural effects of PCP, such as locomotor activity, responded poorly to haloperidol and other D_2 receptor blockers but more completely and at lower doses to clozapine, risperidone, and selective 5-HT_{2A} receptor antagonists.

Research into the causes of NMDA receptor dysfunction (e.g. genetic, environmental) is ongoing, and several 'sub-hypotheses' have emerged (as reviewed in Moghaddam & Javitt, 2012). For example, a glutamate hyperactivity theory posits that excess glutamate activity at non-NMDA receptor sites is the cause of schizophrenia symptoms. On the other hand, the cortical disinhibition theory postulates that inhibition of GABA-ergic interneurons allows for increased firing of cortical pyramidal neurons that in turn produces positive, negative, and cognitive symptoms. Polymorphisms of the genes that code for the various elements that constitute the NMDA receptor have been identified in patients with schizophrenia.

Conclusion

This chapter describes the evolution of neurochemical theories for depression (involving norepinephrine and serotonin) and schizophrenia (involving dopamine, serotonin, and glutamate), the two most well-studied psychiatric disorders. There are neurochemical theories of other disorders, such as bipolar disorder and anxiety disorders, but a discussion of these theories is beyond the scope of this chapter (whilst Chapters 8 and 9 address these briefly). When these theories first emerged, they tantalized the field with the possibility of a simple chemical solution for depression or schizophrenia. Those hopes were inspired by the discovery of 'biologic' treatments for other mental disorders in the early twentieth century (penicillin for syphilis-induced general paresis of the insane; nicotinamide for pellagra) and they were further buoyed by findings in the mid-twentieth century that dopamine repletion reverses symptoms of Parkinson's disease (Carlsson, 1959; Hornykiewitz, 1973). Although these neurochemical theories have allowed us to refine drugs available to treat both mood disorders and psychotic disorders, principally by reducing 'off-target' side-effects, they have not yet yielded a definitive solution to the most severe of all psychiatric disorders.

Modern understandings of the neurochemical underpinnings of mental disorders are becoming more nuanced. As highlighted in the discussions here, the field has shifted from models of simple neurochemical deficiencies or excesses to models of circuit dysfunction caused by the imbalance or dysregulation of several interacting neurotransmitters. The number of known neurotransmitters has grown, and our knowledge of how they participate in micro- and macro-circuits that ultimately drive behaviour has developed. Emerging still are new techniques that can further our knowledge; for example, optogenetic research uses lasers and designer receptors exclusively activated by designer drugs (DREADDs) (Deisseroth, 2015; Roth, 2016) to modulate nerve cell activity in freely moving animal preparations.

The ultimate goal of generating and testing neurochemical theories is to better understand the pathophysiology of psychiatric disorders in order to better treat, if not prevent or cure, them. However, neurochemistry alone cannot accomplish these goals. Neurochemistry illuminates just one facet of brain physiology, and it must be integrated with other disciplines (such as neuroanatomy, neurophysiology, neuropathology, brain imaging, and genetics) to yield a more complete understanding of normal and abnormal behaviour.

References

Arnsten, A. F., Girgis, R. R., Gray, D. L., & Mailman, R. B. (2017). Novel dopamine therapeutics for cognitive deficits in schizophrenia. *Biological Psychiatry*, **81**, 67–77.

Axelrod, J., Herting, G., & Potter, L. (1962). Effect of drugs on the uptake and release of 3H-norepinephrine in the rat heart. *Nature*, **194**, 297.

Baumeister, A. A. & Francis, J. L. (2002). Historical development of the dopamine hypothesis of schizophrenia. *Journal of the History of Neurosciences*, **11**, 265–277.

Brodie, B. B., Olin, J. S., Kuntzman, R. G., & Shore, P. A. (1957). Possible interrelationship between release of brain norepinephrine and serotonin by reserpine. *Science*, **125**, 1293–1294.

Brodie, B. B., Pletscher, A., & Shore, P. A. (1955). Evidence that serotonin has a role in brain function. *Science*, **122**, 968.

Brodie, B. B., Spector, S., & Shore, P. A. (1959). Interaction of monoamine oxidase inhibitors with physiological and biochemical mechanisms in brain. *Annals of the New York Academy of Sciences*, **80**, 609–616.

Bunney Jr, W. E. & Davis, J. M. (1965). Norepinephrine in depressive reactions. A review. *Archives of General Psychiatry*, **13**, 483–494.

Coppen, A. (1967). The biochemistry of affective disorders. *British Journal of Psychiatry*, **113**, 1237–1264.

Deisseroth, K. (2015). Optogenetics: 10 years of microbial opsins in neuroscience. *Nature Neuroscience*, **18**, 1213–1225.

Gaddum, J. (1954). Drug antagonist to 5-hydroxytrypatmine. In: *Ciba Foundation Symposium on Hypertension*, ed. G. Wolstenholme. Boston: Little Brown.

Hornykiewicz, O. (1973). Dopamine in the basal ganglia. Its role and therapeutic implications (including the clinical use of L-DOPA). *British Medical Bulletin*, **29**(2), 172–178.

Horton, R. W. (1992). The neurochemistry of depression: evidence derived from studies of post-mortem brain tissue. *Molecular Aspects of Medicine*, **13**, 191–203.

Javitt, D. C. & Zukin, S. R. (1991). Recent advances in the phencyclidine model of schizophrenia. *American Journal of Psychiatry*, **148**, 1301–1308.

Kane, J., Honigfeld, G., Singer, J., & Meltzer, H. (1988). Clozapine for the treatment-resistant schizophrenic. A double-blind comparison with chlorpromazine. *Archives of General Psychiatry*, **45**, 789–796.

Kegeles, L. S., et al. (2010). Increased synaptic dopamine function in associative regions of the striatum in schizophrenia. *Archives of General Psychiatry*, **67**, 231–239.

Klimek, V., et al. (1997). Reduced levels of norepinephrine transporters in the locus coeruleus in major depression. *Journal of Neuroscience*, **17**, 8451–8458.

Krystal, J. H., et al. (1994). Subanesthetic effects of the noncompetitive NMDA antagonist, ketamine, in humans. Psychotomimetic, perceptual, cognitive, and neuroendocrine responses. *Archives of General Psychiatry*, **51**, 199–214.

Lahti A. C., Koffel, B., Laporte, D., & Tamminga, C. A. (1995). Subanesthetic doses of ketamine stimulate psychosis in schizophrenia. *Neuropsychopharmacology*, **13**, 9–19.

Loomer, H. P., Saunders, J. C., & Kline, N. S. (1957). A clinical and pharmacodynamic evaluation of iproniazid as a psychic energizer. *Psychiatric Research Reports of the American Psychiatric Association*, **8**, 129–141.

Luby, E. D., Cohen, B. D., Rosenbaum, G., Gottlieb, J. S., & Kelley, R. (1959). Study of a new schizophrenomimetic drug: sernyl. *American Medical Association Archives of Neurology & Psychiatry*, **81**, 363–369.

Luby, E. D., Gottlieb, J. S., Cohen, B. D., Rosenbaum, G., & Domino, E. F. (1962). Model psychoses and schizophrenia. *American Journal of Psychiatry*, **119**, 61–67.

Meltzer, H. Y. (1997). Treatment-resistant schizophrenia—the role of clozapine. *Current Medical Research and Opinion*, **14**, 1–20.

Meltzer, H. Y., Matsubara, S., & Lee, J. C. (1989). Classification of typical and atypical antipsychotic drugs on the basis of dopamine D-1, D-2 and serotonin$_2$ pK$_i$ values. *Journal of Pharmacology and Experimental Therapeutics*, **251**, 238–246.

Miller, R. (2014). *Drugged: The Science and Culture Behind Psychotropic Drugs*. Oxford: Oxford University Press.

Moghaddam, B. & Javitt, D. (2012). From revolution to evolution: the glutamate hypothesis of schizophrenia and its implication for treatment. *Neuropsychopharmacology*, **37**, 4–15.

Pletscher, A., Shore, P. A., & Brodie, B. B. (1956). Serotonin as a mediator of reserpine action in brain. *Journal of Pharmacology and Experimental Therapeutics*, **116**, 84–89.

Robinson, J. D. (2001). *Mechanisms of Synaptic Transmission: Bridging the Gaps (1890–1990)*. Oxford: Oxford University Press.

Roth, B. L. (2016). DREADDs for neuroscientists. *Neuron*, **89**, 683–694.

Schildkraut, J. J. (1965). The catecholamine hypothesis of affective disorders: a review of supporting evidence. *American Journal of Psychiatry*, **122**, 509–522.

Selikoff, I. J., Robitzek, E. H., & Ornstein, G. G. (1952). Treatment of pulmonary tuberculosis with hydrazide derivatives of isonicotinic acid. *Journal of the American Medical Association*, **150**, 973–980.

Valenstein, E. S. (2005). *The War of the Soups and the Sparks: The Discovery of Neurotransmitters and the Dispute Over How Nerves Communicate.* New York: Columbia University Press.

van Praag, H. M., Korf, J., & Puite, J. (1970). 5-hydroxyindoleacetic acid levels in the cerebrospinal fluid of depressive patients treated with probenecid. *Nature*, **225**, 1259–1260.

Woolley, D. W. & Shaw, E. (1954). A biochemical and pharmacological suggestion about certain mental disorders. *Proceedings of the National Academy of Sciences of the United States of America*, **40**, 228–231.

Zhu, K., Ou Yang, T. H., Dorie, V., Zheng, T., & Anastassiou, D. (2019). Meta-analysis of expression and methylation signatures indicates a stress-related epigenetic mechanism in multiple neuropsychiatric disorders. *Translational Psychiatry*, **9**, 32.

Chapter 4

Genetics

Marina Bayeva and Edwin H. Cook

Introduction

Soon after the rediscovery of Mendel's pea studies in the beginning of the twentieth century, German psychiatrist and geneticist Ernst Rudin attempted to demonstrate that Mendelian laws also applied to psychiatric disorders. In 1916, he published the first large family study of schizophrenia and concluded that the risk of psychotic illness in offspring was as high as 7.7% and that the disease followed a non-Mendelian segregation pattern in siblings of schizophrenic probands (Rudin, 1916; Propping, 2005). In 1928, Hans Luxenburger from Munich conducted the first systematic twin study of schizophrenia, finding a concordance rate of 58% in monozygotic twins and making a strong argument for a contribution from both genetic and non-genetic factors (Luxenburger, 1928; Propping, 2005). Around the same time, the rise of psychoanalysis pioneered by Sigmund Freud provided a fundamentally different explanation for psychosis as a product of ego's alienation from reality due to disordered family structure, such as being raised by a 'schizophrenogenic mother' (Fromm-Reichmann, 1948; Hartwell, 1996).

The 'nature versus nurture' debate remained controversial throughout most of the twentieth century. Early epidemiological twin studies consistently showed clustering of mental disorders in families but failed to disentangle genetic causes from environmental factors. Providing data in support of a complex genetic contribution to schizophrenia became one of the key achievements in the field of psychiatric genetics. Here, we discuss two landmark papers that helped to establish psychiatric disorders as genetic entities. First, Seymour Kety and colleagues (1968) took advantage of adoption registries in Denmark to show that the risk of schizophrenia in genetic parents of schizophrenic probands raised by adoptive families without mental illness was elevated compared to that of genetic parents of adopted probands who did not develop schizophrenia. Second, Robert Plomin and colleagues (1994), in a fundamental review paper, showed that heritability of psychiatric illnesses and even non-pathological behavioural traits was at least as strong, if not stronger, than heritability of common medical illnesses, while also emphasizing the power of quantitative genetics in elucidating the causes of mental disorders.

Technological advances of the early twenty-first century made it possible to move from indirect heritability studies of twins and adoptees to directly interrogating the genome for risk-conferring elements. In the 1960s, Irving Gottesman and James Shields (1967) proposed that schizophrenia was a polygenic illness and that the disease phenotype was determined by a complex interplay of many genes with various effect sizes. Formation of the Psychiatric Genomics Consortium (PGC) in 2007, by the merger of many existing consortia, promoted multinational collaboration on an unprecedented scale (Sullivan, 2018). We are now beginning to identify individual genes and molecular networks implicated in mental disorders, such as the PGC Schizophrenia Study Group's study (Ripke et al., 2014) that revealed 108 schizophrenia risk loci. Moreover, the important role for *de novo* genetic elements such as copy number variants (CNVs) and loss of function single nucleotide variants (SNVs) that confer a high relative risk is beginning to emerge for many psychiatric illnesses. A study of autism spectrum disorder (ASD) by Stephan Sanders and colleagues (2015) showed how non-inherited *de novo* SNVs can contribute to a complex behavioural phenotype through their effects on distinct molecular networks. Taken together, these studies bring us closer to a comprehensive understanding of the biology of mental disorders.

Mental illness in adopted schizophrenics: genes or psychology?

Main citation

Kety, S. S., Rosenthal, D., Wender, P. H., & Schulsinger, F. (1968). The types and prevalence of mental illness in the biological and adoptive families of schizophrenics. *Journal of Psychiatric Research*, 6, 345–362.

Background

The two most influential early figures in psychiatry, Sigmund Freud and Emil Kraepelin, shared the same birth year of 1856, yet held profoundly different views on the origin and pathophysiology of mental illness (Trede, 2007), a controversy that for over a century remained open for debate. Freud represented the 'psychodynamic school' of thought, and its followers argued that mental illness was a result of 'deviant and pathogenic psychological experiences [derived from] aberrant parenting' (Wender et al., 1974), thus advocating for the familial environment as its causative agent. On the other hand, the 'genetic school' that emerged from Kraepelin's meticulous classifications of psychiatric symptoms proposed the hereditary nature of mental disorders. This controversy was further fuelled by epidemiological studies in the 1940s through to the 1960s (Kringlen, 1966) that documented an increased incidence of psychotic illness in families with schizophrenia, yet did little to resolve the nature versus nurture dispute. A highly influential paper by Kety et al. (1968) was the field's first attempt to disentangle these variables by retrospective family studies.

Methods

Kety et al. aimed at resolving the 'nature versus nurture' controversy in the aetiology of psychotic illness by first identifying adopted individuals with schizophrenia who were raised by non-biological parents, and then retrospectively assessing psychotic symptoms in *biological* families of these individuals. This study design removed 'a disproportionate segment of environmental and interpersonal factors' shared by family members of patients with schizophrenia. The authors took advantage of several population registries in Denmark including: the Adoption Registry to identify adoptees and their adoptive/biological parents; the Folkeregister (Population Registry) to track, longitudinally, each individual's marital status and place of residence within Denmark; and the Psychiatric Registry of the Institute of Human Genetics to obtain psychiatric hospitalization records and diagnosis of each individual. Out of 5,483 children adopted between 1924 and 1947, 507 were admitted to a psychiatric hospital for any reason. From these, 33 index cases with 'definitive schizophrenia' (as determined by four independent physician raters) and 33 carefully matched controls with no history of psychiatric admissions were selected. A comprehensive population registry search was then performed for all of the index and control cases, which identified a total of 483 biological relatives (parents, siblings, and half-siblings), 67 of whom had a history of at least one admission to a psychiatric hospital. The authors calculated the relative prevalence of psychotic illness in biological relatives of adopted schizophrenic index cases versus non-schizophrenic controls.

Results

The retrospective search for biological and adoptive relatives of 33 schizophrenic index cases and 33 matched controls yielded a total of 463 family members, with a similar number and distribution of identified relatives between the index and control cases. As a group, biological parents of both cases and controls differed greatly from adoptive parents in their age and socioeconomic class, which is likely explained by stringent selection criteria that adoptive parents were required to meet prior to being granted an adoption. However, broader comparison of all family members in respect to the above characteristics revealed no significant differences between the adoptive and biological families of both index and control cases, making it feasible to compare prevalence of mental illness between the groups. Out of 150 biological relatives of adoptees with schizophrenia, 8.7% had a diagnosis of 'schizophrenia spectrum illness', while only 1.9% of biological relatives of non-schizophrenic controls carried that diagnosis. Among biological half-siblings of index cases, 10–11% were diagnosed with psychotic illness, while there were no such diagnoses among biological half-siblings of control cases. Moreover, biological relatives of index cases were more likely to carry a diagnosis of 'psychopathy, delinquency or character disorder', and all of the five discovered cases of suicide among biological relatives occurred in families of index cases.

Conclusions and critique

Kety et al. provided the first evidence of a sizeable genetic component in the aetiology of a psychotic illness. There was over a fourfold increase in prevalence of schizophrenia spectrum illness in biological relatives of adoptees with schizophrenia compared to control adoptees without schizophrenia. These findings supported a contribution of heritable factors to the development of schizophrenia. Notable limitations include the collection of data from governmental and hospital records, with no in-person interviews to confirm diagnoses or assess the home environment of the study subjects, a limitation that applies to a majority of other registry studies. The authors note that their study was not designed to look closely at the complexity of environmental factors given the small sample size. Importantly, they did not show that schizophrenia was not transmitted through psychological factors, such as aberrant parenting, independent of an offspring's genetic loading. In later studies, such as the one by Paul Wender and colleagues (1974), genetic factors were further confirmed to be the primary factor in transmission of schizophrenia, opening the door to a number of follow-up studies of genetics, molecular mechanisms, and neurological pathways not only in psychosis, but also in many other psychiatric illnesses.

Quantitative genetics as a launching point for studying human behaviour

Main citation

Plomin, R., Owen, M. J., & McGuffin, P. (1994). The genetic basis of complex human behaviors. *Science*, 264, 1733–1739.

Background

The twentieth century witnessed a dramatic shift in our understanding of the biology of psychiatric illnesses. Mental disorders, which were primarily viewed as a byproduct of one's environment in the 1950s, gradually gained recognition as multifaceted and heritable entities that went beyond 'good' or 'bad' parenting. However, despite abundant evidence from early twin and adoption studies of the 1960s and 1970s (such as Kety et al., 1968, reviewed in the section 'Mental illness in adopted schizophrenics: genes or psychology'), the causes of psychiatric disorders continued to be viewed as fundamentally different from common medical 'afflictions', such as hypertension or cancer. Technological advances only further widened this gap: while many rare non-psychiatric medical disorders were linked to specific genes (Chial, 2008), causative agents for psychiatric disorders remained elusive. Even in the 1990s, the link between genes and behaviour continued to be viewed as 'another flight of fancy that comes with millennium fever' (Plomin, 1995), rather than a credible scientific fact.

In this climate, the landmark review paper by Plomin, Michael Owen, and Peter McGuffin achieved two important goals: first, it questioned the artificial distinction between psychiatric disorders and medical illnesses, emphasizing the comparable heritability of both behavioural and physiological traits; and, second, it laid out a roadmap for future research into the genetics of mental illness.

Methods

This review presents evidence for a genetic contribution to both normal and abnormal behaviour, as indicated by comparison of monozygotic and dizygotic twin concordance. Twin studies have long been a staple in genetic research, since monozygotic twins share 100%

of nuclear DNA compared to fraternal twins who share only 50% of their DNA, with both types of twins also exposed to a common environment of the family. The authors argue for the importance of quantitative genetic studies in furthering our understanding of causes of all mental disorders. The paper is divided into two parts: 'Quantitative Genetics' and 'Molecular Genetics'. The first section compares the heritability of medical versus psychiatric disorders and shows that even non-pathological character traits, such as neuroticism, intelligence, or vocational interests, are largely determined by genes. By examining the role of genetic factors in various behaviours, the authors aim to dismantle the artificial border between organic and psychological phenomena. In the second section, the authors advocate for combining molecular and quantitative genetic techniques to identify an array of heritable factors that give rise to complex human behaviours.

Results

In the 'Quantitative Genetics' section of the review, the authors draw marked parallels between the strong heritability of classical mental disorders with that of other common medical conditions. Figures 4.1 and 4.2 show that many psychiatric disorders, such as schizophrenia and autism, are actually more heritable than certain other common medical conditions, including breast cancer and ischaemic heart disease. In fact, the authors claim that 'behavioral disorders on average show greater genetic influence than common medical disorders'. Furthermore, they point out a high degree of heritability even for

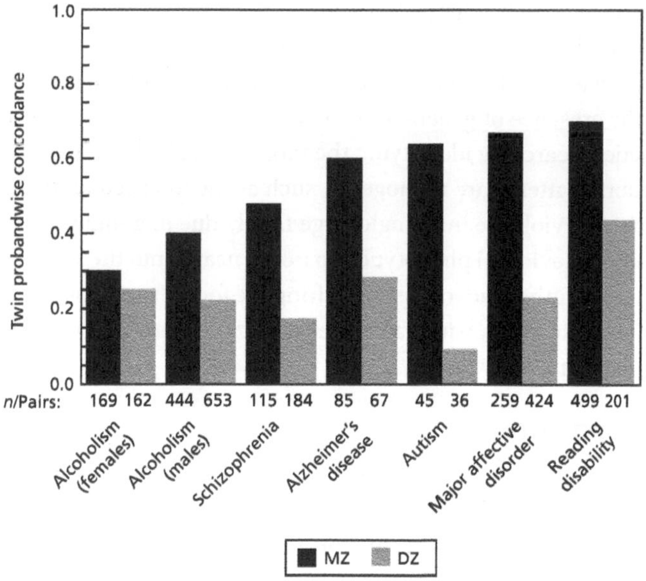

Figure 4.1 Identical, monozygotic (MZ) twin and fraternal, dizygotic (DZ) twin probandwise concordances for behavioural disorders.

Reproduced with permission from Plomin, R., et al. (1994). The genetic basis of complex human behaviors. *Science*, 264(5166), 1733–1739.

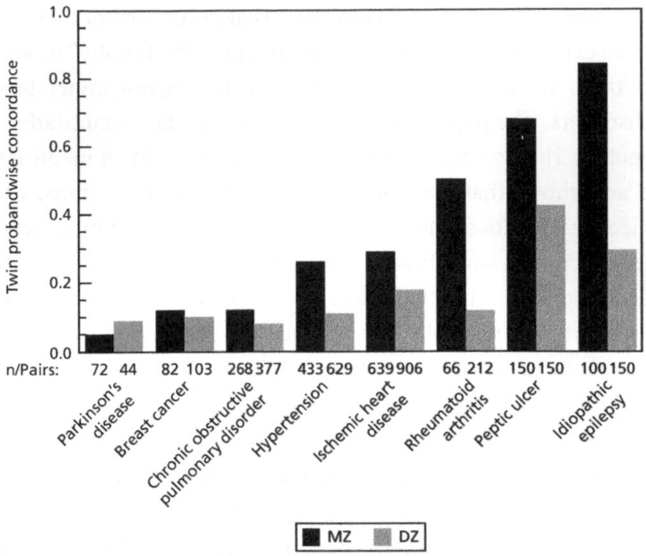

Figure 4.2 Monozygotic (MZ) twin and dizygotic (DZ) twin probandwise concordances for common medical disorders.

Reproduced with permission from Plomin, R., et al. (1994). The genetic basis of complex human behaviors. *Science*, 264(5166), 1733–1739. Copyright © 1994 American Association for the Advancement of Science.

non-pathological personality traits, with both neuroticism and extraversion being 40–50% genetically determined (Figure 4.3).

In the 'Molecular Genetics' section, the authors sketch future directions for genetic studies in behavioural health research, citing a goal of moving 'beyond merely documenting the presence of genetic influence' and using quantitative genetics to 'guide molecular genetic research by identifying the most heritable domains of behavior'. While certain behavioural patterns are monogenic, such as the intellectual disability of phenylketonuria, or risk for violence in a single large family due to a mutated monoamine oxidase B gene, most behavioural phenotypes do not fit neatly into the 'one gene, one disease' paradigm. Thus, the authors advocate for shifting the focus from looking for a single gene to identifying multiple genes with various effect sizes where 'any single gene is neither necessary nor sufficient'.

Conclusions and critique

In seven short pages, Plomin and colleagues achieved two fundamental goals. First, they challenged a commonly held belief that causes of mental disorders were somehow essentially different from those of 'organic' or 'medical' disorders. By drawing together a wealth of genetic research in psychiatry, the authors clearly demonstrated that behavioural disorders, and even healthy character attributes, had a robust heritable component, as strong as 50% for such entities as schizophrenia or the personality trait of extraversion, and up to 80% for late-adult cognitive ability. Indeed, the data presented in this paper

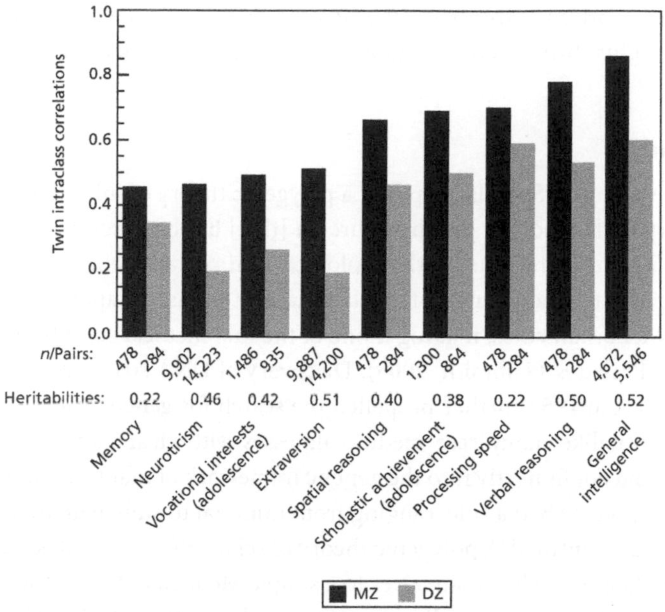

Figure 4.3 Monozygotic (MZ) twin and dizygotic (DZ) twin intraclass correlations for personality (neuroticism and extraversion), vocational interests in adolescence, scholastic achievement in adolescence (combined across similar results for English usage, mathematics, social studies, and natural science), specific cognitive abilities in adolescence (memory, spatial reasoning, processing speed, verbal reasoning), and general intelligence.

Reproduced with permission from Plomin, R., et al. (1994). The genetic basis of complex human behaviors. *Science*, 264(5166), 1733–1739.

convincingly show that mental disorders are as biological as their other medical counterparts. However, as mechanisms of psychiatric disorders become better understood, there is a tendency to reclassify them as neurological conditions, perpetuating an erroneous notion that psychiatric illnesses are somehow caused by nebulous functional factors with no measurable effects on brain physiology, neural networks, molecular pathways, or genes (White et al., 2012).

Important for future research is Plomin's emphasis on quantitative genetics as a tool for studying the biology of behavioural disorders. The authors argue that we should shift our efforts towards large-scale genome-wide studies which proved salient with the expansion of the field towards genome-wide studies.

A polygenic theory of schizophrenia: from concepts to candidate genes

Main citations

Gottesman, I. I. & Shields, J. (1967). A polygenic theory of schizophrenia. *Proceedings of the National Academy of Sciences of the USA*, 58, 199–205.

Schizophrenia Working Group of the Psychiatric Genomics Consortium (2014). Biological insights from 108 schizophrenia-associated genetic loci. *Nature*, 511, 421–427.

Background

In 1967, Gottesman and Shields proposed a polygenic theory of inheritance as a solution to the 'mystery of the etiology of schizophrenia [that] has been refractory to the analytical methods provided thus far by the biological and social sciences'. As early as 1902, British physician Archibald Garrod reported that the disease alkaptonuria was inherited according to Mendelian rules, making it one of the first medical conditions ascribed to a genetic cause (Prasad & Galbraith, 2005). Discovery of DNA structure by James Watson and Francis Crick in 1953 further propelled the search for genetic causes of human diseases. However, unlike many rare medical illnesses with clear patterns of inheritance, schizophrenia did not fit neatly into the genetic framework of that time, and thus the genetic factors were prescribed a role 'ranging from minimal to sufficient' in its aetiology. In the landmark paper entitled 'A polygenic theory of schizophrenia', Gottesman and Shields argued that 'so long as we limit ourselves to a simple Mendelian framework and construe schizophrenia as a homogeneous disease entity, we do not have the "workable concept of heredity"'. Fifty years later, multiple studies have generated ample evidence in support of their argument of schizophrenia being a complex polygenic disease determined by factors such as genetic loading, developmental influences, and pathogenic involvement on multiple molecular and structural levels. In 2014, the largest molecular genetics study of schizophrenia, carried out by the Schizophrenia Working Group of the Psychiatric Genetic Consortium (PGC), employed modern high-throughput genotyping technology in a large sample to go from a concept of schizophrenia as a polygenic disease to identification of over a hundred genetic risk loci.

Methods

Gottesman and Shields' landmark paper started with a hypothesis that schizophrenia was a polygenic disease whose appearance in the next generation was determined by a combination of genetic loading and environmental stress. Using Falconer's analysis for estimating the heritability of the liability to a disease (Falconer & MacKay, 1996), combined with epidemiological data obtained from twin and family studies of patients with schizophrenia, the authors calculated the heritability of schizophrenia (h^2) and contrasted it to that of diabetes (as an example of a medical polygenic disease).

Almost 50 years later, the Schizophrenia Working Group of the PGC used a genome-wide association study (GWAS) that pooled 'all available schizophrenia samples with published or unpublished GWAS genotypes into a single, systematic analysis'. The genome-wide genotype data were used to construct 49 ancestry-matched, non-overlapping, case-control samples and three family-based samples of European ancestry. Altogether, the study examined a total of 36,989 cases with schizophrenia and 113,075 controls, for which disease-associated single nucleotide polymorphisms (SNPs) were identified and validated. The enrichment of candidate genes in specific tissues was assessed by mapping candidate gene sequences onto epigenetic markers for 56 tissues and cell lines. Finally, the newly identified candidate genes were used to construct risk profile scores (RPSs) for various samples and the ability of RPSs to predict the case-control status of a subject was tested.

Results

Gottesman and Shields performed the Falconer's analysis on epidemiological data from several European twin studies to calculate heritability of schizophrenia, h^2, which represents the degree by which genetic factors determine phenotypical variance. In this analysis, disorders primarily caused by environmental factors will have a negligible h^2, while genetically determined conditions will have h^2 approaching 100%. The h^2 for schizophrenia was found to be between 79% and 105% in monozygotic co-twins, and 72% and 106% for dizygotic co-twins, arguing that most of the phenotypical variation seen in schizophrenic families is genetically determined. The validity of these data was supported by a consistency of h^2 values between three different data sets which varied with respect to culture, severity of the disease, and the degree of shared environment between relatives. Moreover, h^2 values were consistent when estimated from data from monozygotic twins, dizygotic twins, non-twin siblings, as well as aunts and uncles.

The major finding of the PGC's study was identification of 108 genetic loci associated with schizophrenia from a pooled sample of almost 37,000 cases and over 110,000 controls using GWAS analysis (Figure 4.4). Of the 108 risk loci, 75% included a protein-coding gene and an additional 8% were within 20 kilobases (kb) of a gene. Eighty-three of the 108 genetic loci associated with schizophrenia had not been known prior to this study. The genes identified by the study segregated into distinct functional classes that included glutamatergic neurotransmission, synaptic plasticity, and voltage-gated calcium channels. Moreover, most of the genes identified by this GWAS were enriched in multiple cortical and striatal tissues, as well as in tissues with important immune functions, particularly B-lymphocytes responsible for acquired immunity.

Conclusions and critique

Gottesman and Shields, in the 1960s, argued for a polygenic aetiology of schizophrenia and used a sophisticated analysis, combined with epidemiological data sets, to show that up to 100% of phenotypical variance between relatives of schizophrenics could be attributed to genetic factors. Importantly, they argued that in order to understand heritability of schizophrenia, the researchers must steer away from focusing on single candidate genes—an approach that proved successful for a number of medical conditions, yet yielded no meaningful results in the mental health field. Half a century later, thanks to the efforts of the PGC, we are finally beginning to understand the genetic underpinnings of schizophrenia. Consistent with the polygenic theory of the disease, the candidate risk loci identified by the GWAS were not randomly distributed, but rather clustered into specific pathways and were expressed in relevant tissues (such as neural and immune lineages).

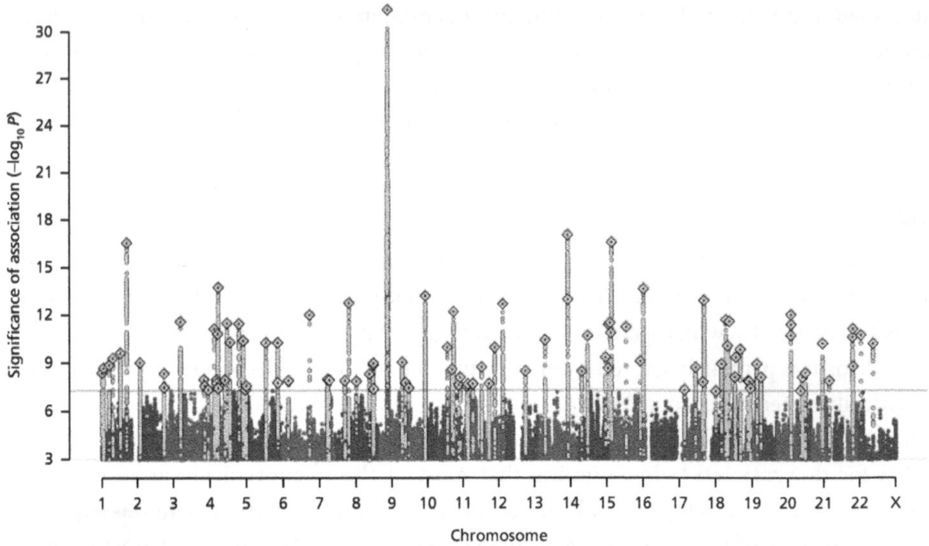

Figure 4.4 Manhattan plot showing schizophrenia associations. Manhattan plot of the discovery genome-wide association meta-analysis of 49 case control samples (34,241 cases and 45,604 controls) and three family-based association studies (1,235 parent affected–offspring trios). The x axis is chromosomal position and the y axis is the significance (-log10 P; 2-tailed) of association derived by logistic regression. The red line shows genome-wide significance levels (5 × 10–8). Single nucleotide polymorphisms (SNPs) in green are in linkage disequilibrium with the index SNPs (diamonds) which represent independent genome-wide significant associations.

Reproduced with permission from Schizophrenia Working Group of the Psychiatric Genomics Consortium. Biological insights from 108 schizophrenia-associated genetic loci. *Nature*, 511, 421–427. Copyright © 2014 Springer Nature. https://doi.org/10.1038/nature13595

It is important to note that identification of a large number of schizophrenia risk loci by the GWAS opened doors to a myriad of mechanistic studies that can help delineate the pathophysiology of this disease on molecular, cellular, tissue, and organism levels. From a methodological standpoint, the GWAS paper proved that this technique can be successfully applied to the study of complex polygenic diseases without reliable biological markers or diagnostic tests, as exemplified by schizophrenia, but generalizable to the majority of psychiatric disorders and behavioural traits, including major depressive disorder (MDD) (Wray et al., 2018), attention deficit hyperactivity disorder (ADHD) (Demontis et al., 2019), and neuroticism (Smith et al., 2016; Nagel, 2018).

Beyond individual genes: contribution of copy number variants to schizophrenia

Main citation

Marshall, C. R., et al. (2017). Contribution of copy number variants to schizophrenia from a genome-wide study of 41,321 subjects. *Nature Genetics*, 49, 27–35.

Background

Studies of psychiatric disorders throughout the twentieth century established a strong genetic component in their aetiology, yet translating heritability into pathophysiological mechanisms only became possible with recent advances in sequencing technologies. GWAS analyses allowed us to search for risk alleles across the entire genome in an unbiased fashion, and over a hundred GWASs of psychiatric diseases have been published since 2007 (Collins & Sullivan, 2013). Single-investigator research gave way to large-scale multinational collaborations, such as the PGC that brought together over 800 investigators from more than 30 countries and collected almost half a million clinical samples (O'Donovan, 2015). The PGC became the largest consortium in the history of psychiatry to date, which enabled identification of rarer risk alleles of modest effect sizes and detection of rarer risk-conferring events, such as CNVs. CNVs are defined as sections of a genome, spanning from 10 kilobases to several megabases, that are deleted or duplicated. Smaller studies had shown that rare CNVs contributed to the risk burden of schizophrenia and that some CNVs conferred risk for schizophrenia. Larger genome-wide studies (whose sample sizes were still typically less than 10,000) remained underpowered for detection of CNVs that either occurred at low frequencies (<0.5%) or had a modest pathogenic effect (odds ratios of 2–10). Creation of the PGC CNV Analysis Group allowed searching for these elements in what became 'the largest genome-wide analysis of CNVs for any psychiatric disorder to date'.

Methods

To conduct a large-scale analysis of CNVs implicated in the pathogenesis of schizophrenia, the CNV Analysis Group used Affymetrix and Illumina platforms to mine the genome for CNVs, and employed several computational algorithms for data analysis. Only those CNVs that were detected by all algorithms were retained for further analysis. CNV burden between cases and controls was compared on multiple levels: genome-wide, select pathways, individual genes, and breakpoint analyses. Data obtained from this study was used to validate CNV risk loci that were identified by previous studies, as well as to calculate the variance in schizophrenia liability that was conferred by CNV risk loci.

Results

The PGC CNV Analysis Group maximized the study's sample size by pooling together all available microarray samples from previous genetic studies of schizophrenia, which added up to a total of over 40,000 subjects. The analysis successfully identified eight novel CNV loci that met stringent quality control protocols and conferred either risk of or protection against schizophrenia. The eight novel CNVs were present in only 1.4% of schizophrenia cases and explained about 0.85% of the variance in schizophrenia liability. The mapping of CNVs against known biological pathways revealed enrichment in synaptic and neuronal components, including presynaptic adhesion molecules, postsynaptic scaffolding proteins, calcium channels, glutamatergic ionotropic receptors and their interacting proteins, as well as pathways that were previously implicated in behavioural phenotypes in mice. A total of eight genome-wide significant loci were identified, most of which included multiple genes, with the exception of neurexin 1 (Table 4.1). Most of the CNV loci identified by the gene-based association test were found at hot spots for non-allelic homologous recombination (NAHR), suggesting that novel CNVs were similar to known pathogenic CNVs in that they tended to occur in regions prone to high rates of recurrent mutation.

Conclusions and critique

Since the beginning of the twenty-first century, over a hundred GWASs with a primary focus on psychiatric disorders have been published, yet overall progress has remained slow. Thus, the significance of this landmark study by the CNV Analysis Group of the PGC is manifold. On a more basic level, the group has identified several novel regions of the genome that either predispose to or protect against schizophrenia. They also show that both rare CNVs and more common genetic alleles converge upon genes that code for functionally relevant brain proteins. A higher rate of *de novo* CNVs in cases, compared to controls, highlights the important role of meiotic genome rearrangement events that confer large risk of the disease but are not inherited from parents, unlike many single genes (such as dopamine receptor D_2 (DRD2) or glutamatergic transmission genes) implicated in schizophrenia (Ripke et al., 2014). Though we are still far from a comprehensive understanding of pathophysiological mechanisms of schizophrenia, these new findings allow for the development of testable hypotheses and open doors to novel treatment options.

The study by the CNV Analysis Group of the PGC showed the importance of large-scale collaborations in psychiatric genetics research. It has been previously postulated that the discovery rate of at-risk alleles remains minimal until a study achieves a breakthrough threshold of 13,000 cases, after which about four independent associations are found per 1,000 added cases (O'Donovan, 2015). While the CNV study was sufficiently powered to detect variants of large effect sizes that occur in >0.1% of cases, it was still underpowered to detect rare CNVs with modest effect sizes or ultra-rare variants regardless of their effect size. Importantly, the combined CNVs and SNP loci identified by the PGC (Ripke et al., 2014) explained only about 5% of the total heritability of schizophrenia, clearly showing that most of the discovery work still lies ahead. Other areas of expanding research include further collaboration, new technologies to detect more subtle genetic variations, and a focus on other non-heritable elements such as chromatin structure and modifications.

Insights into autism spectrum disorder genomic architecture and biology

Main citation

Sanders, S. J., et al. (2015). Insights into autism spectrum disorder genomic architecture and biology from 71 risk loci. *Neuron*, 87, 1215–1233.

Table 4.1 Significant copy number variant (CNV) loci from gene-based association test

Chr.	Start	End	Locus (gene)	Status	Putative mechanism	CNV test	Direction	FWER	BH-FDR	CAS	CON	Regional *P*	OR (95% CI)
22	17400000	19750000	22q11.21	Previously implicated	NAHR	Loss	Risk	Yes	3.54×10^{-15}	64	1	5.70×10^{-18}	67.7 (9.3–492.8)
16	29560000	30110000	16p11.2, proximal	Previously implicated	NAHR	Gain	Risk	Yes	5.82×10^{-10}	70	7	2.52×10^{-12}	9.4 (4.2–20.9)
2	50000992	51113178	2p16.3 (*NRXN1*)	Previously implicated	NHEJ	Loss	Risk	Yes	3.52×10^{-7}	35	3	4.92×10^{-9}	14.4 (4.2–46.9)
15	28920000	30270000	15q13.3	Previously implicated	NAHR	Loss	Risk	Yes	2.22×10^{-5}	28	2	2.13×10^{-7}	15.6 (3.7–66.5)
1	144646000	146176000	1q21.1	Previously implicated	NAHR	Loss + gain	Risk	Yes	0.00011	60	14	1.50×10^{-6}	3.8 (2.1–6.9)
3	197230000	198840000	3q29	Previously implicated	NAHR	Loss	Risk	Yes	0.00024	16	0	1.86×10^{-6}	INF
16	28730000	28960000	16p11.2, distal	Previously reported	NAHR	Loss	Risk	Yes	0.0029	11	1	5.52×10^{-5}	20.6 (2.6–162.2)
7	72380000	73780000	7q11.23	Previously reported	NAHR	Gain	Risk	Yes	0.0048	16	1	1.68×10^{-4}	16.1 (3.1–125.7)
X	153800000	154225000	Xq28, distal	Novel	NAHR	Gain	Risk	No	0.049	18	2	3.61×10^{-4}	8.9 (2.0–39.9)
22	17400000	19750000	22q11.21	Previously reported	NAHR	Gain	Protective	No	0.024	3	16	4.54×10^{-4}	0.15 (0.04–0.52)
7	64476203	64503433	7q11.21 (*ZNF92*)	Novel	NAHR	Loss + gain	Protective	No	0.033	131	180	6.71×10^{-4}	0.66 (0.52–0.84)
13	19309593	19335773	13q12.11 (*ZMYM5*)	Novel	NAHR	Gain	Protective	No	0.024	15	38	7.91×10^{-4}	0.36 (0.19–0.67)

(*continued*)

Table 4.1 Continued

Chr.	Start	End	Locus (gene)	Status	Putative mechanism	CNV test	Direction	FWER	BH-FDR	CAS	CON	Regional *P*	OR (95% CI)
X	148575477	148580720	Xq28 (*MAGEA11*)	Novel	NAHR	Gain	Protective	No	0.044	12	36	1.06×10^{-3}	0.35 (0.18–0.68)
15	20350000	20640000	15q11.2	Previously implicated	NAHR	Loss	Risk	No	0.044	98	50	1.34×10^{-3}	1.8 (1.2–2.6)
9	831690	959090	9p24.3 (*DMRT1*)	Novel	NHEJ	Loss + gain	Risk	No	0.049	13	1	1.35×10^{-3}	12.4 (1.6–98.1)
8	100094670	100958984	8q22.2 (*VPS13B*)	Novel	NHEJ	Loss	Risk	No	0.048	7	1	1.74×19^{-3}	14.5 (1.7–122.2)
7	158145959	158664998	7p36.3 (*VIPR2; WDR60*)	Previously reported	NAHR	Loss + gain	Risk	No	0.046	20	6	5.79×10^{-3}	3.5 (1.3–9.0)

All 17 association signals listed contain at least one gene with false discovery rate (BH-FDR) <0.05 in the gene-based test, with eight containing at least one gene surpassing the family-wise error rate (FWER) <0.05. Genomic positions listed are based on hg18 coordinates. For putative CNV mechanisms, non-homologous recombination (NAHR) and non-homologous end joining (NHEJ) are listed as the likely genomic feature driving CNV formation at each locus. Regional *P* values and odds ratios (ORs) are from a regional test at each locus, where we combine CNV overlapping the implicated region and run the same test as used for each gene (logistic regression with covariates and deviance test *P* value). CNV losses and gains at 22q11.21 are listed as separate association signals, as CNV losses associate with schizophrenia risk, whereas CNV gains associate with protection from schizophrenia. For each association we indicate whether it was previously described in the literature (previously reported) and whether the reported *P* value exceeded the multiple testing correction in this study (previously implicated).

CAS, cases; CON, controls.

Reproduced with permission from Marshall, C. R. et al. Contribution of copy number variants to schizophrenia from a genome-wide study of 41,321 subjects. ***Nature Genetics, 49***:27–35.
 DOI: https://doi.org/10.1038/ng.3725.

Background

As discussed in the section 'Beyond individual genes: contribution of copy number variants to schizophrenia', creation of large consortia in mental health research led to the collection of sufficient sample size to begin identification of individual genes or genetic elements involved in the biology of psychiatric illnesses. *De novo* risk-conferring CNVs in psychiatric disorders typically involve multiple genes and provide a limit to resolution of implication of specific genes. With an earlier report of the role of non-synonymous and particularly loss-of-function (protein truncating due to nonsense mutation) *de novo* SNVs having a role in ASD, specific genes were more directly implicated (Neale et al., 2012). Moreover, it was established that *de novo* germline mutations played a key role in ASD. In this paper, Sanders and colleagues (2015) combined large-scale CNV and exome sequencing studies to (1) identify molecular pathways that were affected by ASD; (2) describe how these *de novo* mutations conferred the risk of the disease; and (3) show that affected females harboured a greater share of risk variants as predicted from a complex model in which males would require less strong events to cross a multifactorial risk threshold and express the disease phenotype.

Methods

For the current study, samples from 2,591 families (a total of 10,220 individuals) from the entire Simons Simplex Collection (SSC) were genotyped using the Illumina platform to determine *de novo* CNVs and exome sequenced to identify *de novo* SNVs. These data were pooled with the existing CNV data from the Autism Genome Project (AGP) and exome sequencing data from the Autism Sequencing Consortium (ASC). Presence of *de novo* deletions/duplications versus rare inherited autosomal CNVs was assessed by comparing data from male and female ASD probands and their unaffected siblings. Comparison of CNVs and SNVs between unrelated disease probands was used to identify recurrent ASD risk loci and specific at-risk genes with resolution down to point mutations. Of note, the risk loci were identified through a statistically significant recurrence of *de novo* SNVs within the same gene in unrelated families. Further analysis of the common ASD-associated genes was used to define functional subnetworks, thus connecting genetic data with putative mechanisms.

Results

Genetic analysis of the 10,220 individuals from 2,591 families yielded a total of 175 *de novo* CNVs, with 166 of those used for further analysis. Affected ASD probands harboured significantly more *de novo* CNVs than unaffected siblings (0.052 versus 0.016), and these *de novo* CNVs were larger and more gene-rich in the probands than in siblings. On the other hand, rare inherited autosomal CNVs made little, if any, contribution to the ASD risk in SSC families. On average, *de novo* CNVs and SNVs were found in 10% and 17% of male and female probands, respectively. While *de novo* loss-of-function SNVs and *de novo* CNVs were associated with a reduction in non-verbal IQ (NVIQ), even those probands

Table 4.2 Integrating small *de novo* deletions in 65 TADA-identified autism spectrum disorder (ASD) genes

dnLoF Count	FDR ≤0.01	0.01 <FDR ≤0.05	0.05 <FDR ≤0.1
≥2	*ADNP, ANK2, ARID1B, ASH1L, CHD2 CDH8, CUL3, DSCAM, DYRK1A, GRIN2B KATNAL2, KDM5B, KMT2C, NCKAP1, POGZ, SCN2A, SUV420H1, SYNGAP1 TBR1, TCF7L2, TNRC6B, WAC*	*BCL11A, FOXP1, GIGYF1 ILF2, KDM6B, PHF2, RANBP17 SPAST, WDFY3*	*DIP2A, KMT2E*
1	*NRXN1, PTEN, SETD5, SHANK2, SHANK3, TRIP12*	*DNMT3A, GABRB3, KAT2B, MFRP, MYT1L, P2RX5*	*AKAP9, APH1A, CTTNBP2, ERBB2IP, ETFB, INTS6, IRF2BPL, MBD5, NAA15 NINL, OR52M1, PTK7, TRIO, USP45*
0	–	*MIB1, SLC6A1, ZNF559*	*ACHE, CAPN12, NLGN3*

Genes with a small *de novo* deletion are in bold.

TADA, the transmission and *de novo* association test; FDR, false discovery rate; dnLoF, *de novo* loss of function.

Reproduced with permission from Sanders, S. J. et al. Insights into Autism Spectrum Disorder Genomic Architecture and Biology from 71 Risk Loci. *Neuron, 87*(6):1215–1233. Copyright © 2015 Elsevier Inc. All rights reserved. DOI: https://doi.org/10.1016/j.neuron.2015.09.016.

with NVIQ in the normal range still contained an excess of *de novo* mutations compared with unaffected siblings. Computational analysis of *de novo* CNVs and SNVs identified six ASD risk loci and 65 ASD risk genes (Table 4.2). These 65 genes showed enrichment for protein–protein interactions and clustered into two large subnetworks: chromatin regulation/transcription (6.6-fold enrichment) and synaptic/neuronal pathways (9.5-fold enrichment) (Figure 4.5). Finally, it is well known that ASD prevalence is significantly higher in males than in females, though prior to this paper it was unclear whether this was due to a difference in pathophysiological mechanisms between the genders, or whether the female sex itself was somehow protective against the expression of the ASD phenotype. Sanders et al. showed that female probands harboured increased burden of *de novo* mutations compared to male probands, and that mutations in males and females targeted a common set of genes, thus supporting a hypothesis that female sex was protective against ASD, and that the underlying genetic mechanisms were similar in males and females.

Conclusions and critique

The landmark paper by Sanders et al. (2015) provides the largest aggregation of *de novo* CNV and SNV data in any psychiatric disorder to date. *De novo* CNVs limited to a single gene and SNVs which lead to the loss of function of one copy of a single gene provided higher resolution that allowed for identification of 65 risk genes for ASD, many of which

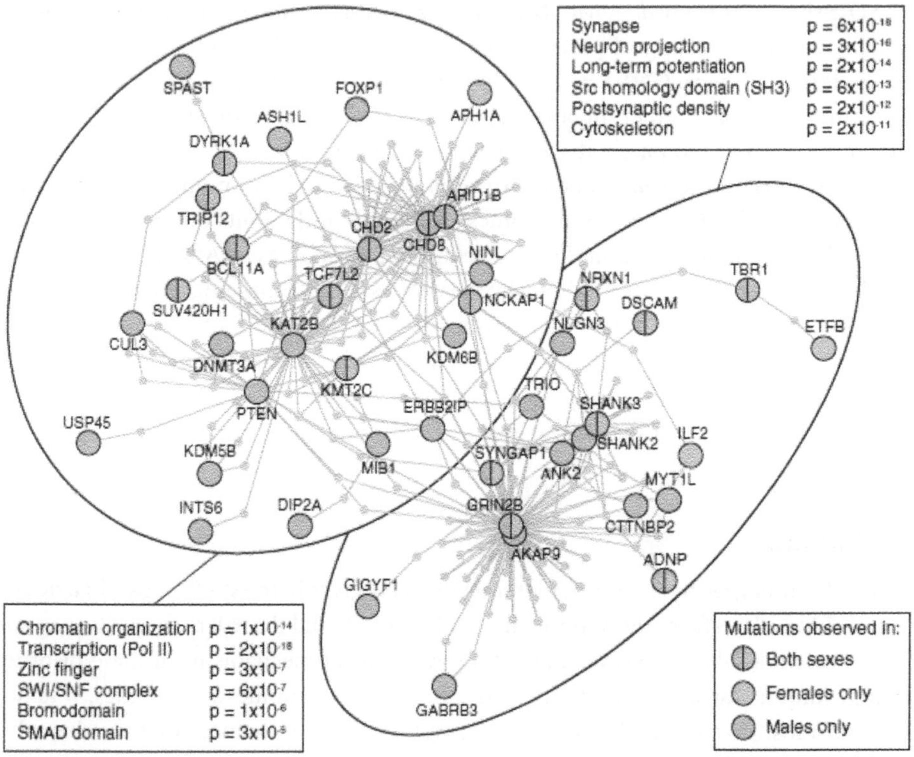

Figure 4.5 Protein–protein interaction (PPI) networks in autism spectrum disorder (ASD). Sixty-five ASD genes identified with a TADA FDR ≤0.01 were submitted as seeds to form a DAPPLE PPI (Rossin et al., 2011). The seed genes are shown as circles in red and/or blue based on the sex of the ASD cases in whom the mutations were identified; the distribution of male and female mutations in the network does not differ from expectation ($p = 0.97$). PPIs are shown as grey lines (edges) and additional genes are pulled into the network to form indirect connections. The network has a clear distinction into two halves (shown by the large ovals). The top gene ontology terms are shown with Benjamini Hochberg corrected *p* values.

TADA: the transmission and *de novo* association test; FDR: false discovery rate

Reproduced with permission from Sanders, S. J., et al. (2015). Insights into autism spectrum disorder genomic architecture and biology from 71 risk loci. *Neuron*, 87(6), 1215–1233. Copyright © 2015 Elsevier Inc. All rights reserved. https://doi.org/10.1016/j.neuron.2015.09.016

have become newly identified single-gene syndromes on the basis of this and related research (e.g. CHD8 deletion). The analysis of ASD risk genes sheds light on molecular mechanisms of ASD, establishing an important role for chromatin regulation and synaptic pathways in its biology.

The approach of Sanders et al. to delineating the genetic architecture of ASD is likely to be applicable to other psychiatric disorders or behavioural phenotypes. The majority of ASD CNV risk loci identified by the current study are broadly associated with other developmental delay phenotypes, and some of the ASD loci are also found to contribute to schizophrenia risk (e.g. 16p11.2 duplication). The finding that a significant portion of ASD risk comes from *de novo* SNVs and CNVs highlights the limited utility of preconception genetic testing of parents, though raises a possibility of screening for large risk-conferring *de novo* CNVs *in utero*. For example, identifying the 16p11.2 deletion *in utero* can potentially predict impairment in social communication skills and a 30-point drop in IQ compared to parental average in the offspring (Moreno-De-Luca et al., 2015). The multifactorial background of cognitive ability and social/communication function of the parents confounds measured outcomes and significantly limits our predictive ability. A much larger sample size would better delineate the genetics of ASD by providing adequate statistical power, as exemplified by the GWAS of schizophrenia (Ripke et al., 2014). Another critique of the study is that it was focused on the impact of larger effect *de novo* variations. Thus, although these *de novo* events may have sizeable individual effects in certain cases of ASD and other psychiatric disorders (such as schizophrenia), it is important to remember that the overall genetic make-up of ASD remains highly polygenic (Gaugler et al., 2014).

Conclusion

In the last century, we have witnessed tremendous progress in the study of psychiatric genetics, making a leap from questioning heritability of mental disorders to identifying specific genes, molecular pathways, and pathophysiological mechanisms of these disorders through multinational collaborations and sophisticated genome-wide studies. It is now clear that most psychiatric illnesses have complex genetic influences that are shaped by interactions between inherited risk alleles and *de novo* mutations. However, many questions remain unanswered. First, even the largest GWAS analysis of more than 100,000 subjects with schizophrenia identified only a small group of risk-conferring elements. The major part of the genetic risk of mental disorders remains to be uncovered, with the first step being the completion of large-scale GWAS in major depressive disorder (Wray et al., 2018), bipolar disorder (Stahl et al., preprint), and ADHD (Demontis et al., 2019), among others. It is likely that further increasing sample sizes of GWAS and exome sequencing analyses will allow for identification of additional genes and CNVs that are both rare and confer a small to moderate risk of a disease.

However, it is also likely that changes in the DNA alone will not explain fully the risk of these disorders, regardless of how large a sample size we can achieve. Thus, it is important to expand our search beyond the DNA itself. Recent studies looking at epigenetic mechanisms of depression, schizophrenia, and bipolar disorder (for a review, see Nestler et al., 2016) highlight the key role of histone modifications, chromatin remodelling, and DNA methylation in these illnesses. These studies also highlight understanding of the interaction between nature and nurture through the study of epigenetic modifications occurring with stress, adverse early life experiences, and even prenatal events. Finally, the role of other non-inherited factors, such as 3D organization of the genome into chromosomal loops and higher-order chromatin structures, is being examined in psychiatric illnesses.

The discovery of the role of *de novo* CNVs and SNVs in psychiatric illnesses shifts our focus from inherited to 'heritable but not inherited' *de novo* risk events in the disease aetiology. In ASD, *de novo* CNVs and *de novo* loss-of-function mutations appear to confer a significantly higher risk of the disease compared to rare mutations that are inherited (Sanders et al., 2015). These findings present a significant challenge to our efforts to predict the risk of psychiatric illnesses through preconception genetic counselling or prenatal testing. A small number of inherited causes of psychiatric phenotypes, such as Fragile X full mutation from a mother or maternal duplication of 15q11-q13, may be identified in parents prior to conception and used to screen the fetus *in utero*. However, most of the genetic variants that alone can sufficiently increase an individual's risk for mental disorders occur *de novo*.

A more complete understanding of the complex genetics of psychiatric disorders, together with technological advances in sequencing and computational biology, will allow us to assess the interplay of many genetic risk factors simultaneously and bring the future of personalized medicine into the field of psychiatry (Prasad & Cook, 2018). Moreover, the development of an increased understanding of the pathophysiology of psychiatric disorders provided by molecular genetics may lead to the development of new treatments that are applicable to those affected.

Finally, it is important to remember that advances in psychiatric genetic research must not overshadow the role of environmental influences and individual psychology in the development of mental illness. Although genetic variations can disrupt multiple brain circuits and signalling pathways, the emergence of a disease phenotype and symptoms specific to each person is likely to depend on the individual's environmental exposures and unique life experiences. Indeed, psychiatric diseases are biopsychosocial entities, and it is our hope that in the future we can embrace all aspects of our field and learn about psychiatric illnesses from many different angles, whether it is genes, neural networks, character structure, family dynamics, or influences of a larger community and culture.

References

Chial, H. (2008). Mendelian genetics: patterns of inheritance and single-gene disorders. *Nature Education*, **1**(1), 63.

Collins, A. L. & Sullivan, P. F. (2013). Genome-wide association studies in psychiatry: what have we learned? *British Journal of Psychiatry*, **202**(1), 1–4.

Demontis, D., et al. (2019). Discovery of the first genome-wide significant risk loci for ADHD. *Nature Genetics*, **51**, 63–75.

Falconer, D. S. & MacKay, T. F. C. (1996). *Introduction to Quantitative Genetics*, 4th edn. Essex, UK: Longmans Green.

Fromm-Reichmann, F. (1948). Notes on the development of treatment of schizophrenics by psychoanalytic psychotherapy. *Psychiatry*, **11**(3), 263–273.

Gaugler, T., et al. (2014). Most genetic risk for autism resides with common variation. *Nature Genetics*, **46**(8), 881–885.

Gottesman, I. I. & Shields, J. (1967). A polygenic theory of schizophrenia. *Proceedings of the National Academy of Sciences of the United States of America*, **58**(1), 199–205.

Hartwell, C. E. (1996). The schizophrenogenic mother concept in American psychiatry. *Psychiatry*, 59(3), 274–297.

Kety, S. S., Rosenthal, D., Wender, P. H., & Schulsinger, F. (1968). Mental illness in the biological and adoptive families of schizophrenics. *Journal of Psychiatric Research*, 6, 345–362.

Kringlen, E. (1966). Schizophrenia in twins. An epidemiological-clinical study. *Psychiatry*, **29**(2), 172–184.

Luxenburger, H. (1928). Vorläufiger bericht über psychiatrische serienuntersuchungen an zwillingen. *Z ges Neurol Psychiat*, **116**, 297–326.

Marshall, C. R., et al. (2017). Contribution of copy number variants to schizophrenia from a genome-wide study of 41,321 subjects. *Nature Genetics*, **49**(1), 27–35.

Moreno-De-Luca, A., et al. (2015). The role of parental cognitive, behavioral, and motor profiles in clinical variability in individuals with chromosome 16p11.2 deletions. *Journal of the American Medical Association: Psychiatry*, **72**(2), 119–126.

Nagel, M., et al. (2018). GWAS meta-analysis of neuroticism (N=449,484) identifies novel genetic loci and pathways. *Nature Genetics*, **50**(7), 920–927.

Neale, B. M., et al. (2012). Patterns and rates of exonic *de novo* mutations in autism spectrum disorders. *Nature*, **485**(7397), 242–245.

Nestler, E. J., et al. (2016). Epigenetic basis of mental illness. *Neuroscientist*, **22**(5), 447–463.

O'Donovan, M. C. (2015). What have we learned from the Psychiatric Genomics Consortium? *World Psychiatry*, **14**(3), 291–293.

Plomin, R. (1995). Molecular genetics and psychology. *Current Directions in Psychological Science*, **4**(4), 114–117.

Plomin, R., Owen, M. J., & McGuffin, P. (1994). The genetic basis of complex human behaviors. *Science*, **264**(5166), 1733–1739.

Prasad, C. & Galbraith, P. (2005). Sir Archibald Garrod and Alkaptonuria–story of metabolic genetics. *Clinical Genetics*, **68**, 199–203.

Prasad, S. & Cook, E. H. (2018). Novel approaches for treating psychiatric disorders of childhood onset. In: *Neurobiology of Mental Illness*, 5th edn, ed. D. S. Charney, J. D. Buxbaum, P. Sklar, & E. J. Nestler. New York: Oxford University Press; pp. 905–914.

Propping, P. (2005). The biography of psychiatric genetics: from early achievements to historical burden, from an anxious society to critical geneticists. *American Journal of Medical Genetics Part B: Neuropsychiatric Genetics*, **136B**(1), 2–7.

Ripke, S., et al. (2014). Biological insights from 108 schizophrenia-associated genetic loci. *Nature*, **511**(7510), 421–427.

Rüdin, E. (1916). *Studien über Vererbung und Entstehung Geistiger Störungen, I. Zur Vererbung und Neuentstehung der Dementia Praecox*. Berlin: Springer.

Sanders, S. J., et al. (2015). Insights into autism spectrum disorder genomic architecture and biology from 71 risk loci. *Neuron*, **87**(6), 1215–1233.

Smith, D. J., et al. (2016). Genome-wide analysis of over 106 000 individuals identifies 9 neuroticism-associated loci. *Molecular Psychiatry*, **21**, 749–757.

Stahl, E., et al. (2018). Genomewide association study identifies 30 loci associated with bipolar disorder. *bioRxiv*, https://www. biorxiv. org/content/early/2018/01/24/173062.

Sullivan, P. F., et al. (2018). Psychiatric genomics: an update and an agenda. *American Journal of Psychiatry*, **175**(1), 15–27.

Trede, K. (2007). 150 years of Freud–Kraepelin dualism. *Psychiatric Quarterly*, **78**(3), 237–240.

Wender, P. H., Rosenthal, D., Kety, S. S., Schulsinger, F. & Welner, J. (1974). Crossfostering. A research strategy for clarifying the role of genetic and experiential factors in the etiology of schizophrenia. *Archives of General Psychiatry*, **30**(1), 121–128.

White, P. D., Rickards, H., & Zeman, A. Z. (2012). Time to end the distinction between mental and neurological illnesses. *British Medical Journal*, **344**, e3454.

Wray, N. R., et al. (2018). Genome-wide association analyses identify 44 risk variants and refine the genetic architecture of major depression. *Nature Genetics*, **50**(5), 668–681.

Chapter 5

Inflammatory mechanisms, the immune system, and psychiatric illness

Ozan Toy, Emmalee Boyle, and Lynn E. DeLisi

Introduction

Emil Kraepelin defined *dementia praecox* as a progressive deteriorating disease and, in one of his texts on this disorder, illustrated what he thought were disintegrating brain neurons characteristic of the underlying pathology that in many ways gave the appearance of 'inflammation' (Kraepelin, 1919). However, in general, research over most of the twentieth century failed to produce any evidence of an association with inflammation. In the 1980s, literature on immunity and autoimmunity in schizophrenia abounded, with reports of elevated antinuclear antibodies, observations of abnormal lymphocytes, and elevated viral antibodies (reviewed in DeLisi, 1984). However, these findings were generally attributed to the effects of medications or chronic institutionalization. Recently, there seems to have been a reintroduction of the possibility that inflammation underlies the disorder, particularly in early stages of the illness, and in addition is related to the genetic tendency for the disorder.

Abnormal immune function has also been attributed to stress and thus is not specific to schizophrenia. A change in immune response is known to occur after stressful life events, such as the loss of a spouse, and has been found to generalize as well to the depressive state. In fact, antidepressants are known to have anti-inflammatory effects. Furthermore, bipolar disorder also has been shown to be associated with deficient immunity, and lithium, its prime treatment, is known to bolster the immune system.

The association of early influenza epidemics with psychosis

Main citation

Menninger, K. A. (1994). Influenza and schizophrenia. An analysis of post-influenzal 'dementia precox', as of 1918, and five years later further studies of the psychiatric aspects of influenza. 1926 [classical article]. *American Journal of Psychiatry*, 151, 182–187.

Background

The Spanish influenza pandemic of 1918–1919 affected more than 500 million individuals worldwide. Between 50 to 100 million individuals died in just one year, and the majority of deaths were among 20- to 40-year-olds (Mamelund et al., 2013). Among survivors, a variety of mental illnesses occurred (Menninger, 1919a, 1921, 1922, 1926). However, a schizophrenia syndrome was the most frequently associated with the 1918 epidemic.

Kraepelin's development of the concept of *dementia praecox* was not formed until the turn of the twentieth century, and thus the influenza outbreak of 1918 was the first time the relationship between influenza and a psychosis was described (Diefendorf & Kraepelin, 1923). This association was highly controversial at the time. Egbert Fell (1919) diagnosed *dementia praecox* in five of twenty post-influenzal cases in 1919. In a study by Fritz Walther (1923), 60 cases of post-influenza psychoses were found. William Sandy (1920) reported that among 70,000 neuropsychiatric cases reported by the army, only 73 were ascribed to influenza, but of those, seven had *dementia praecox*. Sandy concluded that because the patients were in the military, it was unlikely they had psychiatric symptoms before becoming ill with influenza; thus, in the seven cases, influenza was causing the psychosis. In contrast, Isham Harris and David Corcoran (1919) found no cases of *dementia praecox* associated with the influenza epidemic. However, there were other studies describing peculiar catatonic-like symptoms in patients post-influenza (Kirby, 1919).

In 1919, Karl Menninger (who at the time was a psychiatrist in training) reported an association of influenza and psychoses in patients who were admitted to the Boston Psychopathic Hospital in late 1918. Of 80 patients who had been admitted to the hospital for 'mental disturbances' associated with influenza, he diagnosed 16 with delirium, 25 with *dementia praecox*, 23 with 'other types of psychosis', and 16 as unclassified (Menninger, 1919a, 1919b). In 1926, *The American Journal of Psychiatry* published the full case studies by Dr Menninger described in the following sections, in which an infectious/inflammatory cause for some *dementia praecox* was implicated.

Methods

One hundred and seventy-five cases of post-influenza psychosis from Boston Psychopathic Hospital were examined. Inquiries were sent to state hospitals, relatives, and patients five years after the initial observations were made, for updates on their psychiatric condition: 60 cases were found to have *dementia praecox* of which 50 could be followed up after five years and thus were included as case studies.

Results

Of the 175 cases of post-influenza psychosis, one third of all the acute psychoses presented as a schizophrenic syndrome, otherwise known as *dementia praecox*. Of the 50 cases of post-influenza *dementia praecox* included in the follow-up, 21 had the diagnosis of *dementia praecox* confirmed by other hospitals, while 13 went home from the psychiatric hospital and did not have the diagnosis confirmed or contradicted, while in 16 other cases the diagnosis was contradicted by another hospital. The follow-up diagnoses in those 16 cases were: manic depression (9), toxic infections (4), psychosis with mental deficiency (1), and undiagnosable (2). According to Menninger, the most striking results were that 35 of the 50 cases of *dementia praecox* (70%) demonstrated complete recovery within five years, and five cases (10%) showed some improvement in symptoms.

Conclusions and critique

This study suggested that *dementia praecox* was a consequence of influenza in some cases, but association does not prove cause. This was an early epidemiologic study and the technology was not present at the time to study this association further. It should also be noted that the follow-up of some of these patients showed complete recovery, which is unlikely to happen in the majority of cases of schizophrenia. Menninger himself suggested that either the diagnoses of these cases as *dementia praecox* were incorrect, the traditional definition of *dementia praecox* was incorrect, or that influenza produced a specific kind of *dementia praecox* that could self-resolve (Menninger, 1926). Menninger believed that the last conclusion was correct and that the schizophrenia syndrome caused by influenza could vary in its outcome. Thus, the schizophrenia syndrome linked to influenza could be considered a benign process with a good prognosis.

There are several concerns about the diagnostic process in this article that reflect the time in which it was written. It is important to note that American psychiatrists trained from the 1920s through to the late 1960s were taught to diagnose schizophrenia based on the personal feeling evoked by these patients while in their physical presence. Thus, diagnoses varied from clinician to clinician, contrary to the article's assertion that the diagnoses were consistent among staff. Secondly, there was no discussion of what timeline to use when diagnosing post-influenza *dementia praecox*. For example, in case 36, psychosis appeared 10 days after recovering from influenza, while in case 39, the patient developed a psychosis four months later (Menninger, 1926). Thirdly, some of the patients diagnosed with *dementia praecox* would meet criteria for modern-day delirium. (Menninger did diagnose some patients with delirium, but very little was known about delirium at that time.)

There are some limitations associated with the retrospective nature of the study as well. Firstly, the investigator of the case series has to depend on the accuracy and availability of the medical records. Additionally, there is a selection bias present as the investigator is able to self-select the cases. Menninger's article discussed many of the cases in detail, but not all 50 cases were included. Not all family histories were included either. It is likely that the cases demonstrating more significant psychotic symptoms were the ones included in the article. Finally, there is no control group for comparing the incidence of schizophrenia (i.e. in the general population) at that time.

It remains unclear to this date as to whether schizophrenia as we currently know it can be initiated specifically by the influenza virus. Nonetheless, the inflammation caused by such infection could lead to underlying brain pathology associated with schizophrenia and thus to the disease itself. This correlation has been debated in present scientific literature including the idea that schizophrenia occurs more frequently in children born in winter and early spring when viral infections are more prevalent (Battle et al., 1999). In a retrospective study by Bagalkote in 2001, 25 pregnant women who had offspring later diagnosed with schizophrenia were analyzed. About half of the 25 cases reported having contracted influenza during their pregnancy. However, in retrospective studies viral exposure relies on mother's self-reports of influenza, rather than confirmed diagnoses. Given the papers that follow and the renewed interest in inflammation in schizophrenia, the question of an association of influenza with schizophrenia should be revisited.

Evidence of inflammation underlying the neuropathology of schizophrenia

Main citation

Stevens, J. R. (1982). Neuropathology of schizophrenia. *Archives of General Psychiatry*, 39, 1131–1139.

Background

In the 1950s, there was little consensus between pathologists regarding what changes occur in the brains of people with schizophrenia. At that time, most of the histologic studies only focused on the cerebral cortex. Additionally, control specimens were rarely used and staining methods could only test grossly for neurons and myelin. Due to these limitations, it was difficult to differentiate findings specific to schizophrenia from natural ageing or post-mortem changes. Consequently, several post-mortem studies of people with schizophrenia failed to find any gross or cellular evidence of degeneration related to schizophrenia, and thus the disorder was thought to have, as its underlying basis, either neurodevelopmental aberrations or even postnatal adverse family relationship experiences that had no biological effect on the brain. Janice Stevens was one of those investigators who thought 'outside the box', and she continued to search throughout her career for brain evidence of an inflammatory process underlying schizophrenia. This paper was her major contribution that caused much discussion in the field at the time it was published and for years after.

Methods

Histological sections of brains were prepared from 25 patients (ages ranging from 21 to 54 years) known to have schizophrenia who died during their psychiatric hospitalization at St Elizabeth's Hospital in Washington, DC from 1955 to 1963. The death of these patients during hospitalization meant that they were considered to have failed to recover and had most likely suffered the most chronic, severe form of schizophrenia.

The specimens were compared with 28 age-matched deceased patients from the same hospital and time period who did not have schizophrenia. Exclusion criteria included terminal illness or a premorbid state that affected cerebral structure such as malignant hypertension, bacterial endocarditis, miliary tuberculosis, diabetes, meningitis, or hepatic disease. Holzer staining was done to detect glial fibres. Specimens from patients both with and without schizophrenia were examined by pathologists blinded to the clinical diagnosis. The medical records of all patients were examined to ascertain their earliest symptoms of schizophrenia, including any predisposing factors to the illness. The details were documented in case summaries that were created without prior knowledge of the pathology seen in the corresponding brain specimen.

Results

The brains of all 25 patients were found to appear grossly normal. Neuropathological examination showed fibrillary gliosis in three quarters of the brains of the patients with schizophrenia. Gliosis was interpreted as a marker of brain injury and an inflammatory reaction to it. However, the distribution of pathologic changes found in the brains of patients with schizophrenia differed from case to case. Areas of gliosis included periventricular structures of the diencephalon, the periaqueductal regions of the mesencephalon, and the basal forebrain. More specifically, the hypothalamus, midbrain tegmentum, and the substantia innominata were the structures reported to be most affected. Neuronal loss affected the large neurons of the globus pallidus in five specimens. When these areas were stained, they showed altered spiroperidol binding, amine content, and cell loss, which indicates a loss of function in these areas. Lastly, the large multipolar cells of the substantia innominata frequently showed fibrillary gliotic changes and an affinity for IgG and some viral antibodies as well, which can be added evidence of an inflammatory response. Pathologic changes were similar among patients with schizophrenia who received medications and/or electroconvulsive therapy (ECT) compared with those who did not.

Interestingly, the gliosis pattern present in patients with schizophrenia was observed to have a similar distribution in five specimens from controls who did not have schizophrenia but had other neurologic disorders including general paresis, Wernicke's encephalopathy, inclusion body encephalitis, third ventricle colloid cyst, and temporal lobe glioblastoma.

The causes of death varied in patients with the diagnosis of schizophrenia, but 14 patients died unexpectedly from causes such as peritonitis, pneumonitis, or myocardial infarct. The treatments that patients received included insulin coma, ECT, phenothiazines, reserpine, methylphenidate, and cortisone.

Conclusions and critique

This paper found that the areas of the brain most affected in schizophrenia by gliosis included the limbic structures, the basal nuclei, the hypothalamus, and midbrain tegmentum. When these areas are affected by inflammation, changes in perception, cognition, sleep, and appetite can occur. Stevens concluded that her findings represented evidence of low-grade inflammation in people with schizophrenia, although the causes of inflammation could not be determined.

Limitations of the study include a small sample size and restricted generalizability, because the patients represented an extreme end of the schizophrenia spectrum by nature of their institutionalization and hospital death. The author appropriately blinded the examiners to the history of the specimen. However, she did not comment on possible confounders, like the accuracy of the diagnosis of schizophrenia, duration of treatment, race, and sex. Moreover, the study was never independently replicated.

The issue of whether gliosis exists in the brains of people with schizophrenia remains controversial and most investigators dismissed this finding at the time. In the 1980s, the majority of researchers in the field believed that schizophrenia had a developmental component, based on evidence of abnormalities found in the migration of neurons during early brain growth (e.g. Roberts et al., 1987). While gliosis was considered the hallmark of whether an illness is neurodegenerative, it is now clear that degeneration may occur without such evidence (Church et al., 2002). Nevertheless, this issue remained a topic of debate for the following two to three decades (Schnieder & Dwork, 2011).

The association of stress with immune responsivity

Main citation

Keller, S. E., Schleifer, S. J., Liotta, A. S., Bond, R. N., Farhoody, N., & Stein, M. (1988). Stress-induced alterations of immunity in hypophysectomized rats. *Proceedings of the National Academy of Sciences of the USA*, 85, 9297–9301.

Background

The hypothalamic pituitary axis has long been known to modulate the stress-induced immune response via corticosteroid secretion, although stress may also affect immunity in other ways (Keller et al., 1983). The primary aim of this current study was to examine how stress may affect the immune system in an animal model.

Methods

Ninety-six rats were included in this study. The animals were divided into three groups (non-operated, hypophysectomized, and sham hypophysectomized), each of which was further subdivided into two treatment conditions (shocked or not shocked in cage). Animals were sacrificed and their brains and spleens examined. The following analyses were performed:

1) Brains were assayed for pituitary-secreted corticotrophin releasing factor (CRF) and 13-endorphin.
2) Plasma corticosterone and corticotropin (ACTH) were measured.
3) Total leukocyte and differential counts were obtained. T cells, B cells, T-helper cells, and T-suppressor cells were obtained from blood.
4) Stimulation of splenic lymphocytes was examined and natural killer (NK) cell activity was assessed (Shavit et al., 1983).
5) Effector/target ratios were used to assess both peripheral blood and splenic NK cell function.
6) Mitogen-induced lymphocyte stimulation in response to phytohaemagluttin and concanavalin A (Con A) was assessed.

Results

Stress-induced (i.e. shock-induced) production of both ACTH and corticosterone was found in rats with intact pituitaries, and hypophysectomy prevented the release of these hormones. In contrast, multiple measures of immune suppression (as just detailed) were not dependent on pituitary hormone modulation and thus suggest that factors other than the pituitary gland may influence immunosuppression. In addition, the immune response in the spleen is regulated in a different fashion from the peripheral response.

Conclusions and critique

This study showed that the role of the pituitary in response to stress is complex. While it is essential for appropriately modulating the immune system, some aspects of immunity are unaffected. Nevertheless, this was a landmark paper that showed the importance of the interaction between the pituitary and adrenal gland in influencing different components of the immune response during stress. These findings extended previous reports of stress-induced lymphopenia that was dependent on a preserved adrenal gland (Keller et al., 1983), by demonstrating that a similar stress-induced lymphopenia was dependent on an intact pituitary gland.

While this study provided a good animal model for a stress-related response, its generalizability to humans has not been proven, as the stressor (electrical shock) utilized in this study may not be a good model for psychosocial stressors that would occur in human subjects. Overall, it does establish the relationship between neuroendocrine and immunological function, although the lack of a link between these findings and behavioural manifestations in animals is a major limitation. It indirectly suggests that psychological stress produces an immune reaction via the neuroendocrine system. Subsequent studies have shown a relationship between the hypothalamic–pituitary–adrenal (HPA) axis and depression (reviewed in Schule et al., 2009) and novel treatment strategies were proposed by Timothy Dinan (2001). Shinsuke Kito and colleagues (2010) demonstrated changes in the hypothalamic–pituitary–thyroid (HPT) axis following successful treatment with low-frequency right prefrontal transcranial magnetic stimulation in treatment-resistant depression. Given this link, perhaps pituitary hormonal profiles and immune markers should be assessed in patients suffering from depression, followed by possible treatments with medications that either prevent immunosuppression or alter pituitary function.

The association of depression with abnormal immune response

Main citation

Kronfol, Z., Silva Jr, J., Greden, J., Dembinski, S., Gardner, R., & Carroll, B. (1983). Impaired lymphocyte function in depressive illness. *Life Sciences*, 33, 241–247.

Background

Psychosocial stressors, such as bereavement (Bartrop et al., 1977) and sleep deprivation (Palmblad et al., 1979), may be accompanied by an impairment in cell-mediated immunity. Furthermore, studies have demonstrated vulnerability of depressed patients to medical illnesses such as infection (Baldwin, 1979) and neoplasm (Whitlock & Siskind, 1979). Ziad Kronfol and colleagues thus aimed to study the immune response seen in patients with depression. This study was one of the first to identify abnormalities of specific mediators of inflammation in patients with mood disorders.

Methods

Twenty-six moderately depressed individuals and 20 control individuals were assessed. Controls were age and sex matched. All participants were free from medical illness that could influence lymphocyte counts.

Blood samples were collected and lymphocytes cultured with thymidine to measure response to three mitogens: phytohaemagluttinin-P (PHA) and concanavalin A (Con A), both of which stimulate mostly T-lymphocytes (mediators of delayed cellular immunity), as well as pokeweed mitogen (PWM), which stimulates primarily B-lymphocytes (mediators of immunoglobulin production). All participants were free of any type of medication for the two weeks prior to immune testing, and those who did receive medications prior to this drug-free period did not differ significantly from those who had never previously received medications with regard to lymphocyte measures.

Results

Lymphocyte mitogenic activity was decreased among the individuals with depression for all three mitogens. When patients with depression were stratified by severity (mild, moderate, and severe), all three subgroups had significantly lower lymphocyte responses to PWM than the control group. The relationship between depression severity and mitogen response was only studied for PWM because it provided the greatest difference in lymphocyte responsiveness between depressed patients and controls.

Conclusions and critique

This study supported the possibility that impairment in both T-cell mediated immunity and B-cell mediated, antigen-dependent immune function is present in patients with primary depressive illness. This small study was an initial pioneering endeavour that established a connection between psychiatric illness and the immune system and suggested that secondary consequences of depression can lead to physical illnesses resulting from impaired immunity, such as infection and neoplastic disorders. Many studies that followed confirmed these results.

However, the study was limited in several ways. The sample size was small. Measurements of immune function were only obtained once and it is unclear whether decreased immune response would persist if serial measurements were obtained.

Furthermore, there is no mention of which medications the patients were on prior to the two-week medication-free period before immunological testing. Many psychiatric medications have prolonged half-lives, which may or may not contribute to alteration of the lymphocytic response. For example, Margarita Gevorgyan and colleagues (2016) reported effects of antidepressants on immune reactivity in mice and Veerle Gobin and colleagues (2015) showed that fluoxetine suppressed calcium signalling in human T lymphocytes. Others demonstrated the inhibitory effects of antidepressant drugs on the contact hypersensitivity reaction (Curzytek et al., 2015; Kubera et al., 2012). The effects of medication certainly need to be studied further. Particularly it is not clear how long they can last.

Nevertheless, these general findings were confirmed by several other independent studies in major depression (Castle et al., 2008; Cosyns et al., 1989; Darko et al., 1989; Hickie et al., 1993; Kanba et al., 1998; Maes et al., 1989; McAdams & Leonard, 1993; Spurrell & Creed, 1993), although not others. Additional studies expanded this line of inquiry to other populations and immune markers. Marilee Zaharia and colleagues (2000) studied lymphocyte proliferation among major depressive and dysthymic patients. Lymphocyte proliferation in response to mitogens Con A and PHA was reduced to a greater extent among dysthymic than among major depressive patients. Others did not find any change (Andreoli et al., 1993; Bauer et al., 1995; Wodarz et al., 1991; Brambilla et al., 1995). Conversely, two papers found an increase in mitogen lymphocytic stimulation (Kubera et al., 2004; Altshuler et al., 1989). Matthias Rothermundt and colleagues (2001) studied immune patterns in melancholic and non-melancholic major depression and found that melancholic patients had normal cell counts but decreased production of interleukin 2, interferon, and interleukin 10 in acute states of depression. Also, Jaśmina Arabska and colleagues (2018) studied 684 geriatric Caucasian patients with depression and found an increased neutrophil to lymphocyte ratio (NLR) in patients experiencing a first episode of depression, but not in those with recurrent depression. Esra Aydin Sunbul and colleagues (2016) found, in 256 Turkish patients with depression, higher Hamilton Depression Scale (HAM-D) scores associated with higher NLR levels. However, Fatih Kayhan and colleagues (2017) did not find a correlation with NLR in patients with major depressive disorder (MDD). Thus, while overall there is a suggestion in the literature of depressed immune function associated with major depression, there are many inconsistent studies that indicate that there is more research yet to be done on this issue.

Human leukocyte antigen and genetic risk for schizophrenia

Main citation

Sekar, A., et al. (2016). Schizophrenia risk from complex variation of complement component 4. *Nature*, 530, 177–183.

Background

Extensive family, twin, and adoption studies performed throughout the last century have clearly shown that schizophrenia is highly heritable. However, the mechanism for inheritance remained elusive until recently, when results from very large genome-wide association studies (GWAS) showed that many genes of small effect contribute to some of the genetic liability. In the 2014 *Nature* paper resulting from the Schizophrenia Working Group of the Psychiatric Genomics Consortium (PGC), the most significant finding that emerged was an association of schizophrenia to the major histocompatibility complex (MHC) locus on chromosome 6p (Schizophrenia Working Group of the Psychiatric Genomics Consortium, 2014). The MHC locus contains 18 polymorphic human leukocyte antigen (HLA) genes that encode for different antigen-presenting molecules relative to the immune system. The association of schizophrenia to the HLA complex was previously suggested by linkage and association studies, but it was not known which portion of this complex system of immune factors was responsible (Shi et al., 2009). The current paper follows up the PGC report and demonstrates that schizophrenia's association with the MHC arises from structurally diverse alleles of the complement component 4 (C4) genes.

C4 has two isotypes (C4A and C4B) that vary in structure and copy number. There are both long and short forms depending on whether they have a human endogenous retroviral (HERV) insertion. C4A or C4B are commonly present as a tandem array within the MHC class III region and often bind different molecular targets (Carroll et al., 1984; Banlaki et al., 2012).

Methods

A sequence of experiments was performed in order to understand the association of C4 with schizophrenia and how it might explain the underlying basis for high genetic risk for the illness. The authors first identified the 'structural haplotypes' of C4 using a method called 'droplet digital polymerase chain reaction' (ddPCR). They also developed assays to determine the long/short status of each C4A and C4B genotype and then analysed their inheritance in father–mother–offspring trios. Finally, they examined association in the large PGC patient sample to 7,751 single nucleotide polymorphisms (SNPs) that extend across the MHC locus including C4 haplotypes. They also predicted levels of C4A and C4B expression and postulated that C4A expression (based on the association study results) affected risk for schizophrenia. They measured C4A expression, as well as brain distribution of that expression in brains from 35 patients with schizophrenia and 70 controls. To further characterize neuronal C4, they examined human primary cortical neurons for C4 expression, localization, and secretion.

Results

This study identified at least four major haplotypes of the C4 gene that were common enough for population studies. This large association study with schizophrenia PGC samples showed significant association with all SNPs spread throughout the C4 region, with no location being any more significant than another. The associations were also correlated with expression levels, so that the more strongly a particular SNP correlated with the predicted C4A expression, the more strongly it was associated with schizophrenia. Interestingly, despite significance throughout the region, the correlation of each SNP with each other was low, suggesting that more than one independent locus may confer genetic risk for schizophrenia.

The brain expression analyses showed similar expression across all five brain regions analysed.

Conclusions and critique

This paper went beyond genetic linkage and association to the chromosome 6 region of the MHC complex and found that a specific region containing complement C4 was associated with schizophrenia and in proportion to the level of expression of this gene in the brain. Based on their results, the authors suggested that the C4 protein, which has a crucial role in the inflammatory process in aiding the elimination of pathogens, may also contribute in the same way to brain development when synapses are being pruned and reconstructed, particularly during adolescence. Finally, the authors speculated that the inheritance of high-activity C4 alleles could make someone at greater risk for abnormal elimination and pruning of synapses in key regions of the brain.

However, this study needs replication in an independent set of samples. It is unknown what proportion of the genetic risk for schizophrenia can be accounted for by the complement system, but it is estimated to be relatively small, since large numbers of samples were needed to see this effect. Nevertheless, this paper provides further evidence for a clear connection between the immune system and schizophrenia, as well as variation in brain development. Much more research is needed to understand this relationship.

Visualizing inflammation in the brain

Main citation

Pasternak, O., et al. (2012). Excessive extracellular volume reveals a neurodegenerative pattern in schizophrenia onset. *Journal of Neuroscience*, 32, 17365–17372.

Background

The discovery of magnetic resonance imaging (MRI) with diffusion tensor imaging (DTI) enabled the detection of microstructural brain changes *in vivo* (Basser et al., 1994) and helped establish the presence of white-matter deficits in patients with schizophrenia (Kubicki et al., 2007). However, the aetiology of these white-matter abnormalities remains unclear (Assaf & Pasternak, 2008). Assuming this indicates neurodegeneration, its origins could be neuroinflammatory (Potvin et al., 2008; Uranova et al., 2007).

Traditional DTI measures—fractional anisotropy (FA) and mean diffusivity (MD)[1]—fail to differentiate between neuroinflammation and other causes of neurodegeneration; both neuroinflammation and axonal degeneration lead to FA decreases and MD increases (Alexander et al., 2007). A newer method of analysis, called free-water imaging, can measure the diffusion of water molecules into the extraneuronal space near axons (Song et al., 2003), which is thought to be more indicative of neuroinflammation (Schwartz et al., 2006; Sykova & Nicholson, 2008). Thus, free-water imaging can be used to differentiate between pathology related to neuroinflammation and pathology possibly due to axonal degeneration (Pasternak et al., 2009). This paper uses this method to clarify how neuroinflammation and axonal degeneration contribute to the development of white-matter abnormalities and subsequent neurodegeneration seen in patients with schizophrenia.

Methods

Eighteen patients with first-episode psychosis were compared with 20 matched healthy controls. Patients were assessed during their first hospitalization or immediately following discharge. All subjects underwent 3-T MRI with imaging parameters and programs for construction of DTI and free-water maps as detailed in the paper. In order to differentiate between axonal degeneration and neuroinflammation, the authors utilized free-water analysis, which estimates the contribution of freely diffusing water molecules (fractional volume of extracellular water: i.e. water not restricted by cellular membranes) and generates a measure of diffusion fractional anisotropy of water in a tissue (FA_T). The free-water values are expected to increase due to increased accumulation of extracellular fluid. Whilst the FA_T values are expected to be unchanged early on in neuroinflammation, they will decrease with chronic inflammation due to damage of the white-matter tissue. These measurements provide a more specific measurement of neuroinflammation, which FA alone cannot provide. Free-water maps and FA_T maps were generated and white-matter skeleton analysis was done using tract-based spatial statistics. FA, MD, free-water maps, and FA_T maps were then projected onto the skeleton and brain parcellation was calculated using developed computer programs.

Results

Significantly lower FA values throughout the brain on maps of the white-matter skeleton were found in patients compared to controls. The abnormal FA spanned about a third of the left and right hemisphere white matter. Significantly higher MD values were found in areas that overlapped with FA value changes, but also extended beyond those areas. The MD changes covered about half of the right and left hemisphere white matter.

In white matter, the patients showed significantly lower FAT values compared with controls in limited brain areas spanning about 1% of the left and right hemisphere.

[1] Mean diffusivity (MD) is a measurement that reflects the average of tensor eigenvalues within a voxel in a DTI image (O'Donnell & Westin, 2011).

Neuronal connections in the frontal lobe, the superior longitudinal fasciculus bilaterally, the right inferior frontal occipital fasciculus, and the intersection of the callosal fibres within the right superior corona radiata were affected. Furthermore, the patients showed increased free-water values in a diffuse global pattern overlapping with MD and FA value changes spanning about 40% of the left and right hemisphere.

In order to evaluate FAT and mean free-water values in grey-matter regions, four global regions of interest were examined. Mean free-water values in all four regions in patients were significantly higher compared to controls. The difference ranged from a 1.1% to 1.6% increase in extracellular fractional volume. The free-water increase overlapped greatly with MD changes and a slight majority of sections showed significant MD increases. No overall reduced volume in the grey-matter sections were found and global changes of FAT in the grey matter were not evident.

Conclusions and critique

Widespread white-matter abnormalities in patients with first-episode psychosis were observed in comparison to controls. These included an increase in extracellular free-water content that was not present within tissues, as shown by free-water measurements. Thus, this increase in extracellular volume likely reflects neuroinflammation rather than degeneration and that patients with schizophrenia, in their early stages of illness, have evidence of an inflammatory process that may develop into neurodegeneration as a consequence. Evidence for neurodegeneration was in fact already present, as seen by decreased FAT values, particularly in frontal lobe axonal connections. Fibres connecting frontal lobes may be the first to show degeneration in the disease process. This is similar to other neurodegenerative disorders where prolonged inflammation eventually leads to axonal degeneration.

The number of patients evaluated in this study was small and thus these data need replication in a larger study. Additionally, whether the change in DTI indices was influenced by medications is not ruled out. Another possibility is that metabolic disease contributed to alterations in diffusion tensor markers. The prevalence of diabetes is elevated in patients with schizophrenia (Annamalai et al., 2017), and type 2 diabetes mellitus has been associated with reduced white-matter volume and reduced grey- and white-matter FA, with a trend towards increased grey- and white-matter MD (Raffield, 2016).

In summary, this paper was the first to use non-invasive neuroimaging to find evidence of neuroinflammation in living patients with schizophrenia. The authors speculate that their data show that neuroinflammation occurs in patients with a first-episode psychosis, while axonal degeneration occurs later in the course of illness. Future longitudinal studies following this cohort over time, with repeat serial imaging to demonstrate a change in free water and development of neurodegeneration, would be important. If these authors are correct in their conclusions, then introducing anti-inflammatory treatments early in the onset of schizophrenia may lead to better outcomes for this illness and further confirm the neuroinflammation hypothesis of schizophrenia.

Conclusion

The relationship between the immune system and mental illnesses has been studied extensively since the early twentieth century. This chapter highlights studies that were pioneering in the field because their publications opened up new lines of research and new questions about serious mental illness, its risk factors, and its aetiology. Each of the studies used methodology appropriate to the time in which it was written, but not necessarily appropriate by current standards. The first four papers (describing psychotic sequelae to an influenza epidemic, post-mortem gliosis, immune response to stress and in depression) illustrate the methods that needed improvement in psychiatric research, such as better consistency in diagnosis, larger numbers of subjects, and better technology. On the other hand, the last two papers focus on understanding the genetic architecture of schizophrenia in relation to the HLA locus and on using brain imaging to detect inflammation. These are both currently 'state of the art' in study design and methodology. While we have further work to do to understand how altered immunity can affect brain functioning, we clearly have come a long way in the past century and have good confirmatory evidence to begin to target immune abnormalities in new drug development.

References

Alexander, A. L., Lee, J. E., Lazar, M., & Field, A. S. (2007). Diffusion tensor imaging of the brain. *Neurotherapeutics*, **4**(3), 316–329. doi:10.1016/j.nurt.2007.05.011

Altshuler, L. L., Plaeger-Marshall, S., Richeimer, S., Daniels, M., & Baxter Jr, L. R. (1989). Lymphocyte function in major depression. *Acta Psychiatrica Scandinavica*, **80**(2), 132–136.

Andreoli, A. V., Keller, S. E., Rabaeus, M., Marin, P., Bartlett, J. A., & Taban, C. (1993). Depression and immunity: Age, severity, and clinical course. *Brain, Behavior, and Immunity*, 7(4), 279–292.

Annamalai, A., Kosir, U., & Tek, C. (2017). Prevalence of obesity and diabetes in patients with schizophrenia. *World Journal of Diabetes*, **8**(8), 390–396. doi:10.4239/wjd.v8.i8.390

Arabska, J., Lucka, A., Magierski, R., Sobow, T., & Wysokinski, A. (2018). Neutrophil-lymphocyte ratio is increased in elderly patients with first episode depression, but not in recurrent depression. *Psychiatry Research*, **263**, 35–40. doi:S0165-1781(17)30952-6

Assaf, Y. & Pasternak, O. (2008). Diffusion tensor imaging (DTI)-based white matter mapping in brain research: A review. *Journal of Molecular Neuroscience*, **34**(1), 51–61. doi:10.1007/s12031-007-0029-0

Aydin Sunbul, E., et al. (2016). Increased neutrophil/lymphocyte ratio in patients with depression is correlated with the severity of depression and cardiovascular risk factors. *Psychiatry Investigation*, **13**(1), 121–126. doi:10.4306/pi.2016.13.1.121

Baldwin, J. A. (1979). Schizophrenia and physical disease. *Psychological Medicine*, **9**(4), 611. doi:10.1017/s0033291700033948

Banlaki, Z., Doleschall, M., Rajczy, K., Fust, G., & Szilagyi, A. (2012). Fine-tuned characterization of RCCX copy number variants and their relationship with extended MHC haplotypes. *Genes and Immunity*, **13**(7), 530–535. doi:10.1038/gene.2012.29

Bartrop, R. W., Lazarus, L., Luckhurst, E., Kiloh, L. G., & Penny, R. (1977). Depressed lymphocyte function after bereavement. *The Lancet*, **309**(8016), 834–836. doi:10.1016/s0140-6736(77)92780-5

Basser, P. J., Mattiello, J., & LeBihan, D. (1994). MR diffusion tensor spectroscopy and imaging. *Biophysical Journal*, **66**(1), 259–267. doi:10.1016/s0006-3495(94)80775-1

Battle, Y. L., Martin, B. C., Dorfman, J. H., & Miller, L. S. (1999). Seasonality and infectious disease in schizophrenia: The birth hypothesis revisited. *Journal of Psychiatric Research*, **33**(6), 501–509. doi:S0022-3956(99)00022-9

Bauer, M. E., Gauer, G. J., Luz, C., Silveira, R. O., Nardi, N. B., & von Mühlen, C. A. (1995). Evaluation of immune parameters in depressed patients. *Life Sciences*, **57**(7), 665–674. doi:10.1016/0024-3205(95)00318-z

Brambilla, F., Maggioni, M., Cenacchi, T., Sacerdote, P., & Panerai, A. R. (1995). T-lymphocyte proliferative response to mitogen stimulation in elderly depressed patients. *Journal of Affective Disorders*, **36**(1–2), 51–56. doi:0165-0327(95)00059-3

Carroll, M. C., Campbell, R. D., Bentley, D. R., & Porter, R. R. (1984). A molecular map of the human major histocompatibility complex class III region linking complement genes C4, C2 and factor B. *Nature*, **307**(5948), 237–241. doi:10.1038/307237a0

Castle, S., Wilkins, S., Heck, E., Tanzy, K., & Fahey, J. (2008). Depression in caregivers of demented patients is associated with altered immunity: Impaired proliferative capacity, increased CD8+, and a decline in lymphocytes with surface signal transduction molecules (CD38+) and a cytotoxicity marker (CD56+ CD8+). *Clinical & Experimental Immunology*, **101**(3), 487–493. doi:10.1111/j.1365-2249.1995.tb03139.x

Church, S. M., Cotter, D., Bramon, E., & Murray, R. M. (2002). Does schizophrenia result from developmental or degenerative processes? *Journal of Neural Transmission Supplementum*, **63**, 129–147.

Cosyns, P., Maes, M., Vandewoude, M., Stevens, W. J., De Clerck, L. S., & Schotte, C. (1989). Impaired mitogen-induced lymphocyte responses and the hypothalamic–pituitary–adrenal axis in depressive disorders. *Journal of Affective Disorders*, **16**(1), 41–48. doi:10.1016/0165-0327(89)90054-2

Curzytek, K., et al. (2015). Inhibitory effect of antidepressant drugs on contact hypersensitivity reaction is connected with their suppressive effect on NKT and CD8(+) T cells but not on TCR delta T cells. *International Immunopharmacology*, **28**(2), 1091–1096. doi:10.1016/j.intimp.2015.08.001

Darko, D. F., et al. (1989). Mitogen-stimulated lymphocyte proliferation and pituitary hormones in major depression. *Biological Psychiatry*, **26**(2), 145–155. doi:0006-3223(89)90018-8

DeLisi, L. E. (1984). Is immune dysfunction associated with schizophrenia? A review of the data. *Psychopharmacology Bulletin*, **20**, 509–513.

Diefendorf, A. R. & Kraepelin, E. (1923). *Clinical Psychiatry: A Textbook for Students and Physicians, Abstracted and Adapted from the 7th German Edition of Kraepelin's Lehrbuch der Psychiatrie* (new revised and augmented edn). New York: MacMillan. doi:10.1037/13656-000

Dinan, T. (2001). Novel approaches to the treatment of depression by modulating the hypothalamic–pituitary–adrenal axis. *Human Psychopharmacology*, **16(1)**, 89–93. doi:10.1002/hup.188

Fell, E. W. (1919). Postinfluenzal psychoses. *Journal of the American Medical Association*, **72(23)**, 1658. doi:10.1001/jama.1919.02610230012002

Gevorgyan, M. M., Idova, G. V., Al'perina, E. L., Tikhonova, M. A., & Kulikov A. V. (2016). Effect of antidepressants on immunological reactivity in ASC mice with genetically determined depression-like state. *Bulletin of Experimental Biology and Medicine*, **161**(2), 266–269. doi: 10.1007/s10517-016-3392-4

Gobin, V., et al. (2015). Fluoxetine suppresses calcium signaling in human T lymphocytes through depletion of intracellular calcium stores. *Cell Calcium*, **58**(3), 254–263. doi: 10.1016/j.ceca.2015.06.003

Harris, I. G. & Corcoran, D. (1919). Psychoses following influenza. *State Hospital Quarterly*, IV(4).

Hickie, I., Hickie, C., Lloyd, A., Silove, D., & Wakefield, D. (1993). Impaired in vivo immune responses in patients with melancholia. *British Journal of Psychiatry*, **162**(5), 651–657. doi:10.1192/bjp.162.5.651

Kanba, S., Manki, H., Shintani, F., Ohno, Y., Yagi, G., & Asai, M. (1998). Aberrant interleukin-2 receptor-mediated blastoformation of peripheral blood lymphocytes in a severe major depressive episode. *Psychological Medicine*, **28**(2), 481–484. doi:10.1017/s0033291797006454

Kayhan, F., Gunduz, S., Ersoy, S. A., Kandeger, A., & Annagur, B. B. (2017). Relationships of neutrophil-lymphocyte and platelet-lymphocyte ratios with the severity of major depression. *Psychiatry Research*, **247**, 332–335. doi:S0165-1781(16)30813-7

Keller, S., Weiss, J., Schleifer, S., Miller, N., & Stein, M. (1983). Stress-induced suppression of immunity in adrenalectomized rats. *Science*, **221**(4617), 1301–1304. doi:10.1126/science.6612346

Kirby, G. H. (1919). Psychoses associated with influenza. *State Hospital Quarterly*, **IV**(4).

Kito, S., Hasegawa, T., Fujita, K., & Koga, Y. (2010). Changes in hypothalamic–pituitary–thyroid axis following successful treatment with low-frequency right prefrontal transcranial magnetic stimulation in treatment-resistant depression. *Psychiatry Research*, **175**(1–2), 74–77. doi:10.1016/j.psychres.2008.10.002

Kraepelin, E. (1919). *Dementia Praecox and Paraphrenia*. Chicago, IL: Medical Book Company.

Kubera, M., Basta-Kaim, A., Wrobel, A., Maes, M., & Dudek, D. (2004). Increased mitogen-induced lymphocyte proliferation in treatment resistant depression: A preliminary study. *Neuro Endocrinology Letters*, **25**(3), 207–210.

Kubera, M., et al. (2012). Inhibitory effect of antidepressant drugs on contact hypersensitivity reaction. *Pharmacological Reports: PR*, **64**(3), 714–722.

Kubicki, M., et al. (2007). A review of diffusion tensor imaging studies in schizophrenia. *Journal of Psychiatric Research*, **41**(1–2), 15–30. doi:10.1016/j.jpsychires.2005.05.005

Maes, M., Bosmans, E., Suy, E., Minner, B., & Raus, J. (1989). Immune cell parameters in severely depressed patients: Negative findings. *Journal of Affective Disorders*, **17**(2), 121–128. doi:10.1016/0165-0327(89)90034-7

Mamelund, S., Sattenspiel, L., & Dimka, J. (2013). Influenza-associated mortality during the 1918–1919 influenza pandemic in Alaska and Labrador: A comparison. *Social Science History*, **37**(2), 177–229. doi:10.1215/01455532-2074420

McAdams, C. & Leonard, B. E. (1993). Neutrophil and monocyte phagocytosis in depressed patients. *Progress in Neuro-Psychopharmacology and Biological Psychiatry*, **17**(6), 971–984. doi:10.1016/0278-5846(93)90024-m

Menninger, K. A. (1919a). Influenza and neurosyphilis. *Archives of Internal Medicine*, **24**(1), 98. doi:10.1001/archinte.1919.00090240101008

Menninger, K. A. (1919b). Psychoses associated with influenza. *Journal of the American Medical Association*, **72**(4), 235. doi:10.1001/jama.1919.02610040001001

Menninger, K. A. (1921). Influenza and epilepsy. *The American Journal of the Medical Sciences*, **161**(6), 884–907. doi:10.1097/00000441-192106000-00010

Menninger, K. A. (1922). Reversible schizophrenia. *American Journal of Psychiatry*, **78**(4), 573–588. doi:10.1176/ajp.78.4.573

Menninger, K. A. (1926). Influenza and schizophrenia. *American Journal of Psychiatry*, **82**(4), 469–529. doi:10.1176/ajp.82.4.469

O'Donnell, L. J. & Westin, C. F. (2011). An introduction to diffusion tensor image analysis. *Neurosurgery Clinics of North America*, **22**(2), 185–196, viii. doi:10.1016/j.nec.2010.12.004

Palmblad, J., Petrini, B., Wasserman, J., & Åkerstedt, T. (1979). Lymphocyte and granulocyte reactions during sleep deprivation. *Psychosomatic Medicine*, **41**(4), 273–278. doi:10.1097/00006842-197906000-00001

Pasternak, O., et al. (2012). Excessive extracellular volume reveals a neurodegenerative pattern in schizophrenia onset. *Journal of Neuroscience*, **32**(48), 17365–17372. doi:10.1523/JNEUROSCI.2904-12.2012

Potvin, S., Stip, E., Sepehry, A. A., Gendron, A., Bah, R., & Kouassi, E. (2008). Inflammatory cytokine alterations in schizophrenia: A systematic quantitative review. *Biological Psychiatry*, **63**(8), 801–808. doi:10.1016/j.biopsych.2007.09.024

Raffield, L. M., et al. (2016). Analysis of the relationships between type 2 diabetes status, glycemic control, and neuroimaging measures in the Diabetes Heart Study Mind. *Acta Diabeatologica*, **53**(3), 439–447. doi: 10.1007/s00592-015-0815-z

Roberts, G. W., Colter, N., Lofthouse, R., Johnstone, E. C., & Crow, T. J. (1987). Is there gliosis in schizophrenia? Investigation of the temporal lobe. *Biological Psychiatry*, **22**(12), 1459–1468. doi:0006-3223(87)90104-1

Rothermundt, M., Arolt, V., Fenker, J., Gutbrodt, H., Peters, M., & Kirchner, H. (2001). Different immune patterns in melancholic and non-melancholic major depression. *European Archives of Psychiatry and Clinical Neuroscience*, **251**(2), 90–97.

Sandy, W. C. (1920). The association of neuropsychiatric conditions with influenza in the epidemic of 1918. *Archives of Neurology and Psychiatry*, **4**(2), 171. doi:10.1001/archneurpsyc.1920.02180200036004

Schizophrenia Working Group of the Psychiatric Genomics Consortium. (2014). Biological insights from 108 schizophrenia-associated genetic loci. *Nature*, 511(**7510**), 421–427.

Schnieder, T. P. & Dwork, A. J. (2011). Searching for neuropathology: Gliosis in schizophrenia. *Biological Psychiatry*, **69**(2), 134–139. doi:10.1016/j.biopsych.2010.08.027

Schule, C., Baghai, T. C., Eser, D., & Rupprecht, R. (2009). Hypothalamic–pituitary–adrenocortical system dysregulation and new treatment strategies in depression. *Expert Review of Neurotherapeutics*, **9**(7), 1005–1019. doi:10.1586/ern.09.52

Schwartz, M., Butovsky, O., Brück, W., & Hanisch, U. (2006). Microglial phenotype: Is the commitment reversible? *Trends in Neurosciences*, **29**(2), 68–74. doi:10.1016/j.tins.2005.12.005

Shavit, Y., Lewis, J. W., Terman, G. W., Gale, R. P., & Liebeskind, J. C. (1983). Endogenous opioids may mediate the effects of stress on tumor growth and immune function. *Proceedings of the Western Pharmacology Society*, **26**, 53–56.

Shi, J., et al. (2009). Common variants on chromosome 6p22.1 are associated with schizophrenia. *Nature*, 460, 753–757. doi:10.1038/nature08192

Song, S., Sun, S., Ju, W., Lin, S., Cross, A. H., & Neufeld, A. H. (2003). Diffusion tensor imaging detects and differentiates axon and myelin degeneration in mouse optic nerve after retinal ischemia. *NeuroImage*, **20**(3), 1714–1722. doi:10.1016/j.neuroimage.2003.07.005

Spurrell, M. T. & Creed, F. H. (1993). Lymphocyte response in depressed patients and subjects anticipating bereavement. *British Journal of Psychiatry*, **162**(1), 60–64. doi:10.1192/bjp.162.1.60

Sykova, E. & Nicholson, C. (2008). Diffusion in brain extracellular space. *Physiological Reviews*, **88**(4), 1277–1340. doi:10.1152/physrev.00027.2007

Uranova, N. A., Vostrikov, V. M., Vikhreva, O. V., Zimina, I. S., Kolomeets, N. S., & Orlovskaya, D. D. (2007). The role of oligodendrocyte pathology in schizophrenia. *The International Journal of Neuropsychopharmacology*, **10**(04), 537. doi:10.1017/s1461145707007626

Walther, F. (1923). *Ueber Grippepsychosen*. Berne: Bircher.

Whitlock, F. A. & Siskind, M. (1979). Depression and cancer: A follow-up study. *Psychological Medicine*, **9**(4), 747. doi:10.1017/s0033291700034061

Wodarz, N., et al. (1991). Normal lymphocyte responsiveness to lectins but impaired sensitivity to in vitro glucocorticoids in major depression. *Journal of Affective Disorders*, **22**(4), 241–248. doi:10.1016/0165-0327(91)90070-9

Zaharia, M. D., Ravindran, A. V., Griffiths, J., Merali, Z., & Anisman, H. (2000). Lymphocyte proliferation among major depressive and dysthymic patients with typical or atypical features. *Journal of Affective Disorders*, **58**(1), 1–10. doi:S0165-0327(99)00100-7

Chapter 6

Psychological and social factors

Shaun M. Eack

Introduction

Psychological and social factors have a significant role in our understanding of the aetiology, prognosis, and treatment of many psychiatric conditions. Although the biological basis of mental disorders is arguably only beginning to come into focus, the important role of the social environment and psychological characteristics of the individual affected by mental illness has been documented for more than a century. Early work by Sigmund Freud (1894/1962) identified key psychological defense mechanisms involved in neurotic conditions, such as anxiety and depression, and descriptions of soldiers returning from World War I identified 'shell shock' and the devastating psychological impact of the trauma-laden environment that is the battlefield (Rhein, 1919). Such research increasingly recognized the social environment as a critical factor in the aetiology of mental illness, tempering predominant thought at the time situated around personal responsibility and individual dysfunction. Further, this work underscored the importance of the psychology of the individual in shaping responses to environmental traumas and uncovering the cognitive underpinnings of many psychiatric conditions.

As early descriptions of social and psychological phenomena and their role in mental disorders continued to emerge, scientists from around the world began to conduct focused and landmark investigations into the role of the social environment in the development of mental illness and studies of the cognitive and psychological characteristics that support and maintain psychiatric conditions. The discoveries generated by such research were indeed profound and have shifted our thinking as a field from poorly supported models of personal deficit and biological reductionism to complex and interactive biopsychosocial theories integrating the multifactorial influences of biology, the environment, and the individual on the development of mental illness and its outcome and treatment.

This chapter presents a critical review of six landmark papers on the role of psychological and social factors in the development and maintenance of mental illnesses ranging from schizophrenia to borderline personality disorder to major depression. These landmark papers introduced some of the most groundbreaking and transformational thinking in psychiatry to date regarding the social and psychological foundations of mental disorder, and while each paper is characterized by limitations, the resulting work has had a major lasting impact on how the field views people living with mental illness and the role of the social environment in contributing to mental health.

The landmark paper by George Brown and colleagues (1962) was one of the first empirical investigations of the role of the family environment in post-hospital discharge relapse among patients with schizophrenia. This study showed that living environments, not necessarily familial, characterized by high levels of criticism were strongly predictive of psychotic relapse, and demonstrated the predictive power and importance of low-stress environments in post-hospital adjustment of patients with schizophrenia. The landmark papers by Aaron Beck (1963/1964) revolutionized thinking surrounding major depression, identified core cognitive distortions associated with the condition, and became the foundation for the development of the most effective psychological therapy for the treatment of depression to date—cognitive behavioural therapy. The landmark papers by Judith Herman and colleagues (1989) and Shanta Dube and colleagues (2001) represented some of the most rigorous empirical investigations of the role of childhood trauma in the development of mental illness, and established the significant impact of the social environment on developmental borderline personality disorder and suicidality. Finally, the landmark paper by Michael Rutter (1987) reminds us that the social environment and our cognitive characteristics are not only risk-producing, but can also contribute to resilience and lead to protection against mental illness in the face of significant adversity.

Expressed emotion and schizophrenia

Main citation

Brown, G. W., Monck, E. M., Carstairs, G. M., & Wing, J. K. (1962). Influence of family life on the course of schizophrenic illness. *British Journal of Preventive & Social Medicine*, 16, 55–68.

Background

The role of the social environment in the course and outcome of patients with schizophrenia and other severe mental illnesses has been a topic of much current and historical debate. Systematic investigations of the impact of the social environment on outcome largely began with studies of the family environment, some of which were rooted in negative misconceptions about illness development that have now been discredited. For example, theories of the schizophrenogenic mother were predominant in early conceptualizations of the aetiology of schizophrenia, which served to blame families for the condition. Rooted in psychodynamic conceptualizations of the illness, it was theorized that mothers who were overprotective and rejecting would raise children at risk for developing schizophrenia. This theory has been thoroughly unsupported by the evidence, and ultimately led to iatrogenic attempts to separate patients from one of their largest sources of support, their family.

The interest in families, however, led to the important realization of the significance of the social environment in the course and outcome of patients with schizophrenia who, at the time of this research, most often lived with immediate family after discharge from an institution. The concept of 'expressed emotion' was introduced into the literature by Brown and colleagues (1962) as they attempted to characterize the emotions expressed in family households, both by patients and family members, and their contribution to outcome. The authors recognized that previous conceptualizations of the schizophrenogenic mother were inaccurate, and that tension in the family often resulted from coping with a chronic condition and the troubling behaviour that can accompany schizophrenia. The term 'expressed emotion' therefore specifically described critical, hostile, and emotionally over-involved communication and behaviour on the part of the patient and family, and ultimately evolved to characterize household environments, which were not necessarily familial, that exhibited these patterns of emotion. These social factors that characterize environments high in expressed emotion were hypothesized not as aetiological, but as being predictive of whether patients would experience a psychiatric relapse after returning to the community from the hospital. Brown and colleagues (1962) conducted the landmark investigation examining the role of expressed emotion in predicting psychiatric relapse in patients with schizophrenia living with their families.

Methodology

A total of 128 male individuals diagnosed with schizophrenia who were recently discharged from psychiatric hospitals in London, England, were followed over the course of one year to examine relationships between family members' expressed emotion and patients' psychiatric outcome. The study made use of a naturalistic longitudinal panel design, and key relatives living with the patient were interviewed two weeks post-hospital discharge to elicit the degree of expressed emotion in the family (including hostility and criticism expressed toward the patient). Expressed emotion was assessed two weeks after the patient returned to the family home using a semi-structured interview that asked family members and patients about the return home and relationships with others in the household. From these interviews, ratings were made on overall expressed emotion and hostility by the patient and key family members, as well as the dominant behaviour exhibited by the family. After one year or following re-hospitalization, patient outcome data were collected on psychiatric and functional impairment using basic rating scales of psychiatric and behavioural symptoms.

Results

Primary results regarding the association between expressed emotion and outcome were focused largely on whether the patient had deteriorated since hospital discharge (see Table 6.1).

Findings indicated that as caregiver expressed emotion increased, particularly hostility, the likelihood of patient relapse significantly increased. Nearly 90% of patients living in

Table 6.1 Association between expressed emotion and deterioration in patients with schizophrenia

	Percent deteriorated by domain		
Caregiver expressed-emotion level			
High	89%	80%	77%
Minimal	42%	74%	48%
Low	22%	43%	40%
	p <0.01	*p* <0.01	*ns*
Patient expressed- emotion level			
High	75%	79%	–
Minimal	48%	64%	–
Low	59%	45%	–
	ns	*p* <0.05	–

ns = non-significant finding
Adapted from Brown, Monck, Carstairs, & Wing (1962)
Adapted from Leff J., Kuipers L., Berkowitz R., Eberlein-Vries R., Sturgeon D. (1986) Controlled Trial of Social Intervention in the Families of Schizophrenic Patients. In: Goldstein M.J., Hand I., Hahlweg K. (eds) *Treatment of Schizophrenia*. Springer, Berlin, Heidelberg. Copyright © 1986, Springer-Verlag Berlin Heidelberg. DOI: https://doi.org/10.1007/978-3-642-95496-2_14.

high expressed-emotion households experienced significant psychiatric deterioration compared to 22% of patients living in low expressed-emotion households. Although often overlooked, patient expressed emotion, again particularly hostility, also predicted increased likelihood of deteriorated outcome. Emotional over-involvement did not predict outcome, showing that hostility and criticism are the strongest of the expressed-emotion contributors to deterioration.

Conclusions and critique

Expressed emotion is a social construct that describes the level of hostility, criticism, and emotional over-involvement in the social environment in which a patient with schizophrenia is living. From the landmark study by Brown and colleagues (1962) and the many investigations that followed, it can be concluded that hostility and criticism in the environment in which a patient lives are some of the strongest predictors of whether an individual with schizophrenia will have a successful adjustment to the community after discharge from psychiatric hospitalization. The influence of emotional over-involvement in the course and outcome in schizophrenia has largely not been supported, suggesting that this aspect of expressed emotion is less salient in contributing to patient outcomes.

The study by Brown and colleagues (1962) has a number of important limitations. First, it consisted only of men, which certainly limited its generalizability. Second, it was conducted only in London, England, although many other studies in the United States and other countries have replicated the association between expressed emotion and patient relapse. Third, measurement was admittedly limited, as previously validated standardized assessments were largely not utilized for either expressed emotion or patient outcomes, in some cases because such measures had not been developed. Much of the measurement was rudimentary by current standards, although a standardized interview was conducted and a systematic approach to following patients during the study was employed. Finally, because the study made use of a naturalistic longitudinal design, causal relationships between expressed emotion and outcome could not be determined. Strengths of the study included the prospective follow-up of a sizeable patient sample.

The findings from Brown and colleagues (1962) laid the framework for increasingly recognizing the importance of the family and social environment in the course and outcome of schizophrenia and other psychiatric conditions. In the decades that have ensued since this landmark study, the importance of expressed emotion to patient recovery has been replicated and extended to many other psychiatric conditions, including personality disorder and major mood disorders (Butzlaff & Hooley, 1998). The powerful impact of family expressed emotion on patient outcome served as the impetus for the development of family psychoeducation programmes. These programmes effectively reduced relapse rates by partnering with families and providing them with education and support about mental illness (Hogarty et al., 1986).

It is important to recognize that the concept of expressed emotion is not limited to a certain form of kinship; indeed, the concept has been extended to professional caregivers (Moore et al., 1992), and does not imply that family members are responsible for the development of schizophrenia. Rather, expressed emotion shows just how powerful families can be in supporting the recovery of patients with this condition and how significant the emotional tone of the social environment is in predicting outcome in the disorder.

Cognitive theory and depression

Main citations

Beck, A. T. (1963). Thinking and depression: I. Idiosyncratic content and cognitive distortions. *Archives of General Psychiatry*, 9, 324–333.

Beck, A. T. (1964). Thinking and depression: II. Theory and therapy. *Archives of General Psychiatry*, 10, 561–571.

Background

Major depressive disorder is one of the most common mental disorders experienced throughout the world that results in significant loss of productivity, relationships, and quality of life for many people who experience the condition. Because depression is characterized as an affective disorder with prominent mood symptoms, including sadness, guilt, and feelings of hopelessness, the emphasis of psychotherapeutic treatment in the early and middle twentieth century focused directly, and often solely, on these affective symptoms. Psychotherapies frequently targeted amotivation, difficulties in experiencing pleasure, and low mood, which are all important affective targets of depression treatment. However, such interventions largely ignored the cognitive factors that contribute to the major mood symptoms in depression, and consequently many of the psychological factors and cognitive distortions that maintain the affective symptoms of depression were largely untreated.

To the extent that the thought content of patients with depression was considered in psychotherapy, it was usually interpreted through a psychodynamic lens, with a view to early developmental origins and/or their reflection of unconscious desires. Numerous researchers had begun to uncover the cognitive biases associated with various forms of psychopathology, including depression, but a systematic account of distortions in thinking with a view toward a cognitive approach to the psychotherapeutic treatment of depression had not yet been developed. In Beck's (1963, 1964) landmark papers on the thought content of depressed patients seen in psychotherapy, he provides the evidence and theoretical foundation for a cognitive theory of depression and, ultimately, developed cognitive therapy for patients with major affective disorders.

Methodology

The articles by Beck (1963, 1964) are both empirical and theoretical. The first article of 1963 presents empirical qualitative data on 50 patients with major depression and their thought content during psychotherapy, as compared to 31 patients without major depression who were also receiving psychotherapy. During moderate to severe depressive periods, the psychotherapist used clinical interviews, free association techniques, and retrospective accounts to inquire about the thinking patterns patients experienced, and their verbal responses were recorded via handwritten notes. Thematic analyses were then undertaken to identify consistent patterns of distorted thinking in patients with depression, which were subsequently compared to non-depressed patients. The second article by Beck (1964) then presents the theoretical framework of cognitive therapy for depression, based on the findings reported in the first article of patterns of cognitive distortions elicited from depressed patients during psychotherapy.

Results

The results of Beck's (1963) qualitative analysis of themes of verbalized thought content among depressed patients in psychotherapy resulted in the identification of a number of common cognitive distortions, or illogical patterns of thinking, that were hypothesized to contribute to depressive symptoms. Example cognitive distortions included *filtering* (focusing only on negative aspects of the self, situations, and/or others), *personalization* (believing the actions of others are directed toward you personally; comparing yourself to others), and catastrophizing (seeing the worst possible outcome of a situation, regardless of how minor or the likelihood). An important finding from the identification of these cognitive distortions is that many, if not all of them occur in an automatic fashion in depressed patients, such that they are prepotent and readily available in response to many diverse situations and interpersonal encounters. Further, such aberrant thinking was often observed to be linked to and occur immediately before the emergence or reoccurrence of major affective symptoms.

From Beck's (1963) analysis of cognitive distortions in depressed patients and psychiatric controls, he then went on to develop a theoretical framework describing the cognitive underpinnings of depression and proposing a new treatment approach, cognitive therapy, that would address these distortions in thinking. Beck (1964) proposed that patients with depression have developed a core set of beliefs, or *cognitive schema*, that permeates much of their life experiences. Further, these core beliefs are often faulty, lead to the distorted thinking as described in his 1963 article, and should be the focus of psychotherapeutic treatment for depression. Beck observed that the thoughts of depressed patients relied on negative cognitive schemas about the self and others, which were automatic and needed to be interrupted if the cycle between negative cognitions and affects in depression were to be disrupted. This framework provided new targets for psychotherapeutic intervention in depression and shifted the focus of treatment from motivation, affect, and behaviour to cognition, beliefs, and attitudes about the self and others.

Conclusions and critique

The articles by Beck (1963, 1964) were the first empirical and theoretical foundations of a cognitive theory of depression, and would set the stage for a greater understanding of the relationship between cognition and emotion that would continue to be investigated for the next half century and beyond. The methods reported in his initial studies are limited to retrospective accounts of his own psychotherapy patients, and admittedly are less rigorous than those that would be employed today. Despite these limitations, Beck's analysis and interpretation of his findings remain some of the most insightful and groundbreaking contributions in the field of psychiatry. Because of his insights, we now view depression as a core cognitive disorder with affective consequences, and understand that restructuring distorted thinking is one of the most successful avenues for addressing the major mood components of the condition. These conceptual breakthroughs led to the development of cognitive therapy for depression, one of the most effective psychotherapeutic practices, and laid the framework for the cognitive conceptualization of many other psychiatric disorders (including anxiety, personality disorder, and even psychosis).

Beck's work demonstrated just how influential our thought processes are to our interpretation of the world and to the maintenance of core beliefs that drive our motivational and emotional states, and how these states feedback into our core understanding of the self and the world. In an era that was perhaps overly focused on behaviour, Beck challenged the field to interrogate the 'black box' of cognition, which led to the acknowledgement of its importance in depression and other mental illnesses, as well as the efficacy of changing core cognitive schemas as a means of promoting mental health.

Childhood trauma and risk for mental illness

Main citations

Herman, J. L., Perry, C., & Van der Kolk, B. A. (1989). Childhood trauma in borderline personality disorder. *American Journal of Psychiatry*, 146, 490–495.

Dube, S. R., Anda, R. F., Felitti, V. J., Chapman, D. P., Williamson, D. F., & Giles, W. H. (2001). Childhood abuse, household dysfunction, and the risk of attempted suicide throughout the life span: findings from the Adverse Childhood Experiences Study. *Journal of the American Medical Association*, 286, 3089–3096.

Background

The influence of traumatic events on psychological well-being has been an intense area of theoretical and empirical inquiry since the earliest of psychiatric formulations. Freud and many future psychoanalysts theorized that several different forms of psychopathology stemmed from adverse childhood experiences. Clinical and empirical work during the World Wars further buttressed the significance of trauma to mental health as soldiers returned from the battlefield with 'shell shock' that we now know as post-traumatic stress disorder. As scientific inquiry into the role of childhood experiences and their relationship to mental health grew in the second half of the twentieth century, the importance of early environmental experiences continued to be recognized and supported throughout the psychiatric literature. From the development of personality pathology to depression to psychosis, many psychiatric conditions have shown correlates with childhood adversity. The exact pathways of influence continue to remain unclear and likely interact with underlying genetic vulnerabilities, but what is clear is that early environmental experiences carry significant weight in the development of brain disorders and ultimately in the development of mental disorders.

The two landmark papers by Herman et al. (1989) and Dube et al. (2001) illustrate the importance of the early environment and the role of early childhood trauma in the development of broad-spectrum psychopathology. In Herman et al. (1989) the focus is on the development of borderline personality disorder, and in Dube et al. (2001) the association between childhood adversity and suicide is considered. It is important to recognize that these landmark papers only illustrate the degree to which the childhood environment can contribute to the development of mental illness, as numerous investigations have now been conducted showing the contribution of adverse childhood experiences to the development of various mental health conditions.

Methodology

For their landmark paper, Herman et al. (1989) conducted a 100-item semi-structured interview of childhood history with 21 patients with borderline personality disorder, 11 patients with borderline features, and 23 psychiatric controls with other non-borderline personality or mood pathology. The childhood history interviews were conducted by interviewers who were blind to the patient's diagnosis and who asked questions regarding primary caregivers in childhood, major separations, moves and losses, family discipline, physical and sexual abuse, and other aspects of family and social life as a child. The proportion of traumatic experiences by each diagnostic group was the primary analysis of interest for the study. The landmark paper by Dube et al. (2001) surveyed 17,337 adult members of the Kaiser Permanente Health Insurance Agency about their adverse childhood experiences, family and household dysfunction as a child, and whether the participant had ever attempted suicide. The proportion of participants who had attempted suicide, following different adverse childhood experiences, was the primary analytical focus of the study.

Results

Findings from both Herman et al. (1989) and Dube et al. (2001) showed that adults reporting adverse experiences in childhood, including physical and sexual abuse, were significantly more likely to have borderline personality disorder and to have attempted suicide. Prevalence of childhood trauma was particularly high (81%) in patients diagnosed with borderline personality disorder compared to other psychiatric conditions. Results showed the association between adverse childhood experiences and two different forms of psychopathology—borderline personality and suicidality. Dube et al. (2001) also showed that as the number of adverse childhood experiences accumulates, the likelihood of having made a suicide attempt also increases in a dose–response fashion.

Conclusions and critique

It is clear from the studies of Herman et al. (1989) and Dube et al. (2001) that abuse during childhood and other adverse childhood experiences are associated, retrospectively, with the development of diverse forms of psychopathology. The childhood years are an important time for social, emotional, and cognitive development, and it has been theorized that the introduction of traumatic experiences and abuse during this time may impact healthy development in these areas and thus contribute to the onset of a variety of mental health conditions.

The study by Herman et al. (1989) is limited primarily by sample size. Both studies are also considerably limited by their retrospective and self-report nature. These studies asked adult participants to recall adverse experiences from their childhood, which participants may have been less willing to share or may have under- or overestimated, given the difficulties in accurate recall of events from decades before. In addition, although both studies demonstrate a clear association between childhood trauma and mental illness, the causal mechanisms involved in this relationship are not examined, making it particularly important not to draw causal implications from their findings. Many aspects of adversity co-vary, including with childhood trauma, and it may be unobserved correlates with trauma that contribute most to psychopathological development. Further, it may be that trauma impacts early developmental processes in such a way that genetically vulnerable individuals become more prone to mental illness. Many of these questions remain outstanding today and an important next step for this field is to more clearly delineate the mechanisms by which early adversity increases risk for mental disorder, hence increasing understanding of causality beyond known associations.

Resilience and protective factors from mental illness

Main citation

Rutter, M. (1987). Psychosocial resilience and protective mechanisms. *American Journal of Orthopsychiatry*, 57, 316–331.

Background

In the late twentieth century, psychiatric research was again maturing and had accumulated a significant body of evidence demonstrating the importance of adverse environmental experiences on mental health outcomes. Childhood trauma, exposure to violence, separation from family members, and other adverse experiences were increasingly recognized as 'risk factors' for the development of a variety of psychiatric conditions. At the same time, there was a growing sense that the field was overemphasizing these risk factors, which individually carried modest predictive power at best, and for which there was considerable inter-individual variability regarding their association with mental illness. Some individuals raised in the most challenging of circumstances would emerge from childhood with minimal psychiatric impairment and succeed in adult life. Others with a seemingly nurturing upbringing would suddenly develop schizophrenia and experience considerable disability in adulthood. Such observations increasingly suggested that research focused solely on risk was ignoring an important piece of the equation, and that if we could understand those factors that protected individuals experiencing risk from the development of mental illness, new insights could be gained in terms of prevention and treatment. Rutter's (1987) landmark paper on psychosocial resilience presents a framework for studying and understanding the factors and mechanisms involved in protecting against mental disorder.

Methodology

Rutter (1987) uses a selective literature review method to outline different protective factors and mechanisms involved in the development of mental illness or in buffering against risk for the development of psychopathology. He takes particular care in distinguishing factors from processes, and emphasizes that much of what is to be learned regarding protection lies in understanding the processes or cascade of mechanisms involved in protecting against mental illness. Factors are those protective variables that interact with adversity to confer protection against risk. These are properly conceptualized as moderators of risk and change the association between the risk variable and outcome depending on the level of the moderator. Processes, on the other hand, are mechanisms by which a protective factor exerts its effects. For example, high family cohesion is protective against childhood psychiatric disorders. In such a case, family cohesion is a protective factor. Understanding why family cohesion is a protective factor necessitates uncovering the mechanisms by which it achieves its protective influence, such as facilitating healthy attachment and psychological coping mechanisms. These latter two variables are considered protective processes or mechanisms, and they are the cornerstone of Rutter's framework for understanding risk and resilience in mental illness.

Results

Table 6.2 outlines key points from Rutter's resilience framework. The review and framework outlined by Rutter makes a compelling case for the need to study both protective and risk factors for the development of mental illness. Protective factors may come in the form of interactive or moderating factors, or protective processes that impact the cascade of negative consequences of risk. Numerous protective factors from mental illness have been identified, including temperament, parent–child relationships, and other family factors. Protective mechanisms are less well explored but thought to be perhaps the most important, and include mechanisms to buffer against risk, to reduce negative chain reactions from risk, to enhance self-esteem, and to provide opportunities to offset the negative consequences of risk factors.

Conclusions and critique

Rutter (1989) provided an important and landmark framework for understanding psychosocial protective factors and resilience in psychiatric research. He theorized that by understanding why some individuals face such extreme risk, yet still remain healthy and thrive, we can better understand the protective factors involved in mental health and

Table 6.2 Protective factors and mechanisms from Rutter's (1987) model of psychosocial resilience

Factor/mechanism	Description
Protective factors	
Gender	Female gender may be protective against exposure to some risks for mental disorders, such as aggression
Temperament	High regularity and flexibility in temperament can protect against family discord and other adversities
Parent–child relationships	Healthy parent–child relationships can protect against familial risk factors for mental illness
Marital support	High marital support can result in better parenting behaviour, which reduces mental illness risk
Protective Mechanisms	
Risk buffering	Changes the nature of the risk or reduces exposure to it
Reducing negative chain reactions	Alters the cascading sequence of risk factors or contributors to mental illness
Self-esteem/self-efficacy	High confidence and self-worth helps individuals to cope with risks and adversities related to mental health
Opportunity	The right opportunities can offset risk factors by providing new avenues for growth and accomplishment

Adapted with permission from Rutter, M. Psychosocial resilience and protective mechanisms. *American Journal of Orthopsychiatry, 57*(3):316–331. Copyright © 1987, Global Alliance for Behavioral Health and Social Justice. DOI: https://doi.org/10.1111/j.1939-0025.1987.tb03541.x.

social adjustment. His framework identified both protective factors and mechanisms as well as emphasized the importance of understanding the process by which a protective mechanism exerts its effects. Limitations of Rutter's formulation include an overemphasis on family versus other individual, community, and society-level protective factors. These other protective factors have since been delineated in the literature but, at the time, Rutter had a limited set of data to draw upon, given the novelty of research on protective factors when his paper was published.

Since Rutter's (1989) landmark paper, the landscape of psychiatric research has changed to include serious investigations of both risk and protective factors in the development and outcome of mental illness. More broadly, his work on protective factors called increasing attention to non-individual contributors to mental health, including family, social opportunities, and community cohesion. Although many mental health conditions have a clear biological basis, Rutter's work suggests an important interaction between biological risk and environmental support, which has served, in part, as the basis for many prevention efforts to date. There remains, however, a need for increased use of this framework in treatment development, which continues to emphasize risk more than protection.

Conclusion

Psychological and social factors have an important role in the aetiology, course, and treatment of many psychiatric disorders. The landmark papers reviewed here established some of the first foundational evidence regarding the role of the social environment and psychological characteristics in the development of mental illness. From these papers and the sizeable amount of research that they inspired, we now know that critical and hostile environments, characterized by high expressed emotion, are some of the strongest predictors of re-hospitalization in patients with schizophrenia, regardless of whether such environments involve family members, professionals, or other individuals. We also know that depression (and many other mental illnesses) are characterized by dysfunctional and automatic patterns of thinking, which are possible to correct with great therapeutic benefits. Further, the role of environmental trauma, particularly in early childhood, in the development of mental illness has also been established and highlighted promising avenues for prevention. Finally, and perhaps most importantly, Rutter's (1987) work reminds us that the social environment can not only be risky, but also protective, and that there exist social and psychological factors that can act as equally powerful agents to promote resilience and mental health.

The foundational insights provided by these landmark papers ushered in a new era of social and psychological interventions that dramatically reduced human suffering and improved the lives of individuals with mental illness. These papers became the basis of family psychoeducation interventions for psychosis (Hogarty et al., 1986), cognitive therapy treatments for depression and many other psychiatric conditions (Beck, 2005), trauma-focused prevention programmes for at-risk youth (Cohen et al., 2012), and social and psychological interventions to enhance resiliency and mental health (Meyer et al., 2015). Although the fruits of this early research have clearly been established and contributed to major reductions in the public burden of mental illness, future investigations are challenged with how to continue to build on and extend these early insights into more effective and integrated avenues for treating mental disorders.

Currently, we know a great deal about the psychological and social factors that contribute to the aetiology of mental illness, but comparatively little about how these factors shape treatment responsiveness. Further, most social, psychological, and environmental interventions are not well integrated into the biological mainstays of psychiatric treatment, and remarkably little is known about the interaction between biopsychosocial factors in the treatment of mental illness. As the next century of advances in psychiatry ensues, an important challenge to be met is how to integrate our increasingly complex understanding of social, psychological, and biological factors in the aetiology and treatment of mental disorders. By integrating our evidence, a decidedly more complete picture of the individual will be established, leading to continued advances in identification, prevention, and treatment.

References

Beck, A. T. (2005). The current state of cognitive therapy: A 40-year retrospective. *Archives of General Psychiatry*, **62**(9), 953–959.

Beck, A. T. (1964). Thinking and depression: II. Theory and therapy. *Archives of General Psychiatry*, **10**(6), pp. 561–571.

Beck, A. T. (1963). Thinking and depression: I. Idiosyncratic content and cognitive distortions. *Archives of General Psychiatry*, **9**(4), 324–333.

Brown, G. W., Monck, E. M., Carstairs, G. M., & Wing, J. K. (1962). Influence of family life on the course of schizophrenic illness. *British Journal of Preventative and Social Medicine*, **16**(2), 55–68.

Butzlaff, R. L. & Hooley, J. M. (1998). Expressed emotion and psychiatric relapse: A meta-analysis. *Archives of General Psychiatry*, **55**(6), 547–552.

Cohen, J. A., Mannarino, A. P., Kliethermes, M., & Murray, L. A. (2012). Trauma-focused CBT for youth with complex trauma. *Child Abuse & Neglect*, **36**(6), 528–541.

Dube, S. R., Anda, R. F., Felitti, V. J., Chapman, D. P., Williamson, D. F., & Giles, W. H. (2001). Childhood abuse, household dysfunction, and the risk of attempted suicide throughout the life span: Findings from the Adverse Childhood Experiences Study. *Journal of the American Medical Association*, **286**(24), 3089–3096.

Freud, S. (1894/1962). The neuro-psychoses of defense. In: *The Standard Edition of the Complete Works of Sigmund Freud*, Vol. **3**, ed. and trans. J. Strachey. London: Hogarth Press; pp. 45–61.

Herman, J. L., Perry, C., & Van der Kolk, B. A. (1989). Childhood trauma in borderline personality disorder. *American Journal of Psychiatry*, **146**(4), 490–495.

Hogarty, G. E., et al. (1986). Family psychoeducation, social skills training, and maintenance chemotherapy in the aftercare treatment of schizophrenia: I. One-year effects of a controlled study on relapse and expressed emotion. *Archives of General Psychiatry*, **43**(7), 633–642.

Meyer, P. S., Gottlieb, J. D., Penn, D., Mueser, K., & Gingerich, S. (2015). Individual resiliency training: An early intervention approach to enhance well-being in people with first-episode psychosis. *Psychiatric Annals*, **45**(11), 554–560.

Moore, E., Ball, R. A., & Kuipers, L. (1992). Expressed emotion in staff working with the long-term adult mentally ill. *British Journal of Psychiatry*, **161**(6), 802–808.

Rhein, J. H. W. (1919). Neuropsychiatric problems at the front during combat. *Journal of Abnormal Psychology*, **14**(1–2), 9–14.

Rutter, M. (1987). Psychosocial resilience and protective mechanisms. *American Journal of Orthopsychiatry*, 57(3), 316–331.

Section III

Pharmacotherapy

Chapter 7

Schizophrenia

David V. Braitman and Juan R. Bustillo

Introduction

The term *schizophrenia* originated with Eugen Bleuler in 1911, to identify subjects suffering from insanity (now referred to as psychosis) of unknown cause. These individuals were thought to experience a disintegration of the basic psychic functions of thought, affect, and behaviour, manifested in a multiplicity of symptoms. A few years before, Emil Kraepelin had coined the term *dementia praecox* to identify a similar group of psychotic subjects, but emphasized an early onset and a deteriorating course. At the time of publication of this volume, the current definitions (DSM-5, ICD-10) of schizophrenia emphasize the presence of operationally defined psychotic symptoms (delusions, hallucinations, disorganized thinking, and disorganized behaviour) that are primary and persistent. These descriptors are not necessarily of early onset or with a deteriorating course but have serious functional impact, with clear deficits in interpersonal, leisure, and employment or scholarly activities. Hence the conceptual impact of Bleuler and Kraepelin remains. A reading of their classical monographs is enlightening, but these are not in the form of accessible scientific articles. Today, the cause of schizophrenia remains unknown and there is no cure for it. Still, it is essential to seek to understand the illness in the hope that our treatments improve. Here we discuss five papers that have critically shaped our understanding and treatment of schizophrenia. Two of the articles relate to treatment and the three others involve the mechanisms of the disorder.

Jonathan Cole and colleagues affiliated with the National Institute of Mental Health Psychopharmacology Service Center Collaborative Study Group (1964) conducted the first large, multi-centre, randomized controlled trial (RCT) of phenothiazines, establishing their efficacy as the standard of care for schizophrenia. However, many patients who initially benefit become resistant to phenothiazines and other related medications. John Kane and members of the Clozaril Collaborative Study Group (1988) implemented the first controlled trial comparing clozapine to chlopromazine in chronically ill, treatment-resistant schizophrenia patients. This study established clozapine as the treatment of choice for schizophrenia patients who failed to respond to previous antipsychotic therapy. At the time of publication of this volume, it remains the only drug with such an indication.

The neurobiology underlying schizophrenia and response to clozapine or standard antipsychotics requires further studying. Richard Suddath and colleagues (1990) studied monozygotic twins discordant for schizophrenia with structural magnetic resonance imaging (MRI) of the brain. This study confirmed consistent neuropathological features in schizophrenia (e.g. reduced hippocampal volume) and documented that their cause is at least in part not genetic. Alan Breir and colleagues (1997) used positron emission tomography (PET) [^{11}C]raclopride striatal binding, before and after an amphetamine infusion. Striatal presynaptic dopamine release was greater in schizophrenia than controls. This study demonstrated that an increment in dopamine release is fundamental to the pathophysiology of the illness and provides a disease-related substrate for the mechanism of action of antipsychotic medications.

Though the heritability of schizophrenia had been established through multiple family studies, credible identification of specific genes did not take place until the twenty-first century. Stephan Ripke and members from the Schizophrenia Working Group of the Psychiatric Genomics Consortium (2014) implemented the largest genome-wide association study in schizophrenia, with enough power to examine potential small effects across millions of common alleles. One hundred and eight loci, including genes involved in glutamatergic, synaptic, calcium channels, and immune function, met genome-wide significance. This study demonstrated that schizophrenia, though strongly heritable, is a highly polygenic illness likely involving many hundreds of common variants.

An efficacious treatment for schizophrenia

Main citation

Cole, J. O. & the NIMH Psychopharmacology Service Center Collaborative Study Group. (1964). Phenothiazine treatment in acute schizophrenia: effectiveness. *Archives of General Psychiatry*, 10, 246–261.

Background

Prior to the publication of this paper, several phenothiazines were available for the treatment of schizophrenia, supported by a number of small, variously controlled trials. Indeed, the term 'major tranquillizers' (in contrast to 'minor tranquillizers', for example benzodiazepines) was still commonly used to refer to these agents. Clinicians recognized phenothiazines to be helpful, but doubts remained regarding the robustness and specificity of their anti-schizophrenia effects. This paper represented the first careful undertaking to ascertain whether phenothiazines were efficacious for the acute treatment of schizophrenia symptoms. (The title term 'effectiveness' is closer to the current use of the term 'efficacy': an efficacy trial strives to control as many critical variables as possible; an effectiveness trial aims to be generalizable to meaningful clinical contexts.)

Methods

This was a randomized, double-blind clinical trial in a large number (344) of patients with schizophrenia recently hospitalized for an exacerbation of symptoms. It included a variety of settings: four state hospitals, two municipal general hospitals, and three private psychiatric hospitals. The variety of settings were used to increase the generalizability of findings. Patients were randomized to chlorpromazine, thioridazine, fluphenazine, or a placebo for a period of six weeks, and were assessed on the severity of their illness using a number of clinical measures. Dosages were flexibly adjusted by treating physicians to optimize response and tolerability. The clinical assessments used to judge patients' improvement were systematic and included ratings from both blinded psychiatrists and nurses at regular intervals.

Results

Of the placebo-assigned patients, 29% were terminated early from the study due to treatment failure, versus 2% of the phenothiazine-assigned subjects. Of the patients who completed the six weeks of treatment, 75% of those in the phenothiazine group were much or very much improved, versus 40% of the placebo group—a significant difference. (This difference was weighted in favour of the placebo, given the high proportion of early terminations in this group.) Phenothiazines resulted in greater improvements in positive symptoms (exaggeration of normal psychological functions) as well as negative symptoms (reduction in psychological functions). Examples of specific effects on positive symptoms included hebephrenic symptoms (disorganization), incoherent speech, auditory hallucinations, and ideas of persecution. Examples of specific effects on negative symptoms included social participation, self-care, slowed speech, and indifference to the environment. However, there were no differences on any clinical outcome measures between any of the three drugs studied.

In terms of tolerability, there were some general differences. Of medication-treated subjects, 3% were terminated early from the study due to severe complications (including jaundice, hypotension, rash, dystonia, severe parkinsonism, and seizures) versus 0% in the placebo group. There were also differences in some drug-specific side-effects including drowsiness and dizziness, which were more frequent with chlorpromazine and thioridazine, while parkinsonism was more common with fluphenazine. Finally, improvement was not related to severity of parkinsonism or other neurological side-effects.

Conclusions and critique

This study clearly demonstrated the efficacy of phenothiazines for the core symptoms of schizophrenia (later referred to as positive and negative symptoms). This was essential to establish that any general tranquillizing effects were separate from the more specific antipsychotic effects of these agents. It also established that potency (in terms of milligrams of the efficacious dose: higher with fluphenazine, lower with chlorpromazine and thioridazine) did not relate to greater efficacy or specificity of beneficial effects. Finally, it suggested that the neuroleptic properties (extrapyramidal effects or 'seizing of the neuron') of these agents were not tightly linked to the antipsychotic effects. These findings were critical to the shift in terminology away from ataractic (tranquillizing) and neuroleptic medication effects. However, the term 'anti-schizophrenia' drug, recommended by Cole et al., never took hold, in part due to the main limitation of the study: the broad definition of acute schizophrenia, which almost certainly included an undetermined proportion of patients with mania and depression. These agents were later found to be efficacious for psychosis in the context of mania and depression, and also in a variety of other conditions like dementia and delirium. It would take other studies to support the shift to the current term, antipsychotic drug.

An efficacious therapy for treatment-resistant schizophrenia

Main citation

Kane, J., Honigfeld, G., Singer, J., Meltzer, H., & the Clozaril Collaborative Study Group. (1988). Clozapine for the treatment-resistant schizophrenic: a double-blind comparison with chlorpromazine. *Archives of General Psychiatry*, 45, 789–796.

Background

By the 1970s, psychiatrists had embraced the use of antipsychotic drugs in the treatment of schizophrenia. However, these failed in up to 20% of cases, and about 30% relapsed following the first year of treatment. Three multisite European studies in the 1980s had detected an advantage of clozapine over chlorpromazine and haloperidol, though there were concerns of underdosing of the reference drug, and these studies were not designed to examine the potential efficacy in previously non-responsive patients. Despite this, clozapine appeared to be the first drug with superior antipsychotic properties. However, a 2% cumulative incidence of agranulocytosis was identified, with eight fatalities from secondary infection in Finland. Hence, clozapine was withdrawn from clinical research in the USA.

Methods

In order to justify the risk of agranulocytosis, this RCT selected cases of treatment-resistant schizophrenia initially defined retrospectively (n = 319). By history, subjects had had at least three periods of treatment in the preceding five years with different antipsychotic agents from at least two different classes, at doses equivalent to or exceeding 1000 mg/day of chlorpromazine. Each period of treatment was for at least six weeks, without significant symptom improvement. Subjects had also had no period of good functioning in the preceding five years. Subsequently, they were treated with open-label haloperidol (up to 60 mg/day) for a six-week period to prospectively confirm a lack of response and persistent psychotic symptoms.

Subjects were then randomized to double-blinded treatment with clozapine (target dose 500 mg/day, maximum 900 mg/day) or chlorpromazine (target dose 1000 mg/day, maximum 1800 mg/day) for six weeks. Blinded benztropine (6 mg/day) was given to the chlorpromazine group. All subjects had weekly symptom ratings and weekly blood counts to monitor for leucopenia.

Results

Over 80% of patients who met retrospective definition of 'treatment resistance' failed to improve with haloperidol treatment. Of the 268 randomized patients, clozapine-treated patients achieved statistical improvement in positive symptoms by week one, and in negative symptoms by week two, compared with chlorpromazine-treated patients. These advantages were sustained through the six-week period. Furthermore, 30% of patients on clozapine achieved the *a priori*-defined clinically meaningful threshold of improvement (20% decrease in Brief Psychiatric Rating Scale (BPRS) total score *plus* a 'mildly ill' or lower clinical global impression (CGI) score, or a BPRS total score of 35 or lower) versus just 4% of patients treated with chlorpromazine.

In terms of safety, despite use of benztropine, the chlorpromazine-treated subjects had higher reports of extrapyramidal syndrome (EPS), hypotension, and dry mouth compared to the clozapine group. The clozapine-treated subjects had higher reports of hypersalivation, fever, and hypertension. There were no differences in leucopenia.

Conclusions and critique

This study clearly documented the efficacy of clozapine for an important minority of patients with schizophrenia who have failed multiple previous antipsychotic trials. It was the first and, to date, is the only agent that meets this indication for treatment-resistant schizophrenia and is approved by the American Food and Drug Administration for this indication. The very stringent treatment-resistance requirement selected was necessary due to the documented risk of agranulocytosis which limited the generalizability of their findings. Later it became clear that this risk could be managed with weekly blood monitoring. Clozapine was also studied in outpatients partially responsive to antipsychotics, where its superiority was again demonstrated. Interestingly, in first-episode schizophrenia, no advantage was seen with clozapine, perhaps because of the very high rate of antipsychotic response in this population.

Another major consequence of this study was the pharmaceutical industry's massive effort to develop other 'atypical' antipsychotics that would not have a risk of agranulocytosis. The early definition of 'atypical' was thought to include antipsychotic superiority, including the absence of EPS, as well as potential advantages for negative symptoms and cognition (found in later studies to be another advantage of clozapine). Several atypical agents exhibited a lower EPS profile, especially the ones with receptor-blocking profiles most similar to clozapine (for example, quetiapine and olanzapine). However, none of the new drugs at the time demonstrated clozapine's superior efficacy for treatment-resistant patients, and the term 'atypical' has been gradually replaced by 'second-generation' antipsychotic. Hence, clozapine remains the only agent indicated for persistent psychosis in the context of a previous full trial with another antipsychotic agent. However, almost three decades after the landmark Kane et al. paper, it remains greatly underutilized, especially in the USA.

Clear brain-tissue volume reductions in schizophrenia

Main citation

Suddath, R., Christinson, G., Fuller-Torrey, E., Casanova, M., & Weinberger, D. (1990). Anatomical abnormalities in the brains of monozygotic twins discordant for schizophrenia. *The New England Journal of Medicine*, 322, 789–794.

Background

With further development of neuroradiological and neuropathological research techniques, investigators began to train their sights on identifying neuroanatomical differences in major psychiatric disorders to try to better characterize their pathogenesis. Schizophrenia, with its chronic and progressive course and high heritability, became an obvious condition for which to identify brain abnormalities with these new tools. Since its original clinical description, there had been several attempts to examine post-mortem brains in schizophrenia, but results were inconsistent at best. During the 1980s, computerized tomography (CT) and magnetic resonance imaging (MRI) started to be used to examine the brain structure in living patients with schizophrenia compared with healthy volunteers. Not surprisingly, variance within healthy control and schizophrenia groups was much larger than some small mean-group differences in volume detected. In order to try to clarify the magnitude and specificity of structural abnormalities, pairs of twins, one who had developed schizophrenia and the other who had not, were recruited. Healthy twin pairs were also studied as a control.

Methods

Fifteen sets of monozygotic (identical) twins (ages 22 to 44) who were discordant for schizophrenia (DSM-III-R) and seven sets of healthy twins (ages 19 to 44) were studied. The affected twins had been ill for an average of 10.5 years; none were living independently; and 13 of the 15 were taking antipsychotic medication. Hence they were chronically ill. All subjects had a brain MRI at 1.5 tesla with T1-weighted 5 mm thick contiguous coronal slices. The images were inspected both visually and quantitatively (using a computerized image-analysis system). Quantitative measurements were made by two independent raters by manually tracing areas of interest and adding the values for the relevant slices to calculate volumes bilaterally for the prefrontal lobe, temporal lobe, amygdala, hippocampus, temporal horns, and the third ventricle. Through visual inspection of the images, one investigator examined each twin pair, trying to identify the affected twin according to the presence of larger cerebrospinal fluid spaces.

Results

The results showed impressive differences between the twins with and without schizophrenia. In fully 12 of the 15 discordant sets, the affected twin was correctly identified by blinded visual inspection. Of the remaining three twin sets, two were too similar to be distinguished and only one was incorrectly thought to be the affected twin due to abnormally enlarged ventricles.

The results from the quantitative measurement were consistent. In the left hippocampus, 14 of the 15 ($p = 0.006$) twin sets, and in the right, 13 of the 15 ($p = 0.01$) twin sets, had smaller hippocampal size. For the lateral ventricles, 14 of the 15 on the left ($p = 0.03$) and 13 of the 15 on the right ($p = 0.02$) showed larger ventricles. Lastly, the third ventricle was larger in 13 of the 15 ($p = 0.001$) affected twins. There were no significant group differences bilaterally for the grey and white matter in the frontal and temporal lobes' volumes, except for reduced grey matter in the left temporal lobe. Statistical analyses of co-variates suggested that these anatomical differences were unlikely to be related to duration of illness or the extent of exposure to antipsychotic agents.

Conclusions and critique

There are three important findings from this study that have advanced our understanding of schizophrenia. Firstly, there are clear brain-tissue reductions associated with the illness, although the variability related to non-illness factors can muddle the detection of these differences. However, using an ideal control, like in the discordant twin paradigm, these differences were apparent, even with small samples. Secondly, though the global ventricular enlargement suggests a more generalized brain process, the medial temporal lobes seemed to be particularly sensitive to the illness. Lastly, since the illness is about 80% heritable, a large part of the tissue reduction seen in affected twins may be a consequence of the illness or due to an interaction between genetic and environmental factors. Thus, these structural volume changes are in part likely to be environmental and not simply genetic.

The limitations of this study include the confounds of illness chronicity and medication exposure (which were addressed statistically), a small sample size, restricted MRI resolution (which limited the confidence to examine the involvement of multiple other structures), and the absence of an ill control (to ascertain the specificity of the findings to schizophrenia).

In the three decades following this study, there have been further imaging studies—with larger samples, higher field magnets (3T), involving patients (some naive to antipsychotic drugs) very early in the illness, and with longitudinal follow-up—which have verified and refined these original findings. It has been found that these volume reductions go beyond medial temporal grey matter, involving multiple other grey and white matter structures, and are detected in never-treated patients. However, similar reductions are also seen in bipolar and major depressive disorder groups, although they tend to be more severe and progressive in schizophrenia. What underlies the tissue reduction in schizophrenia, and understanding its clinical consequences, is the focus of much current research.

The dopamine hypothesis

Main citation

Brier, A., et al. (1997). Schizophrenia is associated with elevated amphetamine-induced synaptic dopamine concentrations: evidence from a novel positron emission tomography method. *Proceedings of the National Academy of Sciences of the United States of America*, 94, 2569–2574.

Background

The view that dopamine over-activity in some form could explain schizophrenia emerged from two pharmacological observations in humans: (1) the effects of amphetamines (drugs known to increase presynaptic release of dopamine in animals) in causing symptoms that mimic psychosis in healthy individuals and worsen symptoms in patients with schizophrenia; and (2) the effectiveness of dopamine-blocking agents in treating schizophrenia (discussed in the landmark papers of sections 'An efficacious treatment for schizophrenia' and 'An efficacious therapy for treatment-resistant schizophrenia'). In this study, the investigators tested the hypothesis that patients with schizophrenia had alterations in their synaptic dopamine levels. They used a PET brain-imaging method that provided an indirect measure of *in vivo* synaptic dopamine concentration by quantifying the change in dopamine-receptor radiotracer binding produced by amphetamine. This approach was implemented in two complementary studies described here: (1) in non-human primates, to determine the sensitivity of the PET approach compared with a simultaneously derived, more direct measure of striatal extracellular dopamine levels assessed with *in vivo* micro-dialysis; and (2) in humans, to test the hypothesis of elevated amphetamine-induced synaptic dopamine levels in schizophrenia compared to healthy controls.

Methods

In vivo micro-dialysis/PET study

Four adult rhesus monkeys had micro-dialysis probes stereotactically implanted in the head of the caudate nucleus. Under general anaesthesia, extracellular fluid was sampled every 10 minutes from the caudate. Dopamine concentrations were measured from each sample with high-performance liquid chromatography (HPLC). Concurrently, while inside the PET scanner, [^{11}C]raclopride was administered intravenously in a bolus, followed by constant infusion over 90 minutes. Forty minutes later, the first dose of amphetamine, 0.2 mg/kg, was administered intravenously. Thirteen scans were obtained from the onset of the [^{11}C]raclopride bolus, over a period of 90 minutes. Volumes of interest were drawn from images focused on the cerebellum and on the left and right striatum. Specific D_2 binding was computed as a ratio of striatum to cerebellum (a reference region with minimal D_2 binding). Five averaged PET images, before and after amphetamine, were compared to examine the amphetamine-induced displacement of D_2 binding. Following a 90-minute rest, the micro-dialysis/PET procedures were repeated with the second amphetamine dose of 0.4 mg/kg.

Human PET study

Eleven patients with DSM-IV-R diagnosis of schizophrenia and 12 healthy control subjects were studied. Six patients were antipsychotic naive and five had been withdrawn from medication for longer than two weeks. In the PET scanner, $^{[11C]}$raclopride was intravenously administered in a bolus, followed by constant infusion over 120 minutes. Twenty-nine scans were acquired over this two-hour period. Fifty minutes following the raclopride bolus, amphetamine (0.2 mg/kg iv) was infused over 60 seconds. Image processing and analyses were similar to the non-human primate study.

Results

In vivo micro-dialysis/PET study

Amphetamine produced very large increments in dopamine concentrations: the low dose increased dopamine levels 459% from baseline, and the higher dose caused increases of 1365%. However, the concurrent reductions in D_2 binding for the two amphetamine doses were 10.5% and 21.3%. Generally, doubling the amphetamine dose produced a doubling in $^{[11C]}$raclopride binding reductions and in dopamine levels. However, the ratio of percentage mean dopamine increase to percentage mean striatal binding reduction for amphetamine (0.2 mg/kg) was 44:1, demonstrating that relatively small binding changes reflected large changes in dopamine outflow.

Human PET study

In the human study, the baseline striatal D_2 binding did not differ between schizophrenia and control subjects (p = 0.99). Also, amphetamine produced robust reductions in D_2 binding in both groups. However, the schizophrenia group had a greater binding reduction than healthy controls (22.3% versus 15.5% respectively, $p = 0.04$). Potential confounds like differences in age, gender, weight, amphetamine blood level, or previous exposure to antipsychotics did not account for these binding reduction differences.

Conclusions and critique

Greater reductions in striatal-binding ratios with amphetamine, as opposed to increased postsynaptic D_2 striatal binding, were found in unmedicated schizophrenia subjects compared to healthy controls. The very large increments in extracellular dopamine that paralleled reductions in D_2 binding with amphetamine in non-human primates supported the inference that the larger binding changes in schizophrenia subjects reflected increased presynaptic dopamine release.

This study was the most comprehensive test of the hyper-dopaminergic hypothesis of schizophrenia that was not confounded by the effects of antipsychotic medications. Subsequent studies replicated the human findings and a meta-analysis of similar investigations has further consolidated this literature. With the specificity of D_2 blockade in terms of antipsychotic properties and the induction of psychotic symptoms by dopamine-releasing substances, the current study provided a critical mechanism that converged to support the contemporary view that increased striatal dopamine activity represents a final common pathway for psychotic disorders. However, schizophrenia is also characterized by persistent functional and cognitive deficits, which remain in the majority of patients even when psychosis is fully controlled with D_2 blockade. Hence, abnormalities in other neurotransmitter and molecular pathways, in addition to dopamine, are likely to underlie the core functional and cognitive deficits of schizophrenia.

The genetics of schizophrenia

Main citation

Ripke, S. & the Schizophrenia Working Group of the Psychiatric Genomics Consortium. (2014). Biological insights from 108 schizophrenia-associated genetic loci. *Nature*, 511, 421–427.

Background

Over the last 30 years the promise of genetics as a new way to study and understand diseases has been unprecedented. In some conditions, such as Huntington's disease, practitioners are able to perform genetic testing to identify specific variation in a single gene to precisely confirm a diagnosis even years before a disease manifests itself. In most other highly heritable conditions, a single gene or even a multitude of genes are simply not enough to predict a diagnosis. In schizophrenia, researchers have already determined that there is a high degree of heritability, suggesting that genetics plays an important part in the disease process. However, many different genes have been identified to varying degrees in patients with little consistency. One of the difficulties in genetic studies is the required sample sizes which often have to be enormous in order to account for most of the genetic variability that is present in the population. In order to go beyond anything done before, the Schizophrenia Working Group of the Psychiatric Genetics Consortium (PGC) explored group differences amongst millions of common variants across the genome, in the largest study ever undertaken in schizophrenia.

Methods

DNA samples from 36,989 cases and 113,075 controls underwent a genome-wide association study (GWAS). One European and three Asian ancestry-matched, non-overlapping, case-control samples were included. Genotypes from all studies were processed by the PGC using unified quality-control procedures followed by imputation of single nucleotide polymorphisms (SNPs) and insertion-deletions using a standard whole-genome reference panel. In each sample, around 9.5 million variants were tested. For some cases, research-based diagnoses were available, while for others only clinical diagnoses were available (results did not differ depending on diagnostic approach).

Multiple statistical analyses on the genetic data were performed to determine which genes had a significant association with a diagnosis of schizophrenia. The portion of these genes that coded for proteins and that appeared to modify other genes were evaluated. This analysis also examined how these genes matched known enhancer regions in different cell and tissue types to determine if they tended to be expressed in the brain, as would be expected, rather than in other tissues in the body.

Results

In the overall analysis, 128 SNPs surpassed genome-wide significance ($p \leq 5 \times 10^{-8}$). These SNPs were distributed across all chromosomes, with some of the most robust effects found in chromosomes 6, 10, 11, 12, and 14. A risk profile score (RPS) including these SNPs explained about 7% of variation on the liability to schizophrenia, about half of which (3.4%) was accounted for by the significant loci.

To further examine the impact of this overall scoring approach, subjects were grouped into RPS deciles and the odds ratios for having schizophrenia were examined. The odds ratios increased with greater number of schizophrenia risk alleles in each sample, being greatest for the tenth decile across samples: between 7.8 and 20.3, again supporting a 'dose' association with diagnosis. However, the specificity and sensitivity of RPS did not support its use as a predictive test. For example, in the Danish sample, the area under the receiver operating curve, an estimate of the best compromise between sensitivity and specificity, was only 0.62.

These results just focused on SNPs. In order to identify candidate genes, an associated locus was defined as the physical region in the genome containing all SNPs correlated at $r^2>0.6$, for each of the 128 SNPs. This resulted in 108 physically distinct associated loci, 83 of which had not been previously implicated in schizophrenia. Seventy-five percent of these loci included genes that code for proteins. Particularly relevant to schizophrenia were the loci in DRD2 (the target for antipsychotic drugs) as well as various genes involved in synaptic plasticity and glutamatergic neurotransmission (e.g. GRM3, GRIN2A, SRR, GRIA1). Also, several associations at genes encoding voltage-gated calcium channel subunits relevant to synaptic transmission were identified (CACNA1C, CACNB2, and CACNA1I). However, only ten of the associated loci were credibly attributable to a known exonic polymorphism. Hence, the large majority of the 108 loci are more likely to be involved in gene regulation, not in coding for protein structure.

To further examine the regulatory nature of the associations with schizophrenia, the 108 sets were mapped onto sequences with epigenetic markers known to be active enhancers in various tissues. Not surprisingly, the associated loci were significantly related to enhancers present in the brain (e.g. the hippocampus, anterior caudate, cingulate, substantia nigra, middle frontal lobe, angular gyrus, and inferior temporal lobe), but not in other tissues less likely to be relevant to schizophrenia (e.g. bone, cartilage, kidney, and fibroblasts). However, schizophrenia associations were enriched at enhancers active in cells with immune functions, like B-lymphocytes (e.g. CD19 and CD20 lines).

Though this study documented associations with schizophrenia for common genetic variants (SNPs), there was significant overlap between these associated loci and previously identified rare *de novo* mutations in schizophrenia ($p = 0.0061$). Finally, significant overlap was also found between the GWAS loci and those with *de novo* mutations previously reported in autism spectrum disorder (ASD) ($p = 0.035$) and in intellectual disability (ID) ($p = 0.00024$).

Conclusions and critique

In by far the largest sample of psychiatric patients ever collected, a number of genetic loci were found to be associated with a diagnosis of schizophrenia. The sample size, broad genome coverage with GWAS, rigorous standardized sample processing, and a conservative analytical approach provide reassurance for the validity of the results and the low likelihood of type I errors (false positives). In a highly heritable (~0.8) but clinically heterogeneous syndrome like schizophrenia, which involves a very plastic system (the brain), over 100 loci were identified. Hence, schizophrenia is, like many chronic illnesses, a polygenic disorder. Each of these loci has very small contributions in terms of risk, with additive effects, but an RPS based on this data is not ready for individual predictive testing. Very likely, future studies with larger samples and broader genome coverage will identify probably hundreds of other associations.

In terms of pathophysiology, these results clearly support variation in the regulation of genes, not in their actual configuration of protein-coding regions. Several of the genes involved appear to regulate brain and immune function. In terms of brain function, associations with synaptic, glutamatergic, and calcium channel functions are consistent with the post-mortem literature of neuropil retraction and the pharmacological challenge literature of N-methyl-D-aspartate (NMDA) hypofunction in schizophrenia. It is somewhat surprising that no loci associated with GABAergic function were found, because of the robust post-mortem literature involving this system. However, a downstream effect of glutamatergic dysfunction would likely involve gamma-aminobutyric acid (GABA) networks. In terms of the immune-related loci associations, the more plausible ones involve acquired immunity (B-cell lymphocytes), which converge with epidemiological and animal model literature supporting a role for prenatal infections in schizophrenia. Finally, the overlap with previously reported *de novo* mutations in ASD and ID tends to support a pathophysiological relationship between these three neurodevelopmental brain disorders. However, the minute individual loci effects in this study suggest that well-powered tests of the classic Kraepelinian dichotomy (that is, schizophrenia versus bipolar I) will need samples in the tens of thousands to protect against false-negative errors.

Conclusion

If available to comment a century following their classical monographs, Kraepelin and Bleuler would likely be entranced by some of the most significant research in the field of schizophrenia. The confirmation of subtle brain structural abnormalities, documented *in vivo*, would not surprise them (though they would marvel at the MRI tools so widely available). That the familial transmission would be supported with molecular quantification of common genetic variance would thrill them, but they might be as puzzled as we are, by the minuscule effects and the multitude of genes involved. As caring clinicians, they would have welcomed the serendipitous discovery of phenothiazines in the 1940s, but would have wondered why it took two decades to confirm their efficacy and another two to find a treatment for when they failed. Finally, the convergent evidence of increased presynaptic dopamine release in schizophrenia, with the dopamine D_2 blockade mechanism of action of antipsychotic drugs, would provide them some assurance that the psychiatric research enterprise they started in the early 1900s is well poised to find a cure for this devastating disease in the present century.

References

Breier, A., et al. (1997). Schizophrenia is associated with elevated amphetamine-induced synaptic dopamine concentrations: evidence from a novel positron emission tomography method. *Proceedings of the National Academy of Sciences of the USA*, **94**(6), 2569–2574.

Cole, J. O. & the NIMH Psychopharmacology Service Center Collaborative Study Group. (1964). Phenothiazine treatment in acute schizophrenia: effectiveness. *Archives of General Psychiatry*, **10**, 246–261.

Kane, J., Honigfeld, G., Singer, J., Meltzer, H., & the Clozaril Collaborative Study Group. (1988). Clozapine for the treatment-resistant schizophrenic. *Archives of General Psychiatry*, **45**(9), 789–796.

Ripke, S. & the Schizophrenia Working Group of the Psychiatric Genomics Consortium. (2014). Biological insights from 108 schizophrenia-associated genetic loci. *Nature*, **511**(7510), 421–427.

Suddath, R., Christinson, G., Fuller-Torrey, E., Casanova, M., & Weinberger, D. (1990). Anatomical abnormalities in the brains of monozygotic twins discordant for schizophrenia. *The New England Journal of Medicine*, **322**(12), 789–794.

Chapter 8

Pharmacotherapy of mood disorders

Marsal Sanches, Rodrigo Machado-Vieira, and Jair C. Soares

Introduction

Mood disorders are, historically, among the most fascinating psychiatric conditions. Since the early descriptions of melancholia, dating back to Hippocrates, to the nineteenth-century descriptions of *folie circulaire* and *folie à double forme* by Jean-Pierre Falret and Jules Baillarger (later grouped under the denomination of 'manic-depressive illness' and, more recently, bipolar disorder), these conditions have fascinated physicians, psychologists, and the general public (Mason et al., 2016; Campos et al., 2010). Nevertheless, the development of treatment options for mood disorders progressed at a rather slow pace. Up until the advent of electroconvulsive therapy, in the 1930s (see Chapter 17), no effective biological treatment for mood disorders was available (Fink, 2001).

It was only in the late 1940s that the era of the pharmacological treatment of mood disorders was inaugurated, with the description of the anti-manic effects of lithium salts (Cade, 1949). That was followed by the first report on the treatment of depressive disorders with imipramine, in 1957 (Brown & Rosdolsky, 2015). The 1970s saw the development of a new antidepressant (fluoxetine) which was, however, only approved for clinical use more than a decade later (Wong et al., 2005). Also in the 1970s, interest in the potential usefulness of anticonvulsants for the treatment of bipolar illness was ignited, paving the way for the studies in the 1990s that consolidated valproic acid as a first-line treatment for that condition. Finally, the first decade of the 2000s brought a growing concern with the potential discrepancies between the effects of psychotropic medications under controlled conditions during clinical trials and their actual benefit in the clinical setting. That led to the conceptualization of 'real- life' studies of efficacy, such as the Systematic Treatment Enhancement Program for Bipolar Disorder (STEP-BD) and the Sequenced Treatment Alternatives to Relieve Depression (STAR*D) (Sachs et al., 2003; Rush et al., 2004).

When selecting the papers to be included in the present chapter, we attempted to respect the chronology just described, taking into account not only the impact of the paper in question, from a historical standpoint, but also its implications for advancing the field of psychiatry. We discussed the choice of papers with colleagues and also reviewed scholarly papers on the history of mood disorders and their treatment. Yet, choosing which papers to address in the present work was an extremely challenging task. We hereby acknowledge and apologize in advance for the many high-quality, classic papers that could not be included.

Uric acid, guinea pigs, and the impressive effect of a salt on patients with mania

Main citation

Cade, J. F. J. (1949). Lithium salts in the treatment of psychotic excitement. *The Medical Journal of Austalia*, 2, 349–352.

Background

Evidence indicating the potential usefulness of lithium salts in the treatment of mania dates back to the nineteenth century. At the time, imbalances in uric acid were putatively considered to be involved in the pathophysiology of several medical conditions, as well as mental illnesses (Shorter, 2009; Mitchell & Hadzi-Pavlovic, 2000). Since lithium dissolves uric acid *in vitro*, it was utilized in the treatment of gout, and several authors (such as William Hammond, in the United States, and Frederik Lange, in Denmark) described its apparent effectiveness in the treatment of mania and depression (Shorter, 2009). The abandonment of the uric acid theory led to an apparent discredit in the use of lithium for the treatment of mental disorders, which was not mentioned in scientific literature during the first half of the twentieth century. John Cade, a psychiatrist at the Bundoora Repatriation Hospital, a veterans' hospital in the outskirts of Melbourne, Australia, was responsible for resurrecting the interest in lithium as a therapeutic tool in psychiatry (Cade, 1949).

Methods

In the introduction of his seminal paper, Cade describes in detail the animal experiments that led him to use lithium for the management of symptoms in patients with mania. While analysing the toxic effects of urea in guinea pigs, he decided to utilize lithium urate to dissolve uric acid salts. Cade noticed that, in addition to decreasing the toxicity of uric acid, lithium salts also had a sedative effect on the animals. That eventually led to an attempt to use lithium salts for the treatment of ten hospitalized manic patients, as well as three patients with unipolar depressive disorder ('chronic depressive psychosis') and six patients with schizophrenia ('*dementia praecox*'). The clinical presentation of each case, the lithium salts dose, and the individual outcomes were reported in the form of a case series.

Results

The ten manic patients were all male, with ages ranging from 40 to 63 years. All patients experienced marked improvement in their mood symptoms after treatment with lithium salts, although the doses utilized varied considerably. The author described careful adjustments in the doses of the medication, sometimes aiming at achieving a better response while, at others, trying to minimize side-effects. In some cases, lithium citrate was replaced with lithium carbonate, aiming at better tolerability. The most common side-effects reported were gastrointestinal discomfort, dizziness, and unsteady gait. In cases where the medication was discontinued, recurrence of manic symptoms was observed. Several patients could be discharged from the hospital and resumed their regular activities, often achieving premorbid levels of functioning. Patients with depression did not show response to the treatment with lithium salts (although Cade emphasized that there was no worsening in their condition). Similarly, no significant response was observed among the patients with *dementia praecox*, although the three who experienced some degree of agitation and excitement showed some improvement specifically in these symptoms.

Conclusions and critique

Despite the non-systematic nature of his study, Cade seemed extremely concerned about the methodological strengths and limitations of his research. He emphasized that the strong temporal association between treatment with lithium salts and improvement in manic symptoms did represent evidence that the medicine in question was effective in the treatment of mania. He also highlighted the fact that, for the purpose of his study, chronic patients were of particular interest, since spontaneous improvement was less likely among those. However, only three of his patients suffered from chronic mania, while the remaining seven had a history of recurrent symptoms. Moreover, he did address the fact that the controlled study of a large number of treated and untreated patients would allow the performance of statistical analyses and would likely be able to generate more robust conclusions. Yet, he did state that such a study would probably take 'some years' to be performed, since mania was a relatively uncommon condition.

Applying our current methodological standards to the critical analysis of Cade's paper, several other issues could be raised, including the lack of a control group, the lack of blindness, and the non-randomized nature of his study. Nevertheless, Cade's paper is, undoubtedly, considered one of the most important landmarks in the pharmacological treatment of mood disorders. It represented the first evidence in medical literature supporting the use of a medication for the treatment of mental illnesses, having preceded, by several years, the advent of other psychotropic medicines, such as antipsychotics and antidepressants.

His paper did not produce an immediate significant impact, having been authored by an unknown psychiatrist and published away from the centres of excellence for research at the time concentrated in the United States and Europe. Cade never pursued further investigations regarding the potential benefits of lithium for mania, but his paper inspired other authors, such as Mogens Schou (who, in 1954, published a detailed report describing the use of lithium in 21 females and 17 males with mania), to carry out larger and better-controlled studies focusing on the efficacy of the medication in question (Schou et al., 1954; Baastrup & Schou, 1967). Nevertheless, only in 1970 did the American

Food and Drug Administration (FDA) formally approve lithium salts for the treatment of bipolar disorder ('manic-depressive disorder'). Despite some decline in its popularity after the advent of anticonvulsants for the treatment of mania, it remains one of the most effective pharmacological agents for the treatment of bipolar disorder.

A 'miraculous cure' for depressive states

Main citation

Kuhn, R. (1957). Über die behandlung depressiver zustände mit einem iminodibenzylderival (G22355). *Schweizerische Medizinische Wochenschrift*, 87, 1135–1140.

Related reference

Brown, W. A., & Rosdolsky, M. (2015). The clinical discovery of imipramine. *American Journal of Psychiatry*, 172, 426–429.

Background

In the 1950s, the aetiology of depressive states was mainly attributed to psychodynamic processes. Despite the well-described efficacy of electroconvulsive therapy (at the time called 'shock therapy'), the possibility of medications or other biological agents being able to modify the course of illness (rather than just producing some relief in symptomatology) was at the time disregarded by most experts (Lopez-Munoz & Alamo, 2009). Roland Kuhn, a Swiss psychiatrist (and also a psychoanalyst), was the medical director at the Psychiatric Clinic of Thurgau Canton, near Basel. Following the recent discovery of chlorpromazine a few years earlier, drug companies had been working with physicians to test different compounds chemically related to chlorpromazine to enhance their antipsychotic properties. Kuhn had been testing a compound produced by Geigy, an iminodibenzyl derivative named G22355 (Brown & Rosdolsky, 2015). Kuhn noticed that G22355 lacked antipsychotic properties, but it did ameliorate depressive symptoms in patients with schizophrenia, even precipitating hypomania in some. In a letter to Geigy, Kuhn hypothesized that G22355 (later named imipramine) could have antidepressant properties and, with their support, conducted a study.

It is important to emphasize that the original paper authored by Kuhn and published in the *Schweizerische Medizinische Wochenschrift* was never published in English. However, a recent article published in the *American Journal of Psychiatry* (Brown & Rosdolsky, 2015) described the paper's content in detail, after translating it from German into English. Most of the information regarding the methodology and results of Kuhn's original work was obtained from there.

Methods

Kuhn's paper initially addresses the limited options at the time in terms of biological treatments for depression. It then describes the author's experience with G22355. The medication was given in doses equivalent to chlorpromazine, ranging from 75 to 250 mg. Even though the author stated the medication was given to hundreds of patients, including 200 patients with schizophrenia and 100 patients with depressive disorder, the paper focused on the 40 patients who had a good treatment response. Most of his patients were inpatients and severely depressed. Outcomes were reported in a non-standardized way, even though the author described the different dimensions of depressive states with great detail, as well as the side-effects observed.

Results

The author indicated that, even though some patients would show full improvement after a few days of treatment, often several weeks were necessary until a response was observed. The patients experienced improvement not only in their depressed mood but also in the somatic symptoms of depression, such as insomnia. In many cases, improvement was dramatic, and patients and their families considered the treatment 'miraculous'. Kuhn mentioned the increased risk of suicide during treatment, secondary to disinhibition, specifically among those individuals with a slow response to the medicine. He also described, in detail, anticholinergic side-effects. In consonance with the adopted nosology at the time, which classified depressive states as endogenous (i.e. without an obvious trigger) or reactive (i.e. secondary to a stressful event), the author stated that G22355 was particularly effective in patients with 'typical endogenous depression', but also seemed to produce positive effects in cases of 'reactive depression'. He briefly described the effects of the drug on patients with schizophrenia, highlighting that, despite some improvement in terms of mood, no effect was observed in regard to psychotic symptoms.

Kuhn seems to have included very little information about the patients who did not respond to the treatment, although he did include estimates of the response rate to imipramine: 25% to 50% of the depressed patients seemed to show full remission, 20% to 25% did not seem to respond to the treatment, and the remaining patients showed only partial response. Finally, Kuhn also emphasized that, in some cases of depression, which seemed to have a more 'neurotic' basis, the response to the medicine appeared to be limited, with symptoms quickly recurring once the drug was discontinued. These cases, as per the author, should likely be treated with psychotherapy, although the medication might still play a role in the management of depressive and anxious symptoms that could emerge during the treatment.

Conclusions and critique

Kuhn's study was basically observational; there was no statistical analysis. Many methodological issues may be raised, including the lack of a control group, the absence of randomization or structured assessments, and the fact that only patients with severe depression were included in the study, which likely maximized the rates of response to the medication, due to increases in the effect size. The author presented his findings in the Second World Congress of Psychiatry, in Zurich, shortly after the publication of his paper. The results were received with scepticism by the medical community at the time. Yet, imipramine was released in the Swiss market later that year, and in the rest of Europe in 1958. In North America, the medication was introduced due to the work of Heinz E. Lehmann, who had been present at Kuhn's lecture in Zurich and carried out a study in Canada assessing the efficacy of imipramine in 48 patients with depression (Lehmann et al., 1958). The study in question played a significant role in the approval of the drug for use in the United States.

Despite its serendipitous discovery, imipramine formally inaugurated the era of the pharmacological treatment of depression and remains, up until the present, one of the most effective pharmacological treatments for depressive states. Following the success of imipramine, other tricyclic antidepressants were developed, such as amitriptyline (which was approved by the FDA for the treatment of depression in 1961), nortriptyline, desipramine, and clomipramine. Moreover, imipramine had its mechanism of action clarified by the studies of Bernard Brodie and Julius Axelrod, in the early 1960s. That discovery, in addition to the 1952 description of the antidepressant properties of iproniazid (a monoamine oxidase inhibitor initially tested for the treatment of tuberculosis), served as the basis for the eventual formulation of the monoaminergic theory of depression (Lopez-Munoz & Alamo, 2009; Schildkraut, 1965) (see also Chapter 3).

The onset of a new era in the treatment of depression

Main citation

Wong, D. T., Horng, J. S., Bymaster, F. P., Hauser, K. L., & Molloy, B. B. (1974). A selective inhibitor of serotonin uptake: Lilly 110140, 3-(p-trifluoromethylphenoxy)-N-methyl-3-phenylpropylamine. *Life Sciences*, 15, 471–479.

Background

In the 1960s, several authors, inspired by the therapeutic effects of tricyclic antidepressants and monoamine oxidase inhibitors, became interested in what was later coined 'the monoaminergic theory of depression'(Lopez-Munoz & Alamo, 2009). Basically, this theory suggested that deficiencies in the noradrenergic and serotonergic neurotransmission in certain areas of the brain were responsible for the development of depressive symptoms. The noradrenergic hypothesis of depression was first postulated in 1965 by Joseph Jacob Schildkraut, in his classic paper 'The catecholamine hypothesis of affective disorders: a review of supporting evidence' (Schildkraut, 1965) (discussed in Chapter 3). Similarly, a possible relationship between serotonergic dysfunction and depression was initially proposed by Herman M. van Praag in 1964, but was based on peripheral indicators of serotonergic dysfunction, mainly in platelets (Lopez-Munoz & Alamo, 2009). It was not until 1968 that another group, led by Arvid Carlsson, described the effect of tricyclic antidepressants in inhibiting the reuptake of serotonin in the brain (Carlsson et al., 1968). These findings, combined with the reports of decreased levels of serotonin and its metabolite 5-hydroxy-indoleacetic acid in autopsy brain samples of depressed patients who had committed suicide (Shaw et al., 1967), were the main sources of inspiration for the development of a molecule able to inhibit the reuptake of serotonin in the synaptic cleft, therefore increasing the serotonergic transmission and, ultimately, producing improvement in depressive symptoms (Wong et al., 2005). That task was accomplished by a research group led by David Wong, a young biochemist at Lilly Pharmaceuticals, whose extensive work resulted in the development of fluoxetine, which was approved by the FDA in 1987 and released in the United States in 1988 under the brand name Prozac (Wong et al., 2005).

Methods

This is a basic psychopharmacology article describing the effects of a new compound, named Lilly 110140, on the uptake of monoamines in the brain of rats, compared to other monoamine uptake inhibitors. It actually reports the findings of different studies describing *in vitro* and *in vivo* evidence of the selective effect of 110140 on the reuptake of serotonin.

In the first analysis, the authors measured the effects of different compounds on the reuptake of serotonin, norepinephrine, and dopamine, through the *in vitro* analysis of synaptosomes (pinched-off nerve endings) of rat brains. Synaptosomal preparations were obtained from the fractionation of rat brain homogenate in a sucrose gradient, through differential centrifugation techniques. The uptake of neurotransmitters was then measured using a specific method, whereby synaptosomes were incubated in a solution of Krebs bicarbonate buffer containing one of the monoamines (serotonin, norepinephrine, or dopamine) and one of the compounds analysed (Lilly 110140, clomipramine, imipramine, or nortriptyline).

In the second analysis, rats were treated with two doses of 110140, clomipramine, or desipramine, followed by an infusion of tracer-labelled norepinephrine (^{14}C-NE). The rats were then euthanized, their hearts were removed, and the reuptake of ^{14}C-NE in the heart was measured.

In the third analysis, rats were treated with 110140 or clomipramine at equimolar concentrations. The rats were later euthanized and their brains were removed, so that synaptosomal preparations could be obtained.

Results

The first analysis demonstrated that compound 110140 strongly inhibited serotonin uptake into synaptosomes, as indicated by its Ki (inhibitor constant) value. The inhibitory effects of 110140 on the uptake of norepinephrine and dopamine were much weaker. Clomipramine was similar to 110140 in inhibiting serotonin and norepinephrine uptake, but much stronger in inhibiting the uptake of dopamine. Imipramine was four times less effective than 110140 in inhibiting the uptake of serotonin. Nortriptyline displayed a much stronger effect on the inhibition of the uptake of norepinephrine than of serotonin and dopamine. Comparing the Ki of the different compounds with respect to the inhibition of serotonin uptake, the authors concluded that, among the four compounds in question, Lilly 110140 was the most selective competitive inhibitor of serotonin uptake.

The second analysis indicated that the administration of clomipramine or desipramine reduced the uptake of ^{14}C-NE in the heart by 50% and 83%, respectively, while Lilly 110140 did not seem to affect norepinephrine uptake in rat hearts.

Finally, in the third analysis, the synaptosomal preparations of Lilly 110140-treated rats were found to display a 56% inhibition in the uptake of serotonin, whereas in the preparations from clomipramine-treated rats, serotonin reuptake was found to be less than half as effective. In summary, the authors concluded that the results indicated that 110140 had strong effects on the reuptake of serotonin, but not on the central or peripheral uptake of catecholamines.

Conclusions and critique

In their discussion, the authors address some of the evidence pointing to the involvement of serotonin in different mental disorders, including depressive disorders. They mention that the discovery of an agent able to specifically inhibit the uptake of serotonin should be of benefit in not only understanding the pathophysiology of depression, but also treating it. Of note, the results were presented to the Neuroscience (CNS) Research Committee at Lilly in 1973 (prior to the publication of this paper in 1974), and a project team was formed to lead Lilly 110140 (later named fluoxetine) into product development. Following the completion of safety studies in animals, an investigational new drug application was submitted to the FDA in 1976, and Phase I clinical studies were initiated (Wenthur et al., 2014). Phase II studies started in 1978 and, one year later, evidence of the clinical efficacy of fluoxetine in the treatment of depression was first identified. Phase III studies were started in 1981 (Wong et al., 2005). Two years later, a new drug application was submitted to the FDA and, in 1985, the FDA Advisory Committee issued a recommendation for the new medication to be approved. Prozac was approved and launched in Belgium in 1986, but the final approval by the FDA only took place in the last weeks of 1987 (Wong et al., 2005).

In contrast to other psychopharmacological agents, often discovered serendipitously, fluoxetine probably represents the first case, in the history of psychiatry, of a medication that was developed targeting a specific (albeit putative) pathophysiological factor, with a core team of researchers taking responsibility for its development from the early stages of basic psychopharmacology to the characterization of its clinical efficacy and its eventual approval. After its release, fluoxetine quickly became an extremely popular choice among clinicians for the treatment of depression, due to its relatively mild side-effect profile when compared to tricyclic antidepressants and monoamine oxidase inhibitors, and it paved the way for the discovery and launching of other selective-serotonin reuptake inhibitors, such as sertraline and paroxetine. Thirty years after its approval by the FDA, fluoxetine has revolutionized the treatment of depression, having become one of the most utilized medications worldwide. Its indications were expanded to the treatment of several psychiatric conditions other than depressive disorders, such as anxiety disorders, obsessive-compulsive disorder, eating disorders, and premenstrual dysphoric disorder. As of early 2018, a search through PubMed using the MeSH term 'fluoxetine' elicits more than 8,000 papers. Nevertheless, the widespread use and relatively mild side-effect profile of this medication has led to concerns about possible excesses in its utilization and the over-diagnosis of depressive conditions.

The end of lithium supremacy in the management of bipolar disorder

Main citation

Bowden, C. L., et al. (1994). Efficacy of divalproex vs lithium and placebo in the treatment of mania. *Journal of the American Medical Asociation*, 271, 918–924.

Background

In the early 1990s, lithium was the only FDA-approved medicine for the treatment of mania. Despite its well-demonstrated effectiveness, several factors would, at times, limit its use. Those include lack of tolerability, risk of toxicity due to its narrow therapeutic index, and, finally, lack of response: at that time, at least one third of manic patients were unresponsive to or unable to tolerate treatment with lithium salts (Harrow et al., 1990). Since the late 1970s and early 1980s, some authors had pointed to the possible benefits of anticonvulsants in the pharmacological management of bipolar disorder (Ballenger & Post, 1978; Post & Uhde, 1983). The first randomized, double-blind study comparing valproic acid and placebo for the treatment of mania was published in 1991 (Pope et al., 1991). However, that study utilized a small sample size and lacked a lithium comparison group. Charles Bowden, from the University of Texas Health Science Center at San Antonio, led the Depakote Mania Study Group Program, which designed and implemented a study analysing the efficacy of divalproex sodium (an oligomeric complex of sodium valproate and valproic acid) compared with lithium and placebo in the treatment of mania (Bowden et al., 1994). The study was partially funded by a grant from Abbot Laboratories.

Methods

This was a multi-centre, randomized, double-blind study carried out in eight different academic departments across the United States. The sample consisted of 149 inpatients with mania (age range: 18 to 65 years) who met the Research Diagnostic Criteria for manic disorder. After a washout period, patients were randomly assigned to a 21-day treatment period with divalproex (69 patients), lithium (36 patients), or placebo (74 patients). Patients assigned to the medication groups received initially a total daily dose of 750 mg of divalproex or 900 mg of lithium, and after three days the doses were increased to 1000 mg and 1200 mg, respectively. At each centre, an unblinded physician was responsible for reviewing the serum concentration of the medicines and adjusting their doses, aiming at a concentration of 150 micrograms/ml of divalproex or 1.5 mEq/L of lithium, respectively, if tolerated by the participants. The protocol allowed the use of lorazepam or chloral hydrate for agitation, but not antipsychotics. Outcome was primarily measured by the Mania Rating Scale (including two subscales, the Manic Syndrome subscale and the Behaviour and Ideation subscale) based on the Schedule for Affective Disorders and Schizophrenia (SADS) items.

Results

A significant number of patients (64% in the placebo group, 61% in the lithium group, and 48% in the divalproex group) did not complete the study (mainly due to lack of efficacy), and the authors utilized an intent-to-treat analysis. Clinical characteristics of all three groups at baseline were similar, except for the fact that eight patients with a history of four or more manic episodes per year for the previous two years had been randomized to the divalproex group, but results remained basically unchanged when the patients in question were removed from the analysis. Patients in the divalproex group had a greater decrease in the Manic Syndrome subscale scores at day five (and in the Manic Rating Scale at day ten) when compared to placebo. At the end of the study period, marked improvement (defined as at least a 50% decrease in the Manic Syndrome subscale scores) was similar in the two medication groups (49% of the patients in the divalproex group, and 48% of the lithium group) against 25% of the placebo group. Divalproex was found to be equally effective for patients with and without rapid cycling, as well as those with and without a past history of good response to lithium.

Conclusions and critique

Some methodological issues of the study have been pointed out: the lithium group was considerably smaller than the divalproex group, and almost half of the participants assigned to it (48%) had a past history of either non-response or intolerance to lithium (Kravitz & Fawcett, 1994). That factor may have made the lithium group serve more as a placebo group than a benchmark treatment group, potentially maximizing the efficacy of divalproex compared to lithium. The fact that the study results focused on the efficacy of divalproex only in regard to improvement in manic symptoms, providing no findings in regard to remission rates (likely due to the short treatment period), and the high rate of patients who did not complete the study may be considered additional methodological limitations. Finally, the paper provided no data on the efficacy of divalproex as a maintenance treatment for bipolar disorder. Nevertheless, the paper by Bowden et al. inspired a large amount of research on its efficacy and had considerable impact on the consolidation of valproic acid as one of the most prescribed mood stabilizers for the treatment of bipolar disorder.

A huge 'step' for the understanding of bipolar disorder treatment

Main citation

Sachs, G. S., et al. (2003). Rationale, design, and methods of the systematic treatment enhancement program for bipolar disorder (STEP-BD). *Biological Psychiatry*, 53, 1028–1042.

Related references

Sachs, G. S., et al. (2007). Effectiveness of adjunctive antidepressant treatment for bipolar depression. *New England Journal of Medicine*, 356, 1711–1722.
Miklowitz, D. J., et al. (2007). Psychosocial treatments for bipolar depression: a 1-year randomized trial from the Systematic Treatment Enhancement Program. *Archives of General Psychiatry*, 64, 419–426.
Nierenberg, A. A., et al. (2006). Treatment-resistant bipolar depression: a STEP-BD equipoise randomized effectiveness trial of antidepressant augmentation with lamotrigine, inositol, or risperidone. *American Journal of Psychiatry*, 163, 210–216.

Background

In the late 1990s, despite the large number of clinical trials addressing the efficacy of different agents and interventions in the treatment of mental illnesses, little was known about patients' long-term response and outcomes associated with these treatments. Furthermore, given the strict study design, stringent inclusion criteria, and controlled conditions of traditional clinical trials, there was growing concern regarding whether a patient's response to treatment in controlled trials correlated with that observed in daily routine practice. In response, the National Institute of Mental Health (NIMH) encouraged and requested the conceptualization of studies aimed at providing practical answers regarding treatment effectiveness, not only at a doctor–patient level but also from a public health perspective. The Systematic Treatment Enhancement Program for Bipolar Disorder (STEP-BD), funded through a research contract between the NIMH and the Massachusetts General Hospital in 1998, and led by Harvard professor Gary Sachs, was one of those studies.

Methods

This paper provides the justification and methodology for the STEP-BD. As explained by the authors, STEP-BD was not formulated as a single study, but as a 'platform or infrastructure designed to carry out a variety of clinical trials and other studies that require a cohort of well-characterized bipolar subjects' (Sachs et al., 2003).

In order to optimize the generalizability of the findings, inclusion criteria for participants were remarkably broad, with any patients older than 15 years who were seeking outpatient treatment potentially qualifying for study participation, regardless of their bipolar subtype (bipolar disorder I, II, not otherwise specified (NOS), or cyclothymia) or phase of illness. Substance use disorder was not an exclusion criteria, unless patients needed immediate inpatient detoxication at the time of enrolment.

Different sites nationwide participated in the programme, with site selection taking into account not only the availability of the necessary infrastructure and experience with bipolar disorder research but also the need for geographic and demographic balance. Standardized evaluations were performed at the time of enrolment, and model practice procedures, including procedures regarding therapeutic interventions, outcome measurement, and record keeping, were developed, and the treating psychiatrists received specific training in those procedures. Moreover, clinicians were provided with a series of 'menus of reasonable choices': a list of therapeutic options for the management of clinical situations displayed by the patients over the course of the study. For each clinical situation, a sequence of decision points was available, comprising a so-called 'standard care pathway'. The study offered clinicians nine standard care pathways: acute depression, refractory depression, acute mania, refractory mania, rapid cycling, relapse prevention, pregnancy, substance abuse, and other comorbidity (Sachs et al., 2003).

Although, as previously explained, all subjects included in the study were automatically assigned to one of the standard care pathways, at any point during study participation the patients could become eligible for one of the study's randomized care pathways, which included pathways for acute depression, refractory depression, and relapse prevention. The acute depression randomized pathway compared the efficacy of paroxetine, bupropion, and placebo (in combination with a mood stabilizer) in the treatment of acute bipolar depression and also analysed the efficacy of different intensive psychosocial approaches compared with a three-session psychosocial intervention (collaborative care plus). The refractory depression randomized pathway compared the efficacy of different pharmacological adjunctive strategies (inositol versus risperidone, or risperidone versus lamotrigine, or lamotrigine versus inositol) among patients with bipolar depression who failed to respond to two trials with antidepressants. Finally, the relapse prevention randomized pathway focused on patients who had displayed relapse in their mania or hypomania while receiving lithium or valproic acid; they were randomized to either continuing with a single mood stabilizer at a higher dose or receiving a combination of both mood stabilizers. It also assessed the role of psychosocial interventions in relapse prevention, in a similar fashion to the one described in the acute depression randomized pathway. Finally, STEP-BD offered the opportunity of several pilot/ancillary studies and secondary outcome analyses.

Results

The original 2003 paper does not include results, and a detailed description of the findings of STEP-BD is beyond the scope of the present chapter. From 1999 to 2005, the study enrolled a total of 4,361 participants, from 21 sites across the United States. A large number of publications, addressing different clinical and therapeutic aspects of bipolar disorder, have resulted from STEP-BD data analysis, including factors associated with suicidality, functional status, treatment compliance, and relapse risk (Parikh et al., 2010; Bowden et al., 2012), as well as the burden of caregivers (Perlick et al., 2007) and the role of psychosocial interventions in the management of bipolar depression (Deckersbach et al., 2016).

The results of the randomized trial for the treatment of acute bipolar depression indicated that adding bupropion or paroxetine to a mood stabilizer did not show better results when compared to the addition of placebo, and has brought into question the efficacy of antidepressants in patients with bipolar disorder (Sachs et al., 2007). The randomized study, focusing on the efficacy of psychotherapeutic interventions in bipolar disorder (Miklowitz et al., 2007), indicated that patients in intensive psychotherapy were clinically better over the course of the study when compared to those in collaborative care, although no differences were observed among the three intensive-therapy modalities offered (family-focused therapy, interpersonal and social rhythm therapy, and cognitive behavioural therapy). Further, the trial on refractory depression indicated no statistically significant differences between risperidone, lamotrigine, and inositol as augmentation strategies in patients with bipolar depression with respect to rates of recovery, although post-hoc analysis indicated that patients on lamotrigine had greater improvements in depressive symptoms, overall severity of illness, and functional status at the end of the study (Nierenberg et al., 2006).

Conclusions and critique

STEP-BD remains the largest research programme on bipolar disorder ever carried out. Additional analyses from its findings are still in progress, and new articles directly or indirectly related to the programme continue to be published, more than ten years after enrolment was completed. The programme was very well designed and is considered extremely sophisticated from a methodological standpoint, allowing participants to transition from naturalistic to controlled, randomized study arms. Nevertheless, despite the efforts from STEP-BD in ensuring the generalizability of the results, the under-representation of minorities and possible over-representation of patients who seek treatment in academic settings have been cited as methodological limitations (Strakowski, 2007).

Antidepressant effectiveness in 'real life'

Main citation

Trivedi. M. H., et al. (2006). Evaluation of outcomes with citalopram for depression using measurement-based care in STAR*D: implications for clinical practice. *American Journal of Psychiatry*, 163, 28–40.

Related references

Rush, A. J., et al. (2004). Sequenced treatment alternatives to relieve depression (STAR*D): rationale and design. *Controlled Clinical Trials*, 25, 119–142.
Rush, A. J., et al. (2006). Acute and longer-term outcomes in depressed outpatients requiring one or several treatment steps: a STAR* D report. *American Journal of Psychiatry*, 163, 1905–1917.

Background

The Sequenced Treatment Alternatives to Relieve Depression (STAR*D) trial was the third of the practical clinical trials funded by the NIMH, focusing on treatment effectiveness in a more realistic/naturalistic environment, in contrast with the short-term, controlled conditions strictly followed during randomized clinical trials. While STEP-BD addressed participants with bipolar disorder, and the Clinical Antipsychotic Trials of Intervention Effectiveness (CATIE) study focused on the effectiveness of antipsychotics in the treatment of schizophrenia, the STAR*D trial addressed patients with major depressive disorder. The authors aimed at ultimately answering some of the practical questions commonly asked by clinicians, including questions about the magnitude of response that should be realistically expected over the course of the treatment and considerations about switching medications versus using augmentation strategies in patients with partial or no response (Rush et al., 2004). The multisite clinical trial was primarily led by John Rush, from the University of Texas Southwestern Medical Center, in Dallas, with the participation of several collaborators, as well as study directors in 14 regional centres.

Methods

The trial enrolled 4,041 outpatients with major depressive disorder from 23 psychiatric sites and 18 primary care sites across the United States, of which 1,165 were excluded for not meeting severity requirements or because they declined to participate. Therefore, the paper in question included data on 2,876 participants. Only patients who actively sought outpatient treatment were included (no patients were recruited through advertisement, in order to preserve the generalizability of the findings). For the same reason, very few exclusion criteria were adopted, with any patients with non-psychotic major depressive disorder, aged between 18 and 75 years, and a Hamilton Rating Scale for Depression (HAM-D) score equal or superior to 14 (indicating at least a moderate depressive episode) included in the study, as long as deemed safe by their clinicians to be treated in the outpatient setting.

The STAR*D trial was designed according to a stepwise approach (Rush et al., 2004). Phase one assessed the rates of depression remission associated with treatment with flexible doses of citalopram, over a 12- to 14-week period. The participants who did not achieve remission or could not tolerate the phase one medication (citalopram) were randomized to phase two, which compared different strategies that included either replacing citalopram with another therapeutic strategy (sertraline, bupropion, venlafaxine, or cognitive therapy) or continuing with citalopram in association with an augmentation strategy (bupropion, buspirone, or cognitive therapy). Patients who did not achieve remission during phase two were randomized to phase three, during which they could be either switched to mirtazapine or nortriptyline, or continue with their primary antidepressant while receiving augmentation with lithium or thyroid hormone. Those participants who still did not achieve remission were eligible for phase four. In this final phase, patients were randomly assigned to tranylcypromine or the combination of mirtazapine and venlafaxine. Finally, the patients who achieved remission (regardless of the phase of the study) were included in a naturalistic, 12-month follow-up phase.

Clinicians were assisted by a research clinical coordinator in the measurement of symptoms and side-effects during visits, and also by the use of a treatment manual with recommendations regarding medication changes, based on the patient's condition at the time of the visits. Change on the 17-item HAM-D was the primary outcome measure, and the

Quick Inventory of Depressive Symptomatology, Self-Report (QIDS-SR) was adopted as a secondary outcome.

Results

The mean daily dose of citalopram utilized was 41.8 mg, and was similar for patients who achieved and did not achieve remission. The response rate was 47%, but remission rates were considerably lower, ranging from 27.5% (based on the HAM-D scores) to 32.9% (QIDS-SR). For the patients who achieved remission, the mean time to remission was 6.7 weeks. Rates of discontinuation due to intolerance/adverse events was lower among those patients who achieved remission than among those who did not (2% and 11%, respectively). Pretreatment correlates of non-remission included unemployment, lower income, non-Caucasian ethnicity, male gender, lower educational status, poor functioning and lower quality of life at baseline, anxious depression, and comorbid generalized anxiety disorder. Remission rates were similar in primary care and psychiatric care settings (Trivedi et al., 2006). In the subsequent phases of the study, remission rates were progressively lower (Rush et al., 2006), and withdrawal rates became gradually higher, reaching 42% after phase three. Overall, around 50% of patients became symptom-free after two treatment phases, and 67% of those who did not withdraw from the study achieved remission after four treatment phases (Gaynes et al., 2012). In phases two, three, and four, there were no clear differences between switching and augmentation strategies.

Conclusions and critique

The STAR*D study was praised for its ecological validity and its results. It was the largest 'real-world' clinical trial on the treatment of major depressive disorder ever carried out. The remission rate associated with monotherapy with citalopram (30%) was initially considered 'robust' by the authors, but the overall remission rates in the study clinics were lower than expected (Gaynes et al., 2012). However, given that patients' preferences (switching versus augmentation) were taken into account before randomization, there were differences between groups in regard to severity of depression, with the group that was switched to a new medication in phase two (rather than switching to cognitive behavioural therapy or receiving augmentation) containing patients with more severe depressive states. Moreover, fewer participants than expected selected cognitive behavioural therapy, which limited a better evaluation of its actual role in the treatment of depression in the trial.

The issue regarding the randomization, as already described, as well as the lack of a placebo arm, have been cited as methodological limitations of the study (Blier, 2007). Nevertheless, the STAR*D trial is considered a classic in the history of mood disorder research. A large number of subsequent analyses, involving the most diverse factors related to treatment response in depressive disorders, have been carried out and resulted in a large number of publications. The study's conclusions on the remission rates of major depressive disorder have influenced a whole generation of psychiatrists and are often cited to illustrate the limited efficacy of available treatments for depressive disorders and the urgent need for new therapeutic strategies targeting treatment-resistant depression.

Conclusion

The different landmark papers included in the present chapter comprise more than 50 years of evolution in the field of psychiatry. From the initial study on lithium salts authored by Cade to the more recent papers discussed, a trend can be easily noticed, with studies progressing from craft-like research, with uncontrolled designs and small samples, to highly sophisticated and well-funded multisite clinical trials, including thousands of patients. Nonetheless, the historical meaningfulness of the papers discussed in the present chapter needs to be measured not only by their methodological soundness but also by their pioneering and long-lasting implications for the treatment and better understanding of mental illnesses.

Ongoing research on the treatment of mood disorders seems to be migrating from a pure pharmacological approach to a more integrated model, including the role of pharmacogenetics, neuroimaging, and neuropsychological performance in the conceptualization of more personalized treatments for these conditions. Similarly, non-pharmacological biological interventions, such as different neurostimulation techniques, have been the object of great interest over the last few years regarding their role in the treatment of mood disorders, and are seen as an extremely promising area of study. The future will prove if any of these innovative approaches has the potential to revolutionize the treatment of mood disorders and produce long-lasting impacts. Paraphrasing Edward Teller, 'Today's science is tomorrow's technology' (Teller & Brown, 1975).

References

Baastrup, P. C., & **Schou, M.** (1967). Lithium as a prophylactic agent: its effect against recurrent depressions and manic-depressive psychosis. *Archives of General Psychiatry* **16**(2), 162–172.

Ballenger, J. C., & **Post, R. M.** (1978). Therapeutic effects of carbamazepine in affective illness: a preliminary report. *Communications in Psychopharmacology*,**2**(2), 159–175.

Blier, P. (2007). The usefulness of large studies in psychopharmacology: understanding their strong points and their drawbacks. *Journal of Psychiatry & Neuroscience*, **32**(4), 232.

Bowden, C. L., et al. (1994). Efficacy of divalproex vs lithium and placebo in the treatment of mania. *Journal of the American Medical Association*,**271**(12), 918–924.

Bowden, C. L., et al. (2012). Aims and results of the NIMH systematic treatment enhancement program for bipolar disorder (STEP-BD). *CNS Neuroscience & Therapeutics*, **18**(3), 243–249.

Brown, W. A., & **Rosdolsky, M.** (2015). The clinical discovery of imipramine. *American Journal of Psychiatry*, **172**(5), 426–429.

Cade, J. F. J. (1949). Lithium salts in the treatment of psychotic excitement. *The Medical Journal of Australia*, **2**(10), 349–352.

Campos, R. N., **de Oliveira Campos, J. A.**, & **Sanches, M.** (2010). Historical evolution of mood disorders and personality disorders concepts: difficulties in the differential diagnostic. *Revista de Psiquiatria Clínica*, **37**(4), 162–166.

Carlsson, A., **Fuxe, K.**, & **Ungerstedt, U.** (1968). The effect of imipramine on central 5-hydroxytryptamine neurons. *Journal of Pharmacy and Pharmacology*, **20**(2), 150–151.

Deckersbach, T., et al. (2016). A cluster analytic approach to identifying predictors and moderators of psychosocial treatment for bipolar depression: results from STEP-BD. *Journal of Affective Disorders*, **203**, 152–157.

Fink, M. (2001). Convulsive therapy: a review of the first 55 years. *Journal of Affective Disorders*, **63**(1), 1–15.

Gaynes, B. N., Warden, D., Trivedi, M. H., Wisniewski, S. R., Fava, M., & Rush, A. J. (2012). What did STAR*D teach us? Results from a large-scale, practical, clinical trial for patients with depression. *FOCUS*, **10**(4), 510–517.

Harrow, M., Goldberg, J. F., Grossman, L. S., & Meltzer, H. Y. (1990). Outcome in manic disorders. A naturalistic follow-up study. *Archives of General Psychiatry*, **47**(7), 665–671.

Kravitz, H. M., & Fawcett, J. (1994). Efficacy of divalproex vs lithium and placebo in mania. *Journal of the American Medical Association*, **272**(13), 1005–1006.

Lehmann, H. E., Cahn, C. H., & De Verteuil, R. L. (1958). The treatment of depressive conditions with imipramine (G 22355). *Canadian Journal of Psychiatry*, **3**(4), 155–164.

Lopez-Munoz, F., & Alamo, C. (2009). Monoaminergic neurotransmission: the history of the discovery of antidepressants from 1950s until today. *Current Pharmaceutical Design*, **15**(14), 1563–1586.

Mason, B., Brown, E., & Croarkin, P. (2016). Historical underpinnings of bipolar disorder diagnostic criteria. *Behavorial Science*, **6**(3), 14.

Miklowitz, D. J., et al. (2007). Psychosocial treatments for bipolar depression: a 1-year randomized trial from the Systematic Treatment Enhancement Program. *Archives of General Psychiatry*, **64**(4), 419–426.

Mitchell, P. B., & Hadzi-Pavlovic, D. (2000). Lithium treatment for bipolar disorder. Bulletin of the World Health Organization, **78**(4), 515–517.

Nierenberg, A. A., et al. (2006). Treatment-resistant bipolar depression: a STEP-BD equipoise randomized effectiveness trial of antidepressant augmentation with lamotrigine, inositol, or risperidone. *American Journal of Psychiatry*, **163**(2), 210–216.

Parikh, S. V., LeBlanc, S. R., & Ovanessian, M. M. (2010). Advancing bipolar disorder: key lessons from the Systematic Treatment Enhancement Program for Bipolar Disorder (STEP-BD). *Canadian Journal of Psychiatry*, **55**(3), 136–143.

Perlick, D.A., et al. (2007). Prevalence and correlates of burden among caregivers of patients with bipolar disorder enrolled in the Systematic Treatment Enhancement Program for Bipolar Disorder. *Bipolar Disorder*, **9**(3), 262–273.

Pope, H. G., McElroy, S. L., Keck, E., & Hudson, J. I. (1991). Valproate in the treatment of acute mania: a placebo-controlled study. *Archives of General Psychiatry*, **48**(1), 62–68.

Post, R. M., & Uhde, T. W. (1983). Treatment of mood disorders with antiepileptic medications: clinical and theoretical implications. *Epilepsia*, **24**(Suppl 2), S97–108.

Rush, A. J., et al. (2004). Sequenced treatment alternatives to relieve depression (STAR*D): rationale and design. *Controlled Clinical Trials*, **25**(1), 119–142.

Rush, A. J., et al. (2006). Acute and longer-term outcomes in depressed outpatients requiring one or several treatment steps: a STAR*D report. *American Journal of Psychiatry*, **163**(11), 1905–1917.

Sachs, G. S., et al. (2003). Rationale, design, and methods of the systematic treatment enhancement program for bipolar disorder (STEP-BD). *Biological Psychiatry*, **53**(11), 1028–1042.

Sachs. G. S., et al. (2007). Effectiveness of adjunctive antidepressant treatment for bipolar depression. *New England Journal of Medicine*, **356**(17), 1711–1722.

Schildkraut, J. J. (1965). The catecholamine hypothesis of affective disorders: a review of supporting evidence. *American Journal of Psychiatry*, **122**(5), 509–522.

Schou, M., Juel-Nielsen, N., Strömgren, E., & Voldby, H. (1954). The treatment of manic psychoses by the administration of lithium salts. *Journal of Neurology, Neurosurgery and Psychiatry*, **17**(4), 250.

Shaw, D. M., Camps, F. E., & Eccleston, E. G. (1967). 5-Hydroxytryptamine in the hind-brain of depressive suicides. *British Journal of Psychiatry*, **113**(505), 1407–1411.

Shorter, E. (2009). The history of lithium therapy. *Bipolar Disorder*, **11**, 4–9.

Strakowski, S. M. (2007). Approaching the challenge of bipolar depression: results from STEP-BD. *American Journal of Psychiatry*, **164**(9):1301–1303.

Teller, E., & Brown, A. (1975). *The Legacy of Hiroshima*. Westport, Conn.: Greenwood Press.

Trivedi, M. H., et al. (2006). Evaluation of outcomes with citalopram for depression using measurement-based care in STAR*D: implications for clinical practice. *American Journal of Psychiatry*, 163(1), 28–40.

Wenthur, C. J., Bennett, M. R., & Lindsley, C. W. (2014). Classics in chemical neuroscience: fluoxetine (Prozac). *ACS Chemical Neuroscience*, **5**(1), 14–23.

Wong, D. T., Perry, K. W., & Bymaster, F. P. (2005). Case history: the discovery of fluoxetine hydrochloride (Prozac). *Nature Reviews Drug Discovery*, **4**(9), 764–774.

Chapter 9

Pharmacotherapy of anxiety and related disorders

Dan J. Stein

Introduction

Anxiolytic agents have been used since the dawn of mankind. However, the rigorous use of randomized clinical trials (RCTs) of medications for the pharmacotherapy of anxiety and related disorders is a relatively recent development. This chapter discusses six RCTs that have contributed significantly to the development of the field, including work on generalized anxiety disorder, panic disorder, obsessive-compulsive disorder, and social anxiety disorder. Any such list is necessarily incomplete; these selections may however shed light on early and ongoing challenges in the field and key advances to date.

An immediate question is the optimal classification of anxiety disorders, and there has been an ongoing conversation between nosologists and psychopharmacologists interested in anxiety disorders. Indeed, the first paper discussed here was published in 1964 and provides data from a RCT on panic disorder by Donald Klein (1964), who introduced the notion of 'pharmacological dissection' (that the differential response of mental disorders to psychotropics sheds light on nosological differences) (Klein, 1987). Klein subsequently played a key role in developing the anxiety disorders chapter in the third edition of the *Diagnostic and Statistical Manual of Mental Disorders* (DSM-III) in 1980 (Spitzer et al., 1980), a chapter that carefully delineates panic disorder.

The second paper, published by Joseph Zohar and Thomas Insel in 1987, also contributes to this notion of psychopharmacological dissection by emphasizing that whereas various conditions respond to serotonergic and adrenergic antidepressants, obsessive-compulsive disorder (OCD) responds selectively to serotonin reuptake inhibitors (SRIs), such as clomipramine (Zohar & Insel, 1987). During the development of the DSM-5, data that the neural circuitry and pharmacological response of OCD differ from that of other anxiety disorders contributed to the decision to move OCD out of the chapter on anxiety disorders (Stein et al., 2014). Still, anxiety disorders, obsessive-compulsive and related disorders, and trauma- and stressor-related disorders are listed in adjacent chapters, given their overlap.

The development of operational criteria for anxiety disorders in DSM-III and subsequent DSM editions was crucial in providing reliable inclusion criteria for RCTs; this point is exemplified in the third paper by Michael Liebowitz and colleagues (1992) on social anxiety disorder (SAD) and in the fourth paper by Karl Rickels and colleagues (1993) on generalized anxiety disorder (GAD). In addition, these operational criteria provided important impetus for rigorous epidemiological studies of the prevalence of these conditions. During the past two to three decades it has become clear that anxiety disorders are the most prevalent of the mental disorders throughout the world, and that they are associated with a significant burden of disease (Stein et al., 2017).

The introduction of benzodiazepines was a particularly important advance in the pharmacotherapy of anxiety disorders; despite the drawbacks of these agents, they are fast-acting anxiolytics and safer than a number of older medications (e.g. barbiturates). The demonstration that tricyclic agents and monoamine oxidase inhibitors are effective for particular anxiety disorders was another important step forward. Taken together, the papers by Liebowitz and Rickels provide comparisons between the benzodiazepines and the antidepressants, as well as comparisons of these agents with older medications such as beta-blockers.

A number of subsequent additional advances in the pharmacotherapy of anxiety and related disorders are noteworthy. The introduction of selective serotonin reuptake inhibitors (SSRIs) for the treatment of anxiety disorders has been useful; while these agents may not be more efficacious than older antidepressants, they are better tolerated (Baldwin et al., 2014). A broad range of publications has established the efficacy and safety of SSRIs in GAD, panic disorder, OCD, SAD, and post-traumatic stress disorder. The paper by Lewis Baxter and colleagues, also published in the early 1990s, provides data on the SSRI fluoxetine in OCD and is the fifth paper discussed in this chapter (Baxter et al., 1992). It also made a seminal contribution by using brain imaging to shed light on the mechanisms underlying the effects of pharmacotherapy and psychotherapy, and gave impetus to a range of subsequent work in this area (Brooks & Stein, 2015).

The discovery of the efficacy of tricyclic antidepressants, monoamine oxidase inhibitors, and SSRIs for anxiety and related disorders has led to a wealth of research on the role of monoamine neurotransmitter systems in these conditions. In more recent years, however, investigators have attempted to find new molecular entities that target additional receptors. This work has in turn relied on experimental systems which allow the study of psychobiological processes (e.g. fear conditioning and extinction) across species; a so-called translational neuroscience approach that Thomas Insel has played a key role in promoting (Insel & Quirion, 2005; Insel et al., 2010). The last paper, by Kerry Ressler and colleagues (2004), provides 'proof of principle' of this strategy. The chapter concludes with a discussion of key unanswered questions.

The 'pharmacological dissection' of panic disorder

Main citation

Klein, D. F. (1964). Delineation of two drug-responsive anxiety syndromes. *Psychopharmacologia*, 5, 397–408.

Background

The 1950s and 1960s were a golden age of serendipitous discoveries in psychopharmacology. Tricyclic antidepressants and monoamine oxidase inhibitors (MAOIs) were shown to have positive impacts on mood in depressed patients, while antipsychotic agents were introduced for the treatment of schizophrenia. Rigorous clinical observations also supported a view that antidepressant agents might be useful in patients with phobic or anxiety symptoms. This paper draws on a large RCT of imipramine versus chlorpromazine versus placebo in patients with a range of diagnoses. In so doing, it provides a seminal description of panic disorder and its response to imipramine.

Methods

The data in this paper are drawn from a double-blind RCT of imipramine versus chlorpromazine (administered with procyclidine to counteract extrapyramidal symptoms) versus placebo. One hundred and sixty-eight patients with different diagnoses began medication; these diagnoses included schizophrenia, affective disorders (including those with phobic and anxiety symptoms), and character disorders. A number of measures, including the Lorr Multidimensional Scale for Rating Psychiatric Patients and the Clyde Mood Scale, were administered before medication and five weeks later. This paper describes in more detail 14 of the patients with phobic and anxiety symptoms; they had been randomly assigned to imipramine ($n = 7$), chlorpromazine ($n = 1$), and placebo ($n = 6$).

Results

On the Mann-Whitney U test, comparison of measures in the imipramine group versus the placebo group found that the medication was accompanied by significantly greater reductions in angry demands, melancholy agitation, motor disturbances, affective distress, pain, and cardio-respiratory somatic symptoms. There were no differences between drug and placebo on the Clyde Mood Scale. A retrospective global clinical impression scale supported the efficacy of imipramine.

In the paper, Klein also gave details of his clinical experience with a case series of additional patients who presented with sudden onset of episodic panic and resultant constriction of activities. He noted that taken together, in 28 of 32 patients, imipramine or MAOIs led to alleviation of panic attacks, but that during long-term follow-up medication termination was often followed by symptomatic exacerbation. He also noted that chlorpromazine was associated with symptom exacerbation rather than relief.

On the basis of careful clinical history and examination, Klein delineated two clinical subgroups of patients with panic attacks. The first group had a chronically high level of separation anxiety from childhood and developed panic attacks under conditions of separation or bereavement. The second group had unremarkable developmental histories and developed attacks in a context of altered endocrine functions (e.g. oophorectomy, hysterectomy, post-partum, pre-partum).

Conclusions and critique

Klein's paper was key in demonstrating that imipramine is useful for panic disorder (although this term is not used in the publication). There have been many advances in the conduct of RCTs for anxiety disorders since this work. Nowadays, best practice includes registration and publication of a protocol, obtaining institutional review board approval, appropriately powered sample sizes, use of well-validated standardized symptom measures, following careful Consolidated Standards of Reporting Trials (CONSORT) guidelines for reporting of data, rigorous analysis of a prespecified outcome measure, and making data publicly available for further exploration and inclusion in meta-analysis. Such practices emerged gradually, based on solid foundational work such as Klein's.

Also, nowadays, a team of clinician-scientists might work on a set of related studies, with papers emerging on short-term outcomes, a longer-term discontinuation study, and associated biological studies. It is refreshing and inspiring to read a single paper which brings together rich clinical experience, a RCT, as well as biologically informed observations. Given the current translational neuroscience emphasis, as exemplified in the Research Domain Criteria (RDoC) framework (see Chapter 1), on undertaking clinical science across different diagnoses (Insel et al., 2010), it is humbling to note that this is precisely what was done here. Similarly, a key conceptual conclusion—that patterns of drug response may allow a more refined understanding of psychiatric subpopulations—foreshadows current emphases on personalized medicine.

It is essential to consider, however, whether Klein's key idea of pharmacological dissection was correct. With regards to panic disorder, it turns out that a wide range of different medications, with quite different mechanisms of action, lead to symptom reduction. On the other hand, in other disorders, such as OCD, as discussed next, more selective treatment responses arguably continue to be seen. Indeed, the idea that drug response patterns are important continues to be influential. For example, there do seem to be key differences in symptom response patterns to effective drugs and to placebo—a set of work that was initiated by Klein's group (Quitkin et al., 1991). Similarly, there are ongoing efforts to understand differences between early and later responses to pharmacotherapy (Stein et al., 2009).

Furthermore, a key idea in Klein's paper—that neurobiological characteristics influence treatment outcomes—remains central to efforts in translational neuroscience and personalized medicine. Klein related his findings to John Bowlby's work on the biological function of separation anxiety; he subsequently went on to develop a range of creative approaches to conceptualizing panic disorder and its subtypes, instigating a range of empirical work (Klein, 1993; Preter & Klein, 2014). Still, pharmacotherapy agents have diverse effects and responses to these agents are multi-factorial and polygenic; complexity should not be underestimated (Stein, 2014). Such complexity continues to bedevil contemporary pharmacogenomics; a recent review indicated that genetic testing is not yet useful for predicting outcomes in psychiatric practice (Bousman & Hopwood, 2016). Subtyping disorders continues to be a key aspiration, but here too complexity abounds, with such work only occasionally having clear clinical utility.

Selective response of obsessive-compulsive disorder to serotonin reuptake inhibitors

Main citation

Zohar, J., & Insel, T. R. (1987). Obsessive-compulsive disorder: psychobiological approaches to diagnosis, treatment, and pathophysiology. *Biological Psychiatry*, 22, 667–687.

Background

Although DSM-III included OCD in the chapter on anxiety disorders, this was considered a relatively rare and treatment-refractory disorder. Many clinicians were influenced by psychoanalytical literature which framed OCD in terms of unconscious conflicts. During the 1980s, research undertaken by Insel, Zohar, and others led to a remarkable shift, in which OCD became viewed as a neuropsychiatric disorder, characterized by alterations in specific neuronal circuitry and selective responsiveness to specific pharmacotherapy (Stein, 2002).

Methods

This paper included studies of biological markers of depression (e.g. dexamethasone suppression test (DST), rapid eye movement (REM) latency and density on sleep electroencephalogram, platelet serotonin uptake, platelet ^{3}H-imipramine binding, cerebrospinal fluid 5-hydroxy-indoleacetic-acid) in OCD, a 'pharmacological challenge' study, as well as a RCT.

In the pharmacological challenge, eight adult outpatients who met DSM-III criteria for OCD were administered meta-chlorophenylpiperazine (m-CPP, a serotonergic agonist), metergoline (a serotonergic antagonist), and placebo, on separate days, under double-blind conditions, and OCD symptoms and mood states were then rated during the next few hours.

The RCT comprised a crossover trial in 14 adult outpatients who met DSM-III criteria for OCD, with illness duration of at least one year, with Global-OC rating of least 6 (1–15 scale), and with comorbidity limited to mild secondary depression. The trial compared clomipramine (a serotonergic tricyclic) with desipramine (a noradrenergic tricyclic). Medication was initiated at 50 mg/day and increased at a rate of 50 mg every two days, until a maximum dose of 300 mg/day. Medication was prescribed for six weeks, followed by four weeks on placebo, and then crossover to the alternate drug for six weeks. Several observer rating scales were administered each week.

Results

Biological findings in OCD resembled those found in depression on some measures (e.g. DST, REM latency), but not on others (e.g. REM density, platelet serotonin reuptake, probably platelet ^{3}H-impramine binding, 5-hydroxy-indoleacetic acid); m-CPP (0.5 mg/kg) was found to acutely exacerbate OCD symptoms. The peak response was found in the first three hours after m-CPP administration and was accompanied by anxiety, depression, dysphoria, and 'altered self-reality'. The effects of metergoline on obsessive-compulsive symptoms were generally far less pronounced, but with a decrease noted on one measure.

In the crossover trial, clomipramine (mean dose 235 mg/day) was found to be superior to desipramine (mean dose 290 mg/day) in reducing OCD symptoms, with significance reached at both weeks four and six. On the Comprehensive Psychiatric Rating Scale (Obsessive-Compulsive Subscale), the mean improvement during clomipramine treatment was 28.4%, compared to 4.2% for desipramine. Of ten completers, one patient responded better to desipramine than clomipramine, one patient showed equal response to both drugs, and eight demonstrated a superior response to clomipramine.

Conclusions and critique

This work, suggesting only partial overlap of biological measures in OCD and MDD, worsening of OCD after exposure to a serotonin agonist, and a more robust response of symptoms to a SRI than to a noradrenergic agent, was key for a number of reasons. In general, it provided a foundation for differentiating the neurobiology and pharmacotherapy of OCD from that of major depression, which responds to both SRIs and desipramine. More specifically, it helped develop the so-called serotonin hypothesis of OCD. This in turn advanced clinical practice and research on obsessive-compulsive and related disorders.

From a clinical perspective, it turned out that not only OCD, but also a range of disorders with overlapping phenomenology and psychobiology responded selectively to SRIs (Stein, 2000; Phillips et al., 2010). Like OCD, for example, body dysmorphic disorder, which is characterized by a preoccupation with flawed appearance and consequent rituals, responds better to clomipramine than to desipramine (Hollander et al., 1999). Taken together with growing awareness of the prevalence of these conditions, the introduction of effective pharmatherapies was a major step forward in their management.

Furthermore, this initial work laid the foundation for a great deal of subsequent neurobiological research; the use of brain imaging to explore changes in response to a SSRI and to cognitive-behavioural therapy in OCD is discussed later in this chapter. The field continues to emphasize the importance of the serotonin system in this condition, expanding on this foundation to also consider the role of other alterations, including in the dopaminergic and glutamatergic systems (Kariuki-Nyuthe et al., 2014; Goodman et al., 1992). A range of publications on different SSRIs has emerged, and these continue to be viewed as the first-line pharmacotherapy for OCD, with dopaminergic and glutamatergic agents used for augmentation (Baldwin et al., 2014; Fineberg et al., 2015).

At the same time, the possibility that any common mental disorder is linked to a single specific neurotransmitter across the clinical population seems increasingly remote. In rare cases, specific serotonergic genetic variants may be linked to OCD and other symptoms (Ozaki et al., 2003), but genome-wide association studies of OCD populations have not yielded 'serotonergic hits' (Stewart et al., 2013). Instead, OCD appears to be a polygenic disorder, involving a broad range of genetic risk factors that overlap with those of other mental disorders. The seminal observation of an association between streptococcus and OCD has, analogously, been replaced with an emphasis on a range of environmental insults (Singer et al., 2012). The specificity of disruptions in the neural circuitry of OCD has also been brought into question (Boedhoe et al., 2017). At this stage of our understanding, the complexity of the relevant psychobiology is daunting.

Selective response of social anxiety disorder to monoamine oxidase inhibitors

Main citation

Liebowitz, M. R., et al. (1992). Phenelzine vs atenolol in social phobia: a placebo-controlled comparison. *Archives of General Psychiatry*, 49, 290–300.

Background

While clinicians had long recognized different types of anxiety disorders, the growing awareness of their prevalence, the DSM-III diagnostic criteria, and the availability of new medications all gave impetus to new research. Isaac Marks, a key pioneer, had emphasized the clinical importance of social anxiety in the 1960s (Marks, 1970). Still, research on this particular condition began slowly and, in the 1980s, Michael Liebowitz and colleagues, including Donald Klein, categorized social phobia as a neglected disorder (Liebowitz et al., 1985). They also noted the rationale for studying MAOIs in SAD, including the overlap between SAD and atypical depression (which they had found to respond selectively to these agents).

Methods

Subjects met DSM-III criteria for social phobia, were aged 18–50, and had no comorbid depression or substance abuse. After a one-week placebo run-in, patients were randomized to an eight-week trial comparing phenelzine, atenolol, or placebo. Phenelzine was initiated at 15 mg/d and increased to 60 mg/d by day 15, with an option to increase to 90 mg/d after five weeks. Atenolol was initiated at 50 mg/day and raised to 100 mg/d if tolerated after two weeks. After eight weeks, all those who improved minimally or better entered an eight-week maintenance phase with the same treatments. At the end of week 16, responders to phenelzine or atenolol were randomly assigned to continue medication or to switch to placebo for four weeks. Rating scales during the acute, maintenance, and discontinuation phases included the Liebowitz Social Anxiety Scale (LSAS), and responders were defined as those with a Clinical Global Impression Scale change score of 1 or 2.

Results

One hundred and seventeen patients were entered into the study, and 85 were randomized to treatment. At week 8, response rates were significantly higher for phenelzine (64%) than for both atenolol (30%) and placebo (23%). There were minimal changes between week 8 and week 16 scores, and at week 16 response rates remained significantly higher for phenelzine (52%) than for placebo (19%), with the atenolol response rate (43%) not differing significantly from either phenelzine or placebo. Scores on clinician-rated measures, such as the LSAS, supported these findings at week 8 and 16. Although there was an indication that switching phenelzine responders to placebo led to relapse, the sample size in the discontinuation phase was too small to allow statistical analysis. Findings appeared similar in the smaller group of patients with discrete SAD, and phenelzine also decreased symptoms of avoidant personality disorder.

Conclusions and critique

This RCT provided a firm foundation for the subsequent pharmacotherapy of SAD. It helped raise awareness of SAD and its pharmacotherapy, it provided key elements of strong clinical trial design (e.g. use of standardized symptom severity measures, use of maintenance and relapse prevention analyses), and it set out a number of key questions for future work (e.g. differential response of generalized versus discrete SAD, response of avoidant personality disorder symptoms to pharmacotherapy) (Stein et al., 2004). The introduction of reversible MAOs such as moclobemide was a key next clinical step, but trials were inconsistent and these agents were not approved in the USA (Ipser et al., 2008). A focus on MAOIs in SAD also led to interesting hypotheses about the neurobiology of social anxiety disorder, with Liebowitz and colleagues speculating that the dopaminergic system played a particularly important role in this disorder and in atypical depression.

The subsequent introduction of the SSRIs, with their advantageous safety profile, changed clinical practice and relegated MAOIs to second- or third-line agents in SAD (Baldwin et al., 2014). The larger sample sizes in the SSRI studies also allowed robust relapse prevention analyses (Stein et al., 2002). The introduction of these agents continued to spur interest in the psychobiology of SAD, and a range of neuroimaging and neurogenetic studies of SAD have emerged in recent decades (Hattingh et al., 2012). Indeed, there has been a good deal of progress in delineating the translational neuroscience of social anxiety disorder, with the development of productive links between laboratory studies and clinical research (Fox & Kalin, 2014).

As in the case of panic disorder and OCD, however, it must be acknowledged that much remains to be understood about both the neurobiology and pharmacotherapy of SAD. Informative biological findings have not yielded a specific diagnostic signature; this is perhaps unsurprising given that social anxiety falls on a spectrum from normal/adaptive to dysfunctional/maladaptive (Stein & Bouwer, 1997). Further, while pharmacotherapy is often efficacious, a significant minority of patients are unresponsive to first-line treatments. Explanatory trials conducted in academic settings focus on SAD without comorbidity, but in clinical practice many patients have comorbid substance use disorders, depression, or other conditions, which further impact negatively on treatment outcomes.

Pharmacotherapy of generalized anxiety disorder

Main citation

Rickels, K., Downing, R., Schweizer, E., & Hassman, H. (1993). Antidepressants for the treatment of generalized anxiety disorder: a placebo-controlled comparison of imipramine, trazodone, and diazepam. *Archives of General Psychiatry*, 50, 884–895.

Background

GAD is the most common anxiety disorder in primary care practice. However, psychiatrists rarely see patients with non-comorbid GAD: this reflects the epidemiological finding that GAD is often followed by onset of a range of mood and other disorders, so that by the time individuals present for treatment they have substantial comorbidity (Kessler et al., 2001). Karl Rickels and colleagues have done the field a major service by recruiting patients with GAD, and without comorbidities, for pharmacological trials. Given the availability of both benzodiazepines and antidepressants, a rigorous comparison of their efficacy and safety was key for the field.

Methods

This RCT compared imipramine (up to 200 mg/d) versus trazodone (up to 400 mg/d) versus diazepam (up to 40 mg/d) versus placebo in the treatment of GAD. Two hundred and thirty adult outpatients with a DSM-III diagnosis of GAD, in whom major depression and panic disorder had been excluded and who had a Hamilton Anxiety Scale (HAM-A) total score of at least 18, were included in the study. Seventy-five percent of patients were treated in family practice settings in the community. A range of assessments were used, including the HAM-A.

Results

During the first two weeks of the trial, those treated with diazepam showed the most improvement in anxiety ratings, particularly somatic symptoms. From week three through to week eight, trazodone achieved comparable efficacy and imipramine somewhat better efficacy when compared with diazepam, particularly with regards to psychic symptoms. Predictor analyses did not find specific sociodemographic or clinical predictors (e.g. baseline symptom severity, duration of illness, prior psychotropic therapy) of response to treatment.

In completers, moderate to marked improvement was found in 73% of patients treated with imipramine, 69% of patients treated with trazodone, and 66% of patients treated with diazepam; all significantly higher than the 47% of patients treated with placebo. Individuals treated with antidepressants reported a higher rate of adverse effects than patients treated with diazepam, but retention rates were the same across all treatment arms.

Conclusions and critique

This trial was important in showing that although benzodiazepines have the advantage of decreasing anxiety symptoms in the short term, antidepressants are efficacious for GAD over the longer haul. Benzodiazepines remain one of the most widely prescribed classes of medication. This reflects their significant advantages: they are rapidly acting and they significantly reduce anxiety symptoms. At the same time, there are important concerns. Once a patient has been on benzodiazepine treatment, discontinuation is not entirely straightforward. Furthermore, there are significant adverse events associated with benzodiazepines, particularly in the elderly (Baldwin et al., 2014).

Antidepressants are commonly endorsed as the first-line pharmacotherapy for anxiety disorders such as GAD (Baldwin et al., 2014). This work builds on the foundation laid by early work such as this trial by Rickels and colleagues. The introduction of SSRIs, with their superior safety profile, has meant that these are typically prioritized, while older agents are considered second- or third-line agents. Newer antidepressants such as agomelatine may offer specific advantages (e.g. fewer adverse events) (Stein et al., 2014). A range of other agents have also been introduced (e.g. atypical antipsychotics and pregabalin), but have not replaced the SSRIs (Baldwin et al., 2014).

Many questions remain for the field. A key one is whether early intervention for GAD is efficacious for the prevention of subsequent comorbidity. There is some preliminary evidence for such a view (Goodwin & Gorman, 2002). Current dogma is that a better understanding of the pathophysiology of GAD and other conditions will lead to new treatment targets and ultimately to better pharmacotherapies. Given that so many innovations have been serendipitous, and that systematic biological research has led to relatively few significant 'breakthroughs', it is sometimes difficult to maintain optimism in this view. However, a 'proof of principle' study that encourages some optimism will be presented in the section 'A translational neuroscience approach to anxiety and related disorders'.

Pharmacotherapy and psychotherapy alter brain function in obsessive-compulsive disorder

Main citation

Baxter Jr, L. R., et al. (1992). Caudate glucose metabolic rate changes with both drug and behavior therapy for obsessive-compulsive disorder. *Archives of General Psychiatry*, 49, 681–689.

Background

Given the efficacy of SRIs for many anxiety and related disorders, an immediate question relates to their mechanism of action. Although the SRIs have very specific actions on the serotonin transporter, they also have complex downstream actions, likely affecting multiple pathways and proteins. Brain imaging provides one way of exploring the mechanism of action of these medications, particularly at the circuitry level. Furthermore, brain imaging can be used to determine whether medication and cognitive behavioural therapy (CBT)—the other first-line intervention for many anxiety and related disorders (see Chapter 12)—impact neural circuitry in similar or dissimilar ways, or whether baseline imaging or changes in imaging predict treatment response.

Methods

Twenty adults with OCD were recruited from inpatient and outpatient settings at one institution. Diagnoses were based on DSM-III-R criteria. A small group of normal control subjects ($n = 4$) were also studied. OCD subjects were rated with the Yale-Brown Obsessive-Compulsive Scale (Y-BOCS). Responders to treatment were defined *a priori* as those who were rated as either 'much improved' or 'very much improved' on item 18 of the Y-BOCS (which is taken from the Clinical Global Impression Scale) at the end of the treatment trial.

Patients were allowed to choose between two treatment options: fluoxetine (an SSRI) or behaviour therapy. Ten patients were included in each group, but only nine were suitable for inclusion in the analysis. Patients in the fluoxetine group were started at 20 mg/d and titrated within two weeks to 60 to 80 mg/d, as tolerated. In patients who chose to have behaviour therapy, this consisted of exposure and response prevention, individualized for the patient. These exercises were facilitated by cognitive techniques. Patients met once or twice a week with their therapist, for approximately one hour, to review homework assignments.

Positron emission tomography (PET) of OCD patients was undertaken before treatment and after ten weeks (plus or minus two weeks) of treatment. All subjects were injected with [^{18}F]-fluorodeoxyglucose while in the supine position. The subjects' ears and eyes were open, and they were instructed to look at the white ceiling above the tomograph. Scanning was performed with a PET tomograph. Fifteen transverse sections of the brain were acquired simultaneously. For each subject, an average local cerebral metabolic rate for glucose value (LCMRGlc) was determined for each structure. Structures were chosen for analysis based on existing hypotheses about the neuroanatomy of OCD.

Results

LCMRG1c in the right head of the caudate nucleus divided by that in the ipsilateral hemisphere (Cd/hem) decreased in responders to treatment with either fluoxetine or psychotherapy. Decreases were significantly greater in responders than in non-responders and in normal controls, where there were no changes from baseline. Changes in OCD symptom severity were significantly associated with brain-imaging changes in medication therapy, and tended towards significance in behaviour therapy. Taken together, responders to either fluoxetine or behaviour therapy showed significant correlations between orbital cortex/hem and Cd/hem and thalamus/hem before treatment, but not after.

Conclusions and critique

These data provide a number of seminal insights into OCD and its treatment. In particular, they suggest that a specific neurocircuit, the fronto-striatal-thalamic circuit, is involved in OCD and is impacted by treatment. Second, they suggest that both pharmacotherapy and psychotherapy alter this circuit. Third, they point the way to future work that predicts which individuals might respond to pharmacotherapy versus psychotherapy.

This work continues to influence the field of anxiety and related disorders. Many subsequent studies have explored the impact of pharmacotherapy and of psychotherapy on brain imaging (Brooks & Stein, 2015). Taken together, this work has indicated that different neurocircuits underlie different anxiety and related disorders, and that although interventions are somewhat similar across these conditions, they generally act to normalize specific abnormalities that characterize different entities (Stein, 2006).

That said, many questions remain unresolved. Brain imaging remains a relatively blunt tool, with limited spatial resolution and often poor temporal resolution, and the exact nature of the abnormalities in OCD and other conditions remains ill-defined (Weinberger & Radulescu, 2016). While the research has certainly been informative, brain-imaging data remain insufficiently specific and sensitive to be useful in clinical practice. Imaging-genetic data are gradually emerging, but these may serve to further complicate matters insofar as they emphasize that brain volumes, like other phenotypes, are subject to multifactorial and polygenic influences (Mufford et al., 2017).

A translational neuroscience approach to anxiety and related disorders

Main citation

Ressler, K. J., et al. (2004). Cognitive enhancers as adjuncts to psychotherapy: use of D-cycloserine in phobic individuals to facilitate extinction of fear. *Archives of General Psychiatry*, 61, 1136–1144.

Background

As noted earlier, many experts hold that in order to develop fundamentally novel interventions for mental disorders, a translational neuroscience perspective is key (Insel & Quirion, 2005; Insel et al., 2010). In the case of anxiety and related disorders, including post-traumatic stress disorder, experimental systems that allow the study of fear conditioning and extinction may be particularly valuable (Dias et al., 2013). A wealth of data on the involvement of different neural circuits and neurotransmitter systems in fear conditioning and extinction has been rigorously gathered. In key work, it was found that D-cycloserine, a partial glutamatergic agonist, was able to facilitate fear extinction (Walker et al., 2002). In this seminal translational RTC, D-cycloserine was added to CBT for individuals with specific phobia.

Methods

This RTC examined D-cycloserine versus placebo treatment in the augmentation of exposure therapy. Twenty-eight subjects who met DSM-IV criteria for a specific phobia and who had acrophobia symptoms were enrolled. Subjects were treated with two sessions of behavioural exposure therapy using virtual-reality exposure. D-cycloserine (50 mg) or placebo was administered prior to each of the two sessions. Symptoms were assessed by self-report and by independent assessors prior to treatment and approximately one week and three months post-treatment. Included were measures of acrophobia within the virtual environment, measures of acrophobia in the real world, and general measures of overall improvement. An objective measure of fear, electrodermal skin fluctuation, was also included during the virtual exposure to heights.

Results

Compared to placebo, D-cycloserine resulted in significantly larger reductions of acrophobia symptoms on all main outcome measures, with significantly more improvement within the virtual environment (one week after treatment, $p \leq 0.001$; three months later, $p \leq 0.05$). Subjects receiving D-cycloserine also showed significantly greater decreases in post-treatment skin conductance fluctuations during the virtual exposure ($p \leq 0.05$). Furthermore, subjects receiving D-cycloserine had significantly greater improvement on general measures of real-world acrophobia, clinical global improvement, and number of self-exposures to real-world heights; the improvement was evident early in treatment and was maintained at three months.

Conclusions and critique

This study provides an important 'proof of principle' for the value of a translational neuroscience approach; not merely for anxiety and related disorders, but for psychiatry as a whole. It is remarkable that basic discoveries, based on a solid experimental system for understanding the mechanisms of fear extinction, led to a new therapeutic target, and that this in turn was effectively translated into the clinical setting. A range of promising work in this area has subsequently been undertaken. This includes work not only on D-cycloserine, but also on other pharmacotherapies that may be useful in augmenting psychotherapy.

Further work is needed both to advance the relevant research and to determine the clinical applicability of these sorts of intervention. From a research perspective, not all data have been consistent: this may reflect differences in D-cycloserine activity across disorders, differences in timing and dosing of this agent, or a range of other methodological issues. Further studies are needed to fully delineate and address these issues.

From a clinical perspective, further work seems needed before D-cycloserine and other augmenting pharmacotherapies can be routinely recommended. A Cochrane Review, for example, emphasized the inconsistencies in the findings to date (Ori et al., 2015). On the other hand, a meta-analysis of individualized data led to a more positive view of the existing literature, noting a small treatment effect (Mataix-Cole et al., 2017). Certainly, taken together, this work lays the foundation for future employment of augmentation pharmacotherapy interventions together with CBT.

Conclusion

This chapter has described six landmark papers on the pharmacological treatment of anxiety and related disorders. These papers have not only established treatments for key disorders, but they have also helped elucidate important nosological and pathophysiological principles. That said, many pharmacotherapy questions remain unresolved. Furthermore, the chapter has been able to focus on only a few anxiety and related disorders, neglecting important conditions such as post-traumatic stress disorder. To close the chapter, three key questions for future work in the pharmacotherapy of anxiety and related disorders are outlined.

First, there continues to be some uncertainty about the best approach to evaluating and assessing anxiety symptoms. The DSM and ICD systems provide a symptoms-based approach, which has clear utility in clinical practice. RDoC provides a translational neuroscience approach, which may be more informative in research settings. The incorporation of data from ecological momentary assessment measures, or other digital information including electronic medical records, may also be informative. In the interim, the use of a broad range of approaches and measures seems useful; ultimately a more uniform and focused approach may emerge, with the possible advantage of allowing better meta-analyses of different studies (Stein, 2014).

Second, much remains to be learned about the underlying psychobiology of anxiety and related disorders. Advances in neuroimaging and neurogenetics may prove key to finding new treatment targets. Certainly, advances in 'omic' technologies (e.g. genomics, proteomics) have been breathtaking, and it would be short-sighted to underestimate what might emerge in the next few decades of investigation. That said, biological explanations need to encompass both proximal mechanisms of this sort as well as distal mechanisms which address the evolutionary basis of cognitive-affective processes. Work, such as that done by Isaac Marks and Randolph Nesse (1994), reminds us of the adaptive value of anxiety symptoms and the possibility that, in some cases, the best treatment is no treatment (Frances & Clarkin, 1981).

Third, while many efficacious and safe first-line medications exist, data from real-world effectiveness trials are minimal, as are trials of more complex anxiety disorder patients (e.g. those with comorbidity). There remain questions about how best to scale-up treatment globally to ensure a closing of the treatment gap. In addition, much further work is needed on the pharmacotherapy of treatment-refractory patients and on a range of understudied populations (e.g. child and adolescent anxiety disorders, geriatric anxiety disorders). While the field waits for new treatment targets to emerge from translational neuroscience paradigms, a range of existing molecules are available for trials, and, given the burden of anxiety and related disorders, the study of such agents should be strongly encouraged.

References

Baldwin, D. S., et al. (2014). Evidence-based pharmacological treatment of anxiety disorders, post-traumatic stress disorder and obsessive-compulsive disorder: a revision of the 2005 guidelines from the British Association for Psychopharmacology. *Journal of Psychopharmacology*, **28**, 403–439. doi:10.1177/0269881114525674

Baxter Jr, L. R., et al. (1992). Caudate glucose metabolic rate changes with both drug and behavior therapy for obsessive-compulsive disorder. *Archives of General Psychiatry*, **49**, 681–689.

Boedhoe, P. S., et al. (2017). Distinct subcortical volume alterations in pediatric and adult OCD: a worldwide meta- and mega-analysis. *American Journal of Psychiatry*, **174**, 60–69. doi:10.1176/appi.ajp.2016.16020201

Bousman, C. A., & **Hopwood, M.** (2016). Commercial pharmacogenetic-based decision-support tools in psychiatry. *Lancet Psychiatry*, **3**, 585–590. doi:10.1016/S2215-0366(16)00017-1

Brooks, S. J., & **Stein, D. J.** (2015). A systematic review of the neural bases of psychotherapy for anxiety and related disorders. *Dialogues in Clinical Neuroscience*, **17**, 261–279.

Dias, B. G., **Banerjee, S. B.**, **Goodman, J. V.**, & **Ressler, K. J.** (2013). Towards new approaches to disorders of fear and anxiety. *Current Opinion in Neurobiology*, **23**, 346–352. doi:10.1016/j.conb.2013.01.013

Fineberg, N. A., et al. (2015). Obsessive-compulsive disorder (OCD): practical strategies for pharmacological and somatic treatment in adults. *Psychiatry Research*, **227**, 114–125. doi:10.1016/j.psychres.2014.12.003

Fox, A. S., & **Kalin, N. H.** (2014). A translational neuroscience approach to understanding the development of social anxiety disorder and its pathophysiology. *American Journal of Psychiatry*, **171**, 1162–1173. doi:10.1176/appi.ajp.2014.14040449

Frances, A., & **Clarkin, J. F.** (1981). No treatment as the prescription of choice. *Archives of General Psychiatry*, **38**, 542–545.

Goodman, W. K., **McDougle, C. J.**, & **Price, L. H.** (1992). The role of serotonin and dopamine in the pathophysiology of obsessive compulsive disorder. *International Clinical Psychopharmacology*, 7(Suppl 1), 35–38.

Goodwin, R. D., & **Gorman, J. M.** (2002). Psychopharmacologic treatment of generalized anxiety disorder and the risk of major depression. *American Journal of Psychiatry*, **159**, 1935–1937. doi:10.1176/appi.ajp.159.11.1935

Hattingh, C. J., et al. (2012). Functional magnetic resonance imaging during emotion recognition in social anxiety disorder: an activation likelihood meta-analysis. *Frontiers in Human Neuroscience*, **6**, 347. doi:10.3389/fnhum.2012.00347

Hollander, E., et al. (1999). Clomipramine vs desipramine crossover trial in body dysmorphic disorder: selective efficacy of a serotonin reuptake inhibitor in imagined ugliness. *Archives of General Psychiatry*, **56**, 1033–1039.

Insel, T. R., & **Quirion, R.** (2005). Psychiatry as a clinical neuroscience discipline. *Journal of the American Medical Association*, **294**, 2221–2224. doi:10.1001/jama.294.17.2221

Insel, T., et al. (2010). Research domain criteria (RDoC): toward a new classification framework for research on mental disorders. *American Journal of Psychiatry*, **167**, 748–751. doi:10.1176/appi.ajp.2010.09091379

Ipser, J. C., **Kariuki, C. M.**, & **Stein, D. J.** (2008). Pharmacotherapy for social anxiety disorder: a systematic review. *Expert Review of Neurotherapeutics*, **8**, 235–257. doi:10.1586/14737175.8.2.235

Kariuki-Nyuthe, C., Gomez-Mancilla, B., & Stein, D. J. (2014). Obsessive compulsive disorder and the glutamatergic system. *Current Opinion in Psychiatry*, **27**, 32–37. doi:10.1097/YCO.0000000000000017

Kessler, R. C., Keller, M. B., & Wittchen, H. U. (2001). The epidemiology of generalized anxiety disorder. *Psychiatric Clinics of North America*, **24**, 19–39.

Klein, D. F. (1964). Delineation of two drug-responsive anxiety syndromes. *Psychopharmacologia*, 5, 397–408.

Klein, D. F. (1987). Anxiety reconceptualized. Gleaning from pharmacological dissection–early experience with imipramine and anxiety. *Modern Problems of Pharmacopsychiatry*, **22**, 1–35.

Klein, D. F. (1993). False suffocation alarms, spontaneous panics, and related conditions. An integrative hypothesis. *Archives of General Psychiatry*, **50**, 306–317.

Liebowitz, M. R., et al. (1992). Phenelzine vs atenolol in social phobia: a placebo-controlled comparison. *Archives of General Psychiatry*, **49**, 290–300.

Liebowitz, M. R., Gorman, J. M., Fyer, A. J., & Klein, D. F. (1985). Social phobia: review of a neglected anxiety disorder. *Archives of General Psychiatry*, **42**, 729–736.

Marks, I. M. (1970). The classification of phobic disorders. *British Journal of Psychiatry*, **116**, 377–386.

Marks, I. M., & Nesse, R. M. (1994). Fear and fitness: an evolutionary analysis of anxiety disorders. *Ethology and Sociobiology*, **15**, 247–261.

Mataix-Cols, D., et al. (2017). D-cycloserine augmentation of exposure-based cognitive behavior therapy for anxiety, obsessive-compulsive, and posttraumatic stress disorders: a systematic review and meta-analysis. *Journal of the American Medical Association Psychiatry*, **74(5)**, 501–510. doi:10.1001/jamapsychiatry.2016.3955

Mufford, M. S., et al. (2017). Neuroimaging genomics in psychiatry—a translational approach. *Genome Medicine*, **9**, 102. doi:10.1186/s13073-017-0496-z

Ori, R., et al. (2015).Augmentation of cognitive and behavioural therapies (CBT) with d-cycloserine for anxiety and related disorders. *Cochrane Database of Systematic Reviews*, CD007803. doi:10.1002/14651858.CD007803.pub2

Ozaki, N., et al. (2003). Serotonin transporter missense mutation associated with a complex neuropsychiatric phenotype. *Molecular Psychiatry*, **8**, 933–936. doi:10.1038/sj.mp.4001365

Phillips, K. A., et al. (2010). Should an obsessive-compulsive spectrum grouping of disorders be included in DSM-V? *Depression and Anxiety*, **27**, 528–555. doi:10.1002/da.20705

Preter, M., & Klein, D. F. (2014). Lifelong opioidergic vulnerability through early life separation: a recent extension of the false suffocation alarm theory of panic disorder. *Neuroscience and Biobehavioral Reviews*, **46**(3), 345–351. doi:10.1016/j.neubiorev.2014.03.025

Quitkin, F. M., et al. (1991). Heterogeneity of clinical response during placebo treatment. *American Journal of Psychiatry*, **148**, 193–196. doi:10.1176/ajp.148.2.193

Ressler, K. J., et al. (2004). Cognitive enhancers as adjuncts to psychotherapy: use of D-cycloserine in phobic individuals to facilitate extinction of fear. *Archives of General Psychiatry*, **61**, 1136–1144. doi:10.1001/archpsyc.61.11.1136

Rickels, K., Downing, R., Schweizer, E., & Hassman, H. (1993). Antidepressants for the treatment of generalized anxiety disorder. A placebo-controlled comparison of imipramine, trazodone, and diazepam. *Archives of General Psychiatry*, **50**, 884–895.

Singer, H. S., Gilbert, D. L., Wolf, D. S., Mink, J. W., & Kurlan, R. (2012). Moving from PANDAS to CANS. *Journal of Pediatrics*, **160**, 725–731. doi:10.1016/j.jpeds.2011.11.040

Spitzer, R. L., Williams, J. B., & Skodol, A. E. (1980). DSM-III: the major achievements and an overview. *American Journal of Psychiatry*, **137**, 151–164. doi:10.1176/ajp.137.2.151

Stein, D. J. (2000). Neurobiology of the obsessive-compulsive spectrum disorders. *Biological Psychiatry*, 47, 296–304.

Stein, D. J. (2002). Obsessive-compulsive disorder. *Lancet*, **360**, 397–405. doi:10.1016/S0140-6736(02)09620-4

Stein, D. J. (2006). Advances in understanding the anxiety disorders: the cognitive-affective neuroscience of 'false alarms'. *Annals of Clinical Psychiatry*, **18**, 173–182. doi:10.1080/10401230600801192

Stein, D. J. (2014). An integrative approach to psychiatric diagnosis and research. *World Psychiatry*, **13**, 51–53. doi:10.1002/wps.20104

Stein, D. J., & Bouwer, C. (1997). A neuro-evolutionary approach to the anxiety disorders. *Journal of Anxiety Disorders*, **11**, 409–429.

Stein, D. J., Craske, M. A., Friedman, M. J., & Phillips, K. A. (2014). Anxiety disorders, obsessive-compulsive and related disorders, trauma- and stressor-related disorders, and dissociative disorders in DSM-5. *American Journal of Psychiatry*, **171**, 611–613. doi:10.1176/appi.ajp.2014.14010003

Stein, D. J., et al. (2009). Onset of activity and time to response on individual CAPS-SX17 items in patients treated for post-traumatic stress disorder with venlafaxine ER: a pooled analysis. *International Journal of Neuropsychopharmacology*, **12**, 23–31. doi:10.1017/S1461145708008961

Stein, D. J., Scott, K. M., de Jonge, P., & Kessler, R. C. (2017). Epidemiology of anxiety disorders: from surveys to nosology and back. *Dialogues in Clinical Neuroscience*, **19**, 127–136.

Stein, D., Ono, Y., Tajima, O., & Muller, J. E. (2004). The social anxiety disorder spectrum. *Journal of Clinical Psychiatry*, **65**, 27–33.

Stein, D., Versiani, M., Hair, T., & Kumar, R. (2002). Efficacy of paroxetine for relapse prevention in social anxiety disorder—a 24-week study. *Archives of General Psychiatry*, **59**, 1111–1118. doi:10.1001/archpsyc.59.12.1111

Stein, D. J., et al. (2014). Agomelatine in generalized anxiety disorder: an active comparator and placebo-controlled study. *Journal of Clinical Psychiatry*, **75(4)**, 362–368. doi:10.4088/JCP.13m08433

Stewart, S. E., et al. (2013). Genome-wide association study of obsessive-compulsive disorder. *Molecular Psychiatry*, **18**, 788–798. doi:10.1038/mp.2012.85

Walker, D. L., Ressler, K. J., Lu, K. T., & Davis, M. (2002). Facilitation of conditioned fear extinction by systemic administration or intra-amygdala infusions of D-cycloserine as assessed with fear-potentiated startle in rats. *Journal of Neuroscience*, **22**, 2343–2351.

Weinberger, D. R., & Radulescu, E. (2016). Finding the elusive psychiatric 'lesion' with 21st-century neuroanatomy: a note of caution. *American Journal of Psychiatry*, **173**, 27–33. doi:10.1176/appi.ajp.2015.15060753

Zohar, J., & Insel, T. R. (1987). Obsessive-compulsive disorder: psychobiological approaches to diagnosis, treatment, and pathophysiology. *Biological Psychiatry*, **22**, 667–687.

Chapter 10

Pharmacotherapy in child and adolescent psychiatry

Jenni E. Farrow, Francisco Romo-Nava, and Melissa DelBello

Introduction

The evolution of child and adolescent psychiatry is inextricably linked to changing views of child development. In the eighteenth century, behavioural problems were attributed to amorality and were viewed as deserving of punishment. Moreover, a child's brain was not considered developed enough to exhibit psychopathology. In the nineteenth century, Henry Maudsley's discussion of 'the insanity of early life' inspired a constitutional-hereditary approach to childhood psychiatric disorders, regarding them as static, with little prospect for successful treatment (Rey, 2015). By the early twentieth century, this view was challenged by Sigmund Freud's and Ivan Pavlov's demonstrations of how life experiences influence behaviours. Though psychoanalysis and behaviourism significantly contributed to child psychiatry, their emphasis on the first years of life encouraged an ideology of blame. The terms 'schizophrenogenic mother' and 'refrigerator mother' were commonly used to describe the aetiologies of schizophrenia and autism, respectively. Such unempirical and unidimensional explanations for childhood mental disorders slowed the scientific advancement of child and adolescent psychiatry.

As the 1950s progressed, increasing recognition of the interplay between biology and environment challenged psychoanalytical theory and encouraged implementation of psychopharmacological interventions (Chess, 1988). In 1967, the first National Institute for Mental Health (NIMH)-funded randomized controlled trial in child psychopharmacology demonstrated the efficacy of dextroamphetamine for what is now called attention deficit hyperactivity disorder (ADHD) (Eisenberg, 2007). Since, the growing role of pharmacotherapy has reflected a shift in the conceptualization of childhood psychiatric disorders as brain-based illnesses, which has encouraged research of evidence-based understanding, evaluation, and treatment of pediatric mental illness.

We review six psychopharmacology papers that shaped the prescribing landscape of child and adolescent psychiatry. We begin with the Multimodal Treatment Study of Children With ADHD (MTA), the first long-term trial to evaluate pediatric ADHD treatment. We then review the Treatment for Adolescents With Depression Study (TADS), the largest controlled youth depression outcome study, and the Treatment of Selective Serotonin Reuptake Inhibitor (SSRI)-Resistant Depression in Adolescents (TORDIA) study, the first clinical trial to evaluate depressed adolescents not responding to evidence-based treatment. Additionally, we evaluate the first comparative analysis of the efficacy and safety of second-generation antipsychotics and mood stabilizers in manic youth and adults, and the Child-Adolescent Anxiety Multimodal Study (CAMS), the largest randomized controlled trial of pediatric anxiety. Finally, we examine the US Food and Drug Administration's (FDA) 2004 meta-analysis, (which was not peer reviewed), that precipitated a black-box suicidality warning for antidepressants.

Comparing pharmacological, psychosocial, and combined treatments for children with attention-deficit/hyperactivity disorder

Main citation

MTA Cooperative Group. (1999). A 14-month randomized clinical trial of treatment strategies for attention-deficit/hyperactivity disorder. The MTA Cooperative Group. Multimodal Treatment Study of Children with ADHD. *Archives of General Psychiatry*, 56, 1073–1086.

Background

'ADHD' entered the official lexicon in 1980 with the third edition of the *Diagnostic and Statistical Manual of Mental Disorders* (DSM). Previously, 'brain-damaged child' was used to describe individuals exhibiting signs and symptoms now associated with ADHD; that phrase implied a brain-based aetiology that de-emphasized parental blame and encouraged exploration of pharmacological treatments. 'Brain-damaged child' eventually evolved into 'hyperkinetic reaction of childhood' in the 1968 DSM-II and then into ADHD (Eisenberg, 2007). Prior to the Multimodal Treatment (MTA) Study, extant studies demonstrated the short-term effectiveness of stimulants (the first of which, amphetamine, was reported for use in children in 1937) and some psychosocial interventions, but lacked evidence for long-term treatment effects, cross-setting benefit, and consistent benefit for comorbid and secondary conditions, like academic achievement. The need for a methodologically sound evaluation of long-term, cross-domain treatment strategies for ADHD, reflecting the varying needs of patients with different comorbidities and impairments, was paramount (Richters et al., 1995). The first major clinical trial in the NIMH's history to evaluate a childhood mental disorder (Richters et al., 1995), the MTA study is a long-term, collaborative, multisite study exploring pharmacological, psychosocial, and combined treatments for childhood ADHD.

Methods

In this four-group parallel-design study, 579 children aged 7–9.9 years with DSM-IV ADHD combined type, were randomly assigned to 14 months of medication management, behavioural treatment, combined treatment, or community care. Medication management began with a 28-day double-blinded titration of methylphenidate hydrochloride (MPH) dosed three times daily to find each child's optimal dose based on parent and teacher ratings; the blind was then broken. For those not responding adequately to MPH during titration, alternate medications were titrated openly until a satisfactory one was found. Of those who successfully completed titration, 68.5% were assigned to MPH, with an average initial dose of 30.5 mg/d. Medication was then monitored monthly and adjusted as warranted. Behavioural treatment involved parent training, child-focused treatment in a therapeutic summer camp, and school-based intervention. Combined treatment included medication management and behavioural treatment. Community care involved provision of community health resources, with most participants ultimately receiving medications from their own providers without a specific protocol.

Nineteen outcome measures were evaluated within six main domains:

1. ADHD symptoms: parent-/teacher-completed Swanson, Nolan, and Pelham (SNAP) questionnaire ratings
2. Oppositionality/aggression: parent-/teacher-completed SNAP subscale ratings
3. Social skills: parent-/teacher-completed Social Skills Rating System (SSRS)
4. Internalizing symptoms: parent-/teacher-completed SSRS and child-completed Multidimensional Anxiety Scale for Children
5. Parent–child relations: parent–child relationship questionnaire
6. Academic achievement: Wechsler Individual Achievement Test

Results

All four groups exhibited symptom reduction to varying degrees. For most core ADHD outcome measures (domain 1), combined treatment and medication management were superior to behavioural treatment and to community care, with combined treatment conferring no greater benefit than medication management alone, and behavioural treatment not faring better than community care, while behavioural treatment was not superior to community care. Additionally, combined treatment was superior to community care for all five non-ADHD domains (2–6); in contrast, medication management and behavioural treatment were each superior to community care in one non-ADHD domain only (teacher-rated social skills and parent–child relations, respectively). Notably, the combined treatment group used lower average total daily doses of MPH than the medication management group (31.2 mg versus 37.7 mg).

Conclusions and critique

This study was the first to demonstrate the long-term efficacy and tolerability of medication management in children with ADHD. It was also the first to capture the true benefits of stimulants, because some functional domains, like social skills or academic achievement, require more time for change to occur than can be observed in short-term studies (Richters et al., 1995). It adds to the extant evidence base in demonstrating combined treatment's noteworthy benefit for non-ADHD domains compared to community care. Further, it suggests it is reasonable to consider medication as first-line treatment for children with ADHD and, if carefully monitored, medication alone without intensive behavioural intervention may be adequate. However, the combined group achieved similar outcomes to the MPH group by using 20% lower doses of MPH, indicating the addition of behavioural treatment confers comparable benefit while minimizing stimulant exposure (Murray et al., 2008).

The study's size and scope allowed evaluation of treatment effects across diverse settings, patient groups, and outcome measures. Study limitations include the absence of a no-treatment or placebo group, potentially mitigating the presence of true medication benefit and underestimating the relative effects of behavioural treatment. Additionally, since most subjects in community care received medication, it is unclear which elements of the MTA treatments rendered them more effective than community care.

The MTA study is arguably the most elaborate treatment study in pediatric mental health. It provided crucial information for clinical practice and set a new standard for research, ushering in a new generation of collaborative, multisite, and multimodal treatment trials in child and adolescent psychiatry (Schachar, 1999).

Comparing fluoxetine, cognitive behavioural therapy, and their combination for adolescent depression

Main citation

March, J., et al. (2004). Fluoxetine, cognitive-behavioral therapy, and their combination for adolescents with depression: treatment for adolescents with depression study (TADS) randomized controlled trial. *Journal of the American Medical Association*, 292, 807–820.

Background

Major depressive disorder (MDD) in adolescence is a major risk factor for long-term psychosocial impairment into adulthood and is associated with increased risk of suicide, substance use disorders, and psychiatric and non-psychiatric comorbidities (Glied & Pine, 2002; Thapar et al., 2012). In 1998, when TADS was designed, the literature supported cognitive behavioural therapy (CBT) as a treatment for pediatric depression but was inconclusive for medications (studies of tricyclic antidepressants were unfavourable, whereas Emslie et al.'s 1997 randomized placebo-controlled trial of fluoxetine was positive); moreover, response rates until then were modest (60%). New evidence from adult studies, demonstrating the superiority of combined treatment, inspired the development of TADS.

Methods

TADS was a 12-week, multicentre, randomized, placebo-controlled, parallel-group clinical trial evaluating the efficacy of treatments for adolescents aged 12–17 years with DSM-IV MDD and a baseline Children's Depression Rating Scale-Revised (CDRS-R) total score of ≥45, indicating moderate to severe depression. Notable exclusion criteria were concurrent treatment with psychotherapy or psychotropic medication (other than stable stimulant treatment), a history of two failed selective serotonin reuptake inhibitor (SSRI) trials, and a high risk of 'dangerousness' (as indicated by recent hospitalization for suicidality, recent suicide attempt requiring medical attention, current intent or plan, and current ideation in the absence of sufficient family support). The 439 patients were randomized to four treatment arms: placebo, fluoxetine (10 to 40 mg/day), CBT, or fluoxetine (10 to 40 mg/day) with CBT. The first two groups were double-blinded while the latter two were unblinded.

The main outcome measures were CDRS-R total score change (which was obtained by conducting pairwise comparisons on treatment slopes) and, for responders, the Clinical Global Impressions-Improvement (CGI-I) score at the end of treatment. The CDRS-R total score is based on parent and adolescent interviews. The CGI-I is based on a clinician's view of the patient's overall clinical condition; a positive response was defined as a CGI-I score of one (very much improved) or two (much improved). Harm-related adverse events (AEs) were also assessed and included non-suicidal self-harm, worsening suicidal ideation without self-harm, suicide attempt, violent ideation, and harm to others.

Results

On CDRS-R total score change, planned contrasts on the CDRS-S slope coefficient across 12 weeks demonstrated that fluoxetine with CBT was superior to all groups ($p = 0.02$ against fluoxetine, $p = 0.001$ against CBT, $p = 0.001$ against placebo). Fluoxetine alone and CBT alone were not superior to placebo ($p = 0.1$ and $p = 0.4$, respectively). Fluoxetine was superior to CBT ($p = 0.01$). Response rate was 71.0% in the combined group, 60.6% in the fluoxetine group, 43.2% in the CBT group, and 34.8% in the placebo group.

Suicidality significantly improved in all groups. Odds ratios relative to placebo indicated minimal or no increased risk of AEs (defined as OR ≤ 2) in the CBT-alone group (OR 0.83) and intermediate risk in the combined group (OR 1.62), suggesting a protective effect of CBT on harm-related AEs, including treatment-emergent suicidality. In addition, a statistically significant elevated risk for harm-related AEs was noted in fluoxetine-treated patients compared to non-fluoxetine-treated patients (OR 2.19), suggesting fluoxetine may be associated with suicidality.

Conclusions and critique

TADS demonstrated that combined treatment is best for pediatric depression. In delivering treatment at multiple sites, excluding relatively fewer adolescents with comorbidities, and amassing a patient sample with moderate to severe depression, almost 30% of which had suicidal ideation at baseline, TADS results are generalizable and applicable to clinical practice (Curry et al., 2006; March et al., 2007). Study limitations include the lack of blinding among patients in all treatment arms and the lack of a CBT plus placebo comparison group, which renders it difficult to discern if the superiority of CBT with fluoxetine, relative to fluoxetine alone, reflects improvement associated with expectancy effects and time spent with patients or true treatment effect (March et al., 2006).

TADS represents the state of the art in pediatric depression comparative treatment trials. It informed best-practice guidelines for pediatric depression and identified factors affecting treatment-emergent suicidality. Subsequent analyses addressed practice-relevant questions, such as predictors/moderators of treatment response (Curry et al., 2006), long-term effectiveness of treatment, and suicidality (March & Vitiello, 2009). Finally, TADS provided a model for the systematic collection of suicidality data, informing the FDA's subsequent analyses and conclusions, as discussed later in this chapter (Cook et al., 2009).

Treating SSRI-resistant depression in adolescents

Main citation

Brent, D., et al. (2008). Switching to another SSRI or to venlafaxine with or without cognitive behavioral therapy for adolescents with SSRI-resistant depression: the TORDIA randomized controlled trial. *Journal of the American Medical Association,* 299, 901–913.

Background

Despite advances in the treatment of pediatric depression through TADS, only 60% of youth adequately respond to initial interventions. With pediatric depression increasingly recognized as a recurrent condition associated with significant morbidity and mortality, ongoing development of evidence-based treatment guidelines is paramount. The TORDIA study was developed to provide empirical guidelines for the treatment of depressed adolescents not responsive to an initial SSRI treatment.

Methods

TORDIA was a 12-week, multisite, NIMH-funded, randomized controlled trial. Participants were 334 adolescents aged 12–18 years with DSM-IV MDD who continued to have clinically significant depression (of at least moderate severity based on a CDRS-R score ≥40 and a CGI-S score ≥4) despite at least eight weeks of SSRI treatment. The SSRI had to be at a minimum dosage of 40 mg/day of fluoxetine or its equivalent for the previous four weeks (or 20 mg if 40 mg was not tolerated). Current CBT treatment was an exclusion criterion, but suicidality (notably) was not.

Participants were randomly assigned to one of four treatment arms: switch to a second SSRI (fluoxetine, paroxetine, or citalopram),[1] switch to venlafaxine, switch to a second SSRI plus CBT, or switch to venlafaxine plus CBT. Participants, clinicians, and independent evaluators were blinded to medication treatment assignment and independent evaluators were blinded to CBT assignment. By 12 weeks, the mean SSRI doses were 33.8 mg and the mean venlafaxine dose was 205.4 mg.

Primary outcome measures included adequate clinical response (defined by a CGI-I score of 2 much improved, or less, and an improvement in the CDRS-R score of at least 50%) and the trajectory of the CDRS-R over time. Secondary outcomes included self-reported depression and suicide-related symptoms assessed by the Beck Depression Inventory and the Suicide Ideation Questionnaire-Jr. When testing for the effects of CBT (versus not) and medication (switch to an SSRI versus venlafaxine), response differences were assessed using χ^2 and logistic regression (after adjusting for baseline differences and interactions with treatment). The effect of treatment on the CDRS-R trajectory was assessed by random-effects linear regression.

Results

Adequate clinical response occurred in 54.8% of participants treated with CBT versus 40.5% of participants not receiving CBT ($p = 0.009$). There was no difference in response between switching to a different SSRI or to venlafaxine (47.0% versus 48.2% response, $p = 0.83$). A significant CDRS-R score decrease for time ($p < 0.001$) occurred but not for medication, CBT, site, or any two- or three-way interaction. There were no differences between treatment groups for frequency of AEs. There were 18 suicide attempts among 17 participants; none completed suicide. In the presence of high baseline suicidal ideation, the use of venlafaxine was associated with more non-suicidal self-injury or suicidal events (37.2% versus 23.3%, $p = 0.05$) (Brent, 2009). Discontinuation due to cardiovascular events (prolonged QTc; increased blood pressure or pulse) occurred in one participant taking SSRI and four participants taking venlafaxine ($p = 0.21$). Venlafaxine resulted in significantly greater increases in diastolic blood pressure and pulse.

Conclusions and critique

TORDIA's findings indicate that in moderately severe and chronically depressed adolescents who do not respond to adequate SSRI treatment, adding CBT and switching to another antidepressant results in a higher rate of response than making an antidepressant switch without CBT. There is no difference between switching to another SSRI or to venlafaxine. Considering venlafaxine confers a slightly higher rate of cardiovascular effects and fails to demonstrate superiority to switching to another SSRI, TORDIA supports choosing another SSRI over venlafaxine as a second-line antidepressant. TORDIA's large sample size and inclusion of participants with suicidal ideation confer generalizability to a real-world population. Its limitations include the absence of a control group for greater provider contact in the combined groups and lack of ethnic diversity in the sample.

[1] Midway through the study, paroxetine was replaced by citalopram, given concerns about paroxetine's efficacy and safety.

TORDIA is the first clinical trial to evaluate depressed adolescents not responding to current evidence-based treatment. By uniquely comparing a medication switch plus CBT to a medication switch alone, it helps prescribers select the next best treatment step. This is critical because untreated depression risks episode recurrence, which is associated with depression, anxiety, suicidality, unemployment, and educational and economic underattainment in adulthood (Fergusson et al., 2007). TORDIA extends TADS in its inclusion of chronically depressed adolescents and those with active suicidal ideation, and demonstrates that actively suicidal adolescents can be managed within a clinical trial.

Comparing sertraline, cognitive behavioural therapy, and their combination for paediatric anxiety

Main citation

Walkup, J. T., et al. (2008). Cognitive behavioral therapy, sertraline, or a combination in childhood anxiety. *New England Journal of Medicine*, 359, 2753–2766.

Background

Historically, the diagnosis of paediatric anxiety disorders has been marked by uncertainty. Studies in the 1950s and 1960s evaluated behaviours associated with anxiety, such as school refusal, but this was too heterogeneous to extrapolate to youth. The nosological advances of DSM-III-R (1987) and DSM-IV (1994) recognized the continuity of anxiety disorders from childhood to adulthood by including three childhood anxiety disorders, replacing avoidance disorder of childhood with childhood-onset social phobia, and subsuming overanxious disorder into generalized anxiety disorder. Oft-evolving criteria, however, led to challenges establishing a study population of anxious youth. SSRIs for non-OCD paediatric anxiety were not tested until 1994, when a small study demonstrated fluoxetine's benefit for selective mutism and social phobia (Allen et al., 1995).

By the early 2000s, SSRIs and CBT were established as efficacious for pediatric anxiety. However, response rates for monotherapy were modest (40–50%) and effects of combined therapy were not known (barring one study in OCD). The Child-Adolescent Anxiety Multimodal Study (CAMS) was designed to fill this evidence gap in the treatment of anxiety. The importance of this cannot be understated—anxiety is a common pediatric psychiatric disorder that is often a precursor to adult psychiatric disorders (Compton et al., 2010), rendering treatment optimization of enormous public health consequence.

Methods

CAMS was a 12-week, multicentre, randomized, controlled trial comparing sertraline, CBT, and their combination with placebo. Participants were children and adolescents aged 7–17 years diagnosed with DSM-IV separation anxiety disorder and/or generalized anxiety disorder and/or social phobia. The 488 participants were randomized to sertraline (administered on a fixed-flexible schedule from 25 mg to 200 mg daily), placebo (administered on a fixed-flexible schedule with labelled doses from 50 mg to 200 mg to match sertraline), CBT (14 sessions), and combined treatment (sertraline and CBT). The first two groups were double-blinded, while the latter two were not. The mean dose of study medication at the final visit was 146.0 ± 60.8 mg/day in the sertraline group, 133.7 ± 59.8 mg/day in the combination-therapy group, and 175.8 ± 43.7 mg/day in the placebo group.

The primary outcome measure was treatment response at week 12 defined by a CGI-I score of 1 (very much improved) or 2 (much improved), and by Pediatric Anxiety Rating Scale (PARS) scores. Total PARS scores range from 0 to 30, with a score >13 indicating moderate anxiety and the diagnosis of an anxiety disorder. Overall impairment was assessed using the Children's Global Assessment Scale (CGAS), which estimates level of functioning.

Results

The percentages of children achieving treatment response based on CGI-I were 80.7% in the combination-therapy group, 59.7% in the CBT group, 54.9% in the sertraline group, and 23.7% in the placebo group. Each active treatment was superior to placebo ($p < 0.001$ for all three comparisons). Combination therapy was superior to sertraline alone ($p < 0.001$) and to CBT alone ($p = 0.001$). There was no significant difference in response rate between sertraline and CBT ($p = 0.41$). The same pattern and order of outcomes were noted on the PARS and CGAS. Rates of AEs, including suicidal ($p = 0.36$) and homicidal ($p = 0.54$) ideation were not significantly greater in the sertraline group than the placebo group. There were no suicide attempts. There were fewer reports of insomnia (1.4% versus 8.3%), fatigue (0% versus 6.0%), sedation (0% versus 4.5%), and restlessness or fidgeting (0% versus 3.8%) in the CBT group compared to the sertraline group ($p < 0.05$ for all comparisons).

Conclusions and critique

CAMS was the fifth federally funded, multicentre, large comparative treatment trial for a pediatric mental health disorder. It addressed the dearth of research on the efficacy of psychosocial, psychopharmacological, and combination treatments in the same population of anxious youth and provided evidence for three beneficial treatments for three common paediatric anxiety disorders (Compton et al., 2010). Although combination therapy showed the most benefit, CAMS suggests it is reasonable to consider CBT as an initial treatment option for anxious youth given the lower rates of AEs in the CBT group compared to the sertraline group.

CAMS carries significant public health benefits. Firstly, it informs best-practice guidelines for optimal treatment of pediatric anxiety disorders, which are the most prevalent of pediatric psychiatric disorders and are associated with increased risk of comorbidities, suicidality, sleep problems, and chronic irritability, and, if not adequately managed, may precipitate adult substance misuse and diminished physical functioning and quality of life (Albano et al., 2018). Secondly, it adds to the discussion on antidepressants and suicidality; contrary to the depression studies, CAMS did not demonstrate an increased suicide risk in the sertraline group. Thirdly, additional analyses have informed successive investigations of practice-relevant questions such as those relating to the moderators and predictors of the treatment outcomes (Compton et al., 2014), the durability of study treatments, and the factors affecting remission (Piacentini et al., 2014).

The large sample size, diversity of a multisite study population, and inclusion of subjects with ADHD and other anxiety disorders renders CAMS' results generalizable to most populations. Challenges to generalizability consist of exclusion of children with major depression and developmental disorders, predominant inclusion of young children, and lack of inclusion of the most socioeconomically disadvantaged children (Piacentini et al., 2014). Further, the combination group's lack of control for more visits may have affected AE findings by providing more opportunities for elicitation of AEs compared to the other groups, while its lack of blinding may have led to expectancy effects influencing its superior outcome.

Comparing antipsychotics and mood stabilizers for youth and adults with mania

Main citation

Correll, C. U., Sheridan, E. M., & DelBello, M. P. (2010). Antipsychotic and mood stabilizer efficacy and tolerability in pediatric and adult patients with bipolar I mania: a comparative analysis of acute, randomized, placebo-controlled trials. *Bipolar Disorders*, 12, 116–141.

Background

The epidemiology and treatment of paediatric bipolar disorder were scarcely addressed until the 1990s (Merikangas et al., 2009). The first randomized controlled trial to study the efficacy of lithium in paediatric bipolar disorder was published in 1998 (Geller et al., 1998), almost three decades after lithium was approved by the US FDA for adults with bipolar disorder. Concurrent with the evolution of psychopharmacological treatment for adult bipolar disorder, the study of pediatric bipolar disorder gained momentum. However, indiscriminate use of adult efficacy data to support the use of the same medications in children made it necessary to study differences in the efficacy and tolerability of mood stabilizers (MSs) and second-generation antipsychotics (SGAs) between youth and adults. This paper is the first systematic review comparing MSs and SGAs in the acute treatment of mania in youth and adults.

Methods

The authors used descriptive statistics for pooling outcomes. They weighted the pooled outcomes per medication group in each age group relative to the number of patients in each trial. They identified nine double-blind, randomized, placebo-controlled trials (DB-RPCTs) evaluating pediatric manic or mixed episodes of bipolar disorder, including five industry-sponsored studies of treatment with SGAs and four studies of treatment with conventional MSs (three of which were industry-sponsored). They identified 23 DB-RPCTs evaluating adult manic or mixed episodes, including 14 industry-sponsored studies evaluating SGAs and 11 studies evaluating MSs (ten of which were industry-sponsored).

The primary outcome measure was efficacy defined by last observation carried forward (LOCF) Young Mania Rating Scale (YMRS) score change. Secondary outcomes included LOCF Clinical Global Impressions-Bipolar Disorder (CGI-BP) Overall Illness score change from baseline to endpoint, treatment response (defined as ≥50% YMRS score reduction), remission (defined as endpoint YMRS≤12), all-cause discontinuation, and discontinuation due to inefficacy. Safety and tolerability outcomes included insomnia, somnolence, weight change from baseline, ≥7% weight gain, akathisia, extrapyramidal side effects (EPS), hyperprolactinaemia, and discontinuation due to intolerability.

Results

On the primary outcome, pooled effect sizes (ES) were significantly higher for SGAs than MSs in youth and adults. However, after removing studies with topiramate (which does not have an indication for mania), SGAs had a larger ES than MSs in youth but not in adults. On secondary outcomes, pooled ES for the CGI-BP Overall Illness score were larger for SGAs than MSs in adults, but there was not enough data to report on youth SGA and MS studies. Treatment response using pooled number needed to treat (NNT) did not differ between SGAs and MSs in youth or adults. Further, lithium (ES 0.31, 95% CI: −0.12 to −0.73) and oxcarbazepine (ES 0.11, 95% CI: −0.26 to −0.49) did not separate from placebo in youth, and topiramate did not separate from placebo (ES 0.05, 95% CI: −0.07 to −0.18) in adults. Treatment remission using pooled NNTs did not differ between SGAs and MSs in youth, while SGAs were superior to MSs in adults only when topiramate studies were included. Pooled NNTs for reducing discontinuation for inefficacy and all-cause discontinuation did not differ between medication or age groups, irrespective of topiramate inclusion.

SGAs were associated with more weight gain than MSs relative to placebo in youth but not in adults. However, when topiramate, which was associated with significant weight loss in youth and adults, was excluded from MS studies, weight change from baseline did not differ between MSs and SGAs in youth or adults relative to placebo. Among SGAs, olanzapine conferred the greatest weight gain, with youth gaining more weight than adults. Number needed to harm (NNH) for ≥7% weight gain did not differ among medication or age groups, but an overall significant NNH of 10.0 was noted in youth after only three to four weeks of SGA treatment. SGAs were associated with more somnolence than MSs, and youth treated with SGAs were more likely to experience somnolence than adults. EPS rates and insomnia did not differ across medication and age groups. Youth were less likely to develop SGA-related akathisia and more likely to develop hyperprolactinaemia compared to adults, although aripiprazole, a partial D_2 receptor agonist that does not block dopamine regulation of prolactin, was the sole contributing SGA in adults. There were no significant differences between SGAs and MSs for discontinuation due to intolerability across medication or age groups. However, in youth, relative to placebo, weighted data (including topiramate) suggested SGAs and MSs led to greater discontinuation rates for intolerability. In adults, NNHs were non-significant for all SGAs except ziprasidone (26.3, 95% CI: 14.2–395.5) and, as in youth, weighted data, including topiramate, suggested MSs led to significantly greater discontinuation rates due to intolerability.

Conclusions and critique

This comparative analysis marks the transition of child and adolescent psychopharmacology research into a systematic review and meta-analytical era. Amid controversy regarding the potentially unjustified use of SGAs in youth, it supports the efficacy of SGAs in manic youth while informing the discussion of their risk:benefit ratio (demonstrating that youth are more susceptible to some SGA-related adverse effects including weight gain, somnolence, and hyperprolactinaemia). It provides an evidence base to guide the initial treatment choice for acute mania, placing SGAs ahead of MSs in youth (Fristad & Algorta, 2013). Finally, and more broadly, it supports pediatric mania as a clinical entity warranting medication treatment as with adult mania.

Study limitations include the heterogeneity involved in comparing studies with different populations and designs, particularly considering most paediatric mania studies include outpatients while adult studies include inpatients. Further, due to the unavailability of data in youth, placebo-controlled trials were evaluated, rather than active-controlled SGA versus MS trials, the latter of which would have allowed for a more direct comparison of the two medication classes.

The relationship between psychotropic drugs and paediatric suicidality: the Food and Drug Administration (USA) analysis

Main citation

Food and Drug Administration (USA). (2004). Relationship between psychotropic drugs and pediatric suicidality: review and evaluation of clinical data. Available at: https://www.fda.gov/ohrms/dockets/ac/04/briefing/2004-4065b1-10-TAB08-Hammads-Review.pdf

Background

Concerns about the safety of paediatric antidepressant use emerged in May 2003 when GlaxoSmithKline reported increased suicide-related adverse events (AEs) with paroxetine compared to placebo. In June 2003, the FDA issued a public statement regarding the possible safety risks related to paediatric paroxetine use and expanded its concerns to all antidepressants in public health advisories issued in October 2003 and March 2004 (Busch & Barry, 2009). The FDA then requested that pharmaceutical companies submit their paediatric data for review. The main objective of the subsequent FDA analysis was to evaluate the relationship between psychotropic drugs and paediatric suicidality.

Methods

Eight sponsors of nine antidepressants (fluoxetine, sertraline, paroxetine, fluvoxamine, citalopram, bupropion, venlafaxine, nefazodone, and mirtazapine) submitted datasets from their paediatric MDD, obsessive compulsive disorder, generalized anxiety disorder, social anxiety disorder, and ADHD trials. The result was a pooled analysis of 24 randomized, controlled, short-term (4- to 16-week) paediatric efficacy trials, including TADS, involving over 4,400 children/adolescents ranging from 6 to 18 years old. A fixed-effect meta-analysis was primarily used to provide a weighted average of the treatment effects from the individual trials.

Paediatric suicidality was measured in two ways. The first was suicidality as reported as AEs from the trials. Suicidologists assembled by Columbia University blindly reviewed potential suicide-related events from the trials and coded them as follows:

1. suicide attempt
2. preparatory actions toward imminent suicidal behaviour
3. self-injurious behaviour with unknown intent
4. self-injurious behaviour without suicidal intent (to affect circumstance)
5. self-injurious behaviour without suicidal intent (to affect internal state)
6. suicidal ideation

7-9. other injury events

10. insufficient information
11. self-injurious behaviour without suicidal intent (unspecified type).

The second was suicidality as suggested by scores on the suicidality items in depression rating scales (different scales were used in different trials).

Multiple outcome measures were evaluated, but the primary outcome measure was definitive suicidal behaviour/ideation (codes 1, 2, 6). The primary analysis evaluated the overall risk estimate of definitive suicidal behaviour/ideation by drug across all indications and in MDD trials. Four trials had no events in any treatment group and were excluded from the analysis to avoid the resultant 'zero cell', which renders it impossible to calculate relative risk ratios. The authors submitted that these exclusions should not have affected the overall evaluation of antidepressant suicide risk because three studies represented all available trials for bupropion and nefazodone, and one was not an MDD trial. Additional analyses reviewed trial design attributes for each drug's MDD trials, overall risk estimates of all outcomes across all indications and in the SSRI MDD trials, and the overall risk estimates of treatment-emergent agitation or hostility by drug in the MDD trials.

Results

The primary analysis focused on 120 suicide-related events occurring in the double-blind acute treatment phase (see Table 10.1). Of the 19 trials (excluding TADS' results) evaluated for the primary outcome, eight demonstrated a relative risk (RR) of two or more. There were no completed suicides. The FDA concluded that antidepressants pose a twofold increase in suicidal ideation or behaviour compared to placebo (4% versus 2%), with most events occurring in patients with a baseline history of suicide attempt or ideation.

Table 10.1 Suicide-related adverse events evaluated in the primary FDA analysis of the relationship between psychotropic drugs and paediatric suicidality

Suicide-related adverse events	Total number
Suicide attempt (code 1)	27
Preparatory actions toward suicidal behaviour (code 2)	6
Self-injurious behaviour with unknown intent (code 3)	24
Self-injurious behaviour to affect circumstance (code 4)	2
Self-injurious behaviour to affect internal state (code 5)	5
Suicidal ideation (code 6)	45
Insufficient information (code 10)	7
Self-injurious behaviour, unspecified type (code 11)	4

Modified from Food and Drug Administration (USA). (2004). Relationship between psychotropic drugs and pediatric suicidality: review and evaluation of clinical data. Available at: https://www.fda.gov/ohrms/dockets/ac/04/briefing/2004-4065b1-10-TAB08-Hammads-Review.pdf

Additionally, the FDA concluded that drug treatment is associated with symptoms of hostility or agitation. The overall RRs for all drugs (RR = 1.79) and for all SSRIs (RR = 2.34) in the MDD trials were statistically significant, suggesting an increased risk of developing activation symptoms in the drug group compared to placebo group. However, the likelihood of experiencing suicidal behaviour/ideation among activated patients was not evaluable because information on the timing of the emergence of hostility or agitation was not available in the data.

Conclusions and critique

In October 2004, based on this non-peer-reviewed analysis, the FDA placed a black-box warning label on antidepressants, indicating an increased risk of suicidal thoughts and behaviour in youth. A 2007 meta-analysis confirmed the FDA's overall findings but noted a smaller effect of less than 1%. This difference likely reflects the inclusion of seven additional studies and the use of random-effects rather than fixed-effects models for combining studies, which generate different weighted means of treatment effects[2] (Bridge et al., 2007). In May 2007, the FDA expanded its black-box warning to include young adults of 18–24 years of age, based on age-stratified findings from a similar pooled

[2] The fixed-effects model assumes the estimated drug effect is fixed and that effect differences reflect sampling error; therefore, weights are assigned based on the amount of study information and vary according to individual study size. The random-effects model accepts that the true effect may vary from trial to trial and therefore estimates the mean of a distribution of true effects, so each study's effect size serves as a sample toward the estimated mean, resulting in weight assignments that are more evenly dispersed (Borenstein et al., 2007).

analysis of placebo-controlled, short-term trials in adults; however, the FDA also added a statement explaining that depression and other psychiatric disorders are themselves associated with increased risk of suicide (Friedman, 2014; FDA, 2006).

Limitations of the FDA's investigation include focusing on events occurring in the double-blind acute treatment phase, potentially missing antidepressant-related events occurring later in treatment. In addition, analysis of short-term data potentially missed positive or negative suicidality effects requiring longer medication exposure. Further, with the exception of TADS, the suicidal symptoms evaluated in the analysis were not based on prospective data, but on narrative-based AE reports, which are subject to ascertainment bias (Friedman & Leon, 2007). Finally, use of RR ratios resulted in the exclusion of four studies in which there were no events, which undermines generalizability and risks inaccuracy in understanding the chance of suicidality in the total study population (Bridge et al., 2007).

There are conflicting reports about the pediatric warning's impact. Observational data reveals that paediatric prescription rates for SSRIs dropped 20% between 2003 and 2005, and that primary care antidepressant prescribing decreased by 4.61% annually (Friedman, 2014). Additionally, new diagnoses of pediatric depression decreased by 44% in primary care settings (Friedman, 2014), with a higher proportion of youth being diagnosed by psychiatrists instead, suggesting that clinicians with less experience treating depressed youth deferred management to mitigate negative outcomes and/or malpractice suits (Busch & Barry, 2009). In contrast, a recent analysis of Medical Expenditure Panel Survey data from 2000–2011 demonstrates a decline in pediatric antidepressant use in the early post-warning years (2004–2007), but an increase in the adjusted rates of use to pre-warning levels by 2009 (Kafali et al., 2018). Correlational data, however, cannot establish causality between the warning and diagnostic/therapeutic trends.

The FDA's warning has been criticized as misleading for employing a vague concept of 'suicidality' and basing its conclusions on paediatric data that lacked completed suicides, especially given that untreated depression is the most recognized risk factor for all-age suicide (Lineberry et al., 2007). Amid post-warning declines in diagnosis and prescription rates, concern for an increase in pediatric suicide is paramount. However, there is little evidence of a change in suicide rates correlating with the advisory. While one study demonstrates that post-warning adolescent psychotropic drug poisoning (used as proxy for suicide attempt with unknown intentionality) increased by 21.7% (Friedman, 2014), the Centers for Disease Control and Prevention reports that suicides from poisonings and all causes peaked in 2003 or 2004, then decreased, while the rate of accidental drug poisoning increased in the post-warning period of 2005 and 2006 (Stone, 2014). Further, rates of completed suicides in people of 10–34 years of age increased between 1999 and 2010, without abrupt changes around the time of the FDA warnings (Friedman, 2014), and analysis of Duke University Medical Center Clinical Research Information System psychiatric data from 2000–2009 indicates that overall suicidality decreased after the black-box warning (adjusted OR 0.38) (Gupta et al., 2016).

Conclusion

The landmark papers in child and adolescent psychopharmacology reviewed here have significantly advanced the understanding and treatment of paediatric mental illness. This is of great public health importance given the considerable morbidity and mortality associated with pediatric psychiatric disorders. These papers also promote patient-centred care and collaborative decision-making by providing evidence for multiple treatment options.

In line with the NIMH's Research Domain Criteria Project (see Chapter 1), the future of child and adolescent psychiatry will incorporate integrative research and diagnostic strategies involving neuroimaging, proton magnetic response spectroscopy, biomarker development, and genetics to identify diagnostic markers and individualized predictors of treatment response (Strakowski et al., 2015). Additionally, evaluation of the long-term trajectory of typical and atypical brain development mapped to cognitive and behavioural development will help identify at-risk, presymptomatic, and symptomatic phases of psychiatric disease. This provides the best opportunity for prevention, early diagnosis, and/or time-appropriate provision of therapeutic intervention with potential to transform the trajectory of mental illnesses for children and adolescents (NIMH, 2015).

References

Albano, A. M., et al. (2018). Secondary outcomes from the child/adolescent anxiety multimodal study: implications for clinical practice. *Evidence-Based Practice in Child and Adolescent Mental Health*, 3, 30–41.

Allen, A. J., Leonard, H., & **Swedo, S. E.** (1995). Current knowledge of medications for the treatment of childhood anxiety disorders. *Journal of the American Academy of Child and Adolescent Psychiatry*, 34, 976–986.

Borenstein, M., Hedges, L., & **Rothstein, H.** (2007). *Meta-analysis: fixed effect vs. random effects*. Available at: www.meta-analysis.com (accessed 22 February 2018).

Brent, D., et al. (2008). Switching to another SSRI or to venlafaxine with or without cognitive behavioral therapy for adolescents with SSRI-resistant depression: the TORDIA randomized controlled trial. *Journal of the American Medical Association*, **299**, 901–913.

Brent, D. A. (2009). The treatment of SSRI-resistant depression in adolescents (TORDIA): in search of the best next step. *Depression and Anxiety*, **26**, 871–874.

Bridge, J. A., et al. (2007). Clinical response and risk for reported suicidal ideation and suicide attempts in pediatric antidepressant treatment: a meta-analysis of randomized controlled trials. *Journal of the American Medical Association*, **297**, 1683–1696.

Busch, S. H. & **Barry, C. L.** (2009). Pediatric antidepressant use after the black-box warning. *Health Affairs*, **28**, 724–733.

Chess, S. (1988). Child and adolescent psychiatry come of age: a fifty year perspective. *Journal of the American Academy of Child and Adolescent Psychiatry*, **27**, 1–7.

Compton, S. N., et al. (2010). Child/adolescent anxiety multimodal study (CAMS): rationale, design, and methods. *Child and Adolescent Psychiatry and Mental Health*, **4**, 1–15.

Compton, S. N., et al. (2014). Predictors and moderators of treatment response in childhood anxiety disorders: results from the CAMS trial. *Journal of Consulting and Clinical Psychology*, **82**, 212–224.

Cook, M. N., Peterson, J., & Sheldon, C. (2009). Adolescent depression: an update and guide to clinical decision making. *Psychiatry*, **6**, 17–31.

Correll, C. U., Sheridan, E. M., & DelBello, M. P. (2010). Antipsychotic and mood stabilizer efficacy and tolerability in pediatric and adult patients with bipolar I mania: a comparative analysis of acute, randomized, placebo-controlled trials. *Bipolar Disorder*, **12**, 116–141.

Curry, J., et al. (2006). Predictors and moderators of acute outcome in the Treatment for Adolescents with Depression Study (TADS). *Journal of the American Academy of Child and Adolescent Psychiatry*, **45**, 1427–1439.

Eisenberg, L. (2007). Commentary with a historical perspective by a child psychiatrist: when 'ADHD' was the 'brain-damaged child'. *Journal of Child and Adolescent Psychopharmacology*, **17**, 279–283.

Emslie, G. J., et al. (1997). A double-blind, randomized, placebo-controlled trial of fluoxetine in children and adolescents with depression. *Archives of General Psychiatry*, 54, 1031–1037.

Fergusson, D. M., Boden, J. M., & Horwood, L. J. (2007). Recurrence of major depression in adolescence and early adulthood, and later mental health, educational and economic outcomes. *British Journal of Psychiatry*,**191**, 335–342.

Food and Drug Administration (USA). (2004). Relationship between psychotropic drugs and pediatric suicidality: review and evaluation of clinical data. Available at: https://www.fda.gov/ohrms/dockets/ac/04/briefing/2004-4065b1-10-TAB08-Hammads-Review.pdf

Food and Drug Administration (USA). (2006). Briefing document for the December 13 meeting of the Psychopharmacologic Drugs Advisory Committee. Available at: https://www.fda.gov/ohrms/dockets/ac/06/briefing/2006-4272b1-01-FDA.pdf

Friedman, R. A. (2014). Antidepressants' black-box warning—10 years later. *New England Journal of Medicine*, **371**, 1666–1668.

Friedman, R. A. & Leon, A. C. (2007). Expanding the black box—depression, antidepressants, and the risk of suicide. *New England Journal of Medicine*, **356**, 2343–2346.

Fristad, M. A. & Algorta, G. P. (2013). Future directions for research on youth with bipolar spectrum disorders. *Journal of Clinical Child and Adolescent Psychology*, **42**, 734–747.

Geller, B., et al. (1998). Double-blind and placebo-controlled study of lithium for adolescent bipolar disorders with secondary substance dependency. *Journal of the American Academy of Child and Adolescent Psychiatry*, **37**, 171–178.

Glied, S. & Pine, D. S. (2002). Consequences and correlates of adolescent depression. *Archives of Pediatrics and Adolescent Medicine*, **156**, 1009–1014.

Gupta, S., Gersing, K. R., Alaattin, E., & Burt, T. (2016). Antidepressant regulatory warnings, prescription patterns, suicidality and other aggressive behaviors in major depressive disorder and anxiety diosrders. *Psychiatric Quarterly*, **87**, 329–342.

Kafali, N., Progovac, A., Hou, S. S. Y., & Cook, B. L. (2018). Long-run trends in antidepressant use among youths after the FDA black box warning. *Psychiatric Services*, **69**, 389–395.

Lineberry, T. W., Bostwick, J. M., Beebe, T. J., & Decker, P. A. (2007). Impact of the FDA black box warning on physician antidepressant prescribing and practice patterns: opening Pandora's suicide box. *Mayo Clinic Proceedings*, **82**, 518–520.

March, J., Silva, S.,Vitiello, B., & the TADS Team. (2006). The Treatment for Adolescents with Depression Study (TADS): methods and message at 12 weeks. *Journal of the American Academy of Child and Adolescent Psychiatry*, **45**, 1393–1403.

March, J., et al. (2004). Fluoxetine, cognitive-behavioral therapy, and their combination for adolescents with depression: treatment for adolescents with depression study (TADS) randomized controlled trial. *Journal of the American Medical Association*, **292**, 807–820.

March, J., et al. (2007). The Treatment for Adolescents with Depression Study (TADS): long-term effectiveness and safety outcomes. *Archives of General Psychiatry*, **64**, 1132–1144.

March, J. S. & Vitiello, B. (2009). Clinical messages from the Treatment for Adolescents with Depression Study (TADS). *American Journal of Psychiatry*, **166**, 1118–1123.

Merikangas, K. R., Nakamura, E. F., & Kessler, R. C. (2009). Epidemiology of mental disorders in children and adolescents. *Dialogues in Clinical Neuroscience*, **11**, 7–20.

MTA Cooperative Group. (1999). A 14-month randomized clinical trial of treatment strategies for attention-deficit/hyperactivity disorder. The MTA Cooperative Group. Multimodal Treatment Study of Children with ADHD. *Archives of General Psychiatry*, **56**, 1073–1086.

Murray, D. W., et al. (2008). A clinical review of outcomes of the multimodal treatment study of children with attention-deficit/hyperactivity disorder (MTA). *Current Psychiatry Reports*, **10**, 424–431.

National Institute of Mental Health. (2015). *NIMH strategic plan for research.* Available at: https://www.nimh.nih.gov/about/strategic-planning-reports/index.shtml (accessed 24 March 2018).

Piacentini, J., et al. (2014). 24- and 36-week outcomes for the Child/Adolescent Anxiety Multimodal Study (CAMS). *Journal of the American Academy of Child and Adolescent Psychiatry*, **53**, 297–309.

Rey, J. A., et al. (2015). History of child psychiatry. In: *IACAPAP e-Textbook of Child and Adolescent Mental Health*, ed. J. Rey. Geneva: International Association for Child and Adolescent Psychiatry and Allied Professions.

Richters, J. E., et al. (1995). NIMH collaborative multisite multimodal treatment study of children with ADHD: I. Background and rationale. *Journal of the American Academy of Child and Adolescent Psychiatry*, **34**, 987–1000.

Schachar, R. (1999). The MTA: child and adolescent psychiatry in a new century. *Canadian Journal of Psychiatry*, **44**, 972.

Stone, M. B. (2014). The FDA warning on antidepressants and suicidality—why the controversy? *New England Journal of Medicine*, **371**, 1668–1671.

Strakowsi, S. M., DelBello, M. P., & Adler, C. M. (2015). *Bipolar Disorder in Youth: Presentation, Treatment, and Neurobiology.* Oxford/New York: Oxford University Press.

Thapar, A., Collishaw, S., Pine, D. S., & Thapar, A. K. (2012). Depression in adolescence. *Lancet*, **379**, 1056–1067.

Walkup, J. T., et al. (2008). Cognitive behavioral therapy, sertraline, or a combination in childhood anxiety. *New England Journal of Medicine*, **359**, 2753–2766.

Section IV

Psychosocial interventions

Chapter 11

Psychodynamic therapy

Kevin S. McCarthy and Richard F. Summers

Introduction

Psychodynamic psychotherapy was inaugurated with Sigmund Freud's *Studies on Hysteria* (Breuer & Freud, 1893–1895[1955]). Here, Freud struggled to comprehend a constellation of peculiar symptoms that had their origin in the repression of patients' painful early traumas and unacceptable wishes. When he helped his patients express these memories, their symptoms were ameliorated. In the 125 years since this remarkable discovery, psychodynamic psychotherapy has changed psychiatry, culture, family life, and values. It has resulted in decreased prevalence of certain disorders like the conversion hysteria Freud treated; in changes in attitudes toward children, parenting, and sexuality; in the introduction of the notion of the unconscious into society and the media; and in profound reconsiderations of our understanding of a good life. Dynamic therapy itself has evolved over that time, shedding obsolete notions and incorporating new ones into modern adaptions that are widely taught and practiced (Summers & Barber, 2010). However, the key principles of psychodynamic therapy remain consistent and can be traced across its development: emotional exploration, interpretation, and support; frequent sessions; emphasis on uncovering painful affects and past events; facilitation of affect experiencing and understanding; and a focus on the therapeutic relationship (Summers & Barber, 2010).

In identifying these landmark papers, we concentrated on articles specific to the trajectory of psychodynamic psychotherapy rather than to psychoanalysis proper, the parent method to dynamic therapy typified by very frequent sessions over a longer period of time, a greater intensity in the therapeutic relationship, and greater depth in interpretations. We first nominated major thematic areas representing the content of dynamic treatment or shifts in the way therapy has been conceptualized and practiced: classical theory, brief therapy, object relations, self-psychology, relational models, feminism and multiculturalism, and empirical validation. We then collected articles that either initiated or typified each area, looked at citation counts in major databases (Psychoanalytic Electronic Publishing; Google Scholar) to verify their popularity and impact, and, finally, consulted with colleagues to make certain our selections were comprehensive and informative.

A certain style of reading is required in order to benefit most from psychodynamic writings. First, most articles respond to a dilemma or problem that the community of psychodynamic thinkers and therapists was struggling with at the time, such as a technical problem encountered in practice, personal or theoretical disputes, or outside pressures like sociocultural changes or new practice directives. This context is critical to interpreting the statements of the author, and fortunately the Landmark series format provides just that background and clarification.

Second, psychodynamic writers expend great effort selecting the exact words they use to describe their observations. We offer a quote from each article that encapsulates the author's meaning. Beware, the language in older papers is often insensitive and dated because it reflects cultural values accepted at the time but now repudiated. Do not blame the author for reflecting the times! Many psychoanalysts were quite progressive—Freud advocated for gay and lesbian rights in the 1920s, for instance (Gay, 2006)—and would share current viewpoints were they to be alive now.

Third, psychodynamic writers often assume the role of an expositor of wisdom and regard the readers as responsible for organizing and gathering the meaning of their thoughts. Not every sentence and paragraph will contribute to the main thesis, and there are many elaborate and fascinating tangents. Modern scientific writing is the opposite: concise, linear, and spare to the point of leaving out critical details and assumptions. We will be explicit in guiding readers to the highlights of each article.

Finally, psychodynamic authors invariably perform exquisite gymnastics to trace the lineage of their ideas directly back to Freud and prove their faithful adherence to his words. However, this appeal to authority often minimizes the remarkable advances in thinking and practice that the writer is making. It may be confusing to the reader to grasp the new phenomenon only to find a tortured syllogism applied at the last moment that cements an oblique reference to Freud.

It is with these caveats in mind that we describe the following landmark papers:

- Freud's (1911–1915[1955]) *Papers on Technique* lays out the framework for the practice of psychodynamic psychotherapy based on his successes and failures. The essential mechanism of treatment shifts from memory repression and recovery to awareness of conflicts between instincts and social pressures. Furthermore, Freud unlocks a powerful new tool for therapy, transference, or the tendency to repeat events within the therapeutic relationship.
- Ferenczi and Rank's (1925) *Development of Psycho-Analysis* advocates for one of the first major modifications in psychodynamic techniques. They sought to jumpstart the therapeutic process by accelerating the timeframe of treatment and actively encouraging and working with the patient's interpersonal patterns in therapy.
- Winnicott's (1949) *Hate in the Counter-Transference* is an exposition of the centrality of relationships in psychodynamic therapy, as opposed to drives, and opens the door to the inevitability and potential value of the therapist's own feelings, the countertransference, in treatment.
- Kohut and Wolf's (1978) *Disorders of the Self and Their Treatment* describes the self-psychology movement that arose within psychodynamic psychotherapy, prioritizing empathy and the development of the self. Here, the therapist provides for early deficits in empathy and allows the patient to find healthy new ways to satisfy these longings.

- Chodorow's (1974) *Family Structure and Feminine Personality* is a critique of the psychoanalytic treatment of women, offering a new and unique sociological viewpoint on how family life and relationships explain gender identity development. This work not only blew open antiquated ideas about women in psychodynamic therapy, but also began a broader reconsideration of gender and multicultural issues in dynamic treatment.
- Mitchell's (1984) *Object Relations Theories and the Developmental Tilt* moves beyond both the internal conflict and interpersonal deficit models, and focuses instead on being in a relationship with others. The therapeutic relationship (and indeed every relationship) is a present, ongoing, and negotiated process, and the development of a therapeutic relationship is proposed as the sole and curative motive of dynamic psychotherapy.
- Finally, the empirical article by Leichsenring, Rabung, and Leibing (2004) goes beyond the voluminous clinical observations described by dynamic therapists and quantifies the efficacy of psychodynamic therapy in the face of mounting pressures to demonstrate treatment outcomes.

Establishing the rules of engagement

Main citation

Freud, S. (1911–1915). Papers on technique. In: *The Standard Edition of the Complete Psychological Works of Sigmund Freud, Volume XII*, ed. and trans. J. Strachey (1955). London: Hogarth; pp. 83–171.

Background

At the time of this collection of brief papers, dynamic psychotherapy was 15 years old and had received wide acceptance by the psychiatric community for its stunning ability to help individuals with conversion hysteria and other conditions. At this juncture, psychodynamic therapy was thought to help patients through cathartic recollection of the traumatic experiences they had repressed that were leading to symptoms. Freud, trained as a neurologist, initially used the tools of hypnosis and suggestion to uncover these memories but found more consistent results by employing the 'fundamental rule' of free association. Patients were to express the contents of their mental life regardless of perceived importance or embarrassment, so that the therapist could identify traces in the patients' thinking to memories of these traumatic events. Freud wrote these papers in response to requests for guidance from practitioners about how to practice psychoanalysis and, more importantly, as a recognition of the struggles he had using his technique on different types of patients.

Methods

Freud observed that, for most patients, simply asking them to free associate was not sufficient to alleviate their symptoms. At some point, the patients would become blocked and unable to describe their mental life. Freud saw these moments of silence, unwillingness to cooperate in treatment, or desire to please the therapist as a resistance to the therapy process and getting better. Furthermore, given the repeated contact with the therapist, unlike in other medical treatments, the patient developed a relationship with the therapist and often had strong desires and intentions that were beyond the agreed-upon scope of treatment.

Results

Freud had discovered a phenomenon he had touched up against in earlier works: transference, or the repetition of interpersonal experiences with the therapist. In the first few papers in this series, Freud struggled to reconcile the idea of transference with the early mechanism of dynamic therapy (remembering) because when these instincts and motivations were expressed in the therapeutic relationship, they often interfered with the patient's ability to free associate and recall memories. However, by the end of the series he openly advocated working with the transference, cultivating it through an atmosphere of therapeutic abstinence (not giving any indication of the patient's projected wishes one way or the other), and altering it through interpretation (connecting the motivations back to earlier events in the patient's life).

> But it should not be forgotten that it is precisely [difficulties in therapy from transference] that do us the inestimable service of making the patient's hidden and forgotten erotic impulses immediate and manifest. For when all is said and done, it is impossible to destroy anyone in absentia or in effigie [sic]. (Freud, 1911–1915, p. 108)
>
> Freud, S., 1911–1915. Papers on Technique. In: J. Strachey, ed. and trans. 1955. The Standard Edition of the Complete Psychological Works of Sigmund Freud, Volume XII (1911–1913), pp.83–171

The goal of therapy was to understand the transference as an expression of the unsatisfied early experiences that the patient had never processed. Through greater awareness of this tendency to repeat frustrated wishes, the patient could give up these motivations and satisfy them in more mature ways.

Conclusions and critique

Papers on Technique was a consolidation of the techniques of psychodynamic psychotherapy into one source. The receptive, observant therapeutic stance; the patient's responsibility to produce material; and the judicious use of interpretation continue to typify dynamic therapy to this day. However, these were recommendations for practice, and Freud was famously known to depart from his own advice, chatting with his patients, disclosing about himself, and making suggestions when he thought it helpful (Gay, 2006). Unfortunately, many dynamic therapists reified his recommendations as a series of commandments, rigidly following them with patients who might have benefitted from a little more flexibility, and perhaps inhibiting growth in theory and practice.

The most crucial element of these papers, indeed in all of psychodynamic therapy, is the discovery and use of transference in the therapeutic relationship. Indeed, of his entire work, Freud himself was most proud of the last of these papers (Gay, 2006). Ironically, it is the structural model of the mind (id, ego, and superego) and the psychosexual stages of development (oral, anal, and genital) for which Freud is most remembered: concepts considered no longer current by some. Undergraduate textbooks typically pillory their speculative and insensitive nature (Redmond & Shulman, 2008), rarely focusing on the remarkable discovery of the transference and how to use it.

If you are going to do it, do it right

Main citation

Ferenczi, S. & Rank, O. (1925). *The Development of Psycho-Analysis*, trans. C. Newton. New York: Nervous and Mental Disease Publishing Company.

Background

As an emerging applied field, psychodynamic psychotherapy struggled to integrate two important strands that were developing in parallel: the science of cognitive-affective processes and the actual practice of working with patients. By the time of Sándor Ferenczi and Otto Rank, two influential psychiatrists in the psychoanalytic community and associates of Freud, theory had been given priority in status. There were no formal training opportunities in dynamic treatment at that time, and so new therapists learned their practice by trial and error, from publications and talks, which led them to believe that discussing theory with the patient was how therapy should be conducted. Furthermore, therapy was lengthening in duration as practitioners were viewing it as more of an open academic exploration and theory-building endeavour, sometimes forgetting the needs of the patient in front of them. At a conference, Ferenczi and Rank discovered that they were both presenting similar papers on these practice issues and combined their thoughts together in this monograph.

Methods

Ferenczi and Rank noted characteristic errors in practice that they believed to be a result of the preference toward theory and lack of training experiences. These errors included rigid adherence to technique, incorrect formulation or failure to conceptualize, intellectualization of the therapy process, passivity and inactivity on the part of the therapist, and 'wild analysis' (that is, too great a level of intervention or impulsivity by the therapist). It was to this state of dynamic therapy that they offered their thoughts on how to sharpen and enliven the treatment process.

Results

Several surprising conclusions were drawn in this paper, the foremost being an argument for the re-equalization of practice to theory. Ferenczi and Rank suggested that clinical work be valued for the data it can provide and for the fastest amelioration of symptoms possible. Second, they strongly advocated for the activity of the therapist, which they understood as facilitating the transference through both interpretation and direct suggestion or support, as opposed to waiting for its emergence in the treatment. Third, interventions are not to be withheld or delivered heavy handedly, but administered with competence at opportune times. They implicated the need for a formulation of the patient and a therapeutic focus, suggesting 'the analyst can, on the basis of properly combining his knowledge with the individual material the patient offers, determine exactly the time, the kind and the degree of his intervention' (Ferenczi & Rank, 1925, p. 61). Fourth, patients need to re-experience the transference situation in order to understand it. Ferenczi and Rank gave preference to emotional insight, as they saw psychodynamic practice becoming too didactic to be helpful to patients. Finally, a treatment can and should be brief in nature. Indeed, they fully expected, with the maturation of dynamic psychotherapy, that the best practice would be the most time-efficient.

Conclusions and critique

The views of Ferenczi and Rank were largely ignored at the time by the psychodynamic community in the excitement for scientific progress and in the politics of the psychoanalytic movement. However, their work had pervasive influence, as they foresaw much of the practice of modern therapy. Many treatment developers, like David Malan, Lester Luborsky, Hans Strupp, Habib Davanloo, and Leigh McCullough, explicitly traced the foundation and parameters of their versions of short-term dynamic therapy back to Ferenczi and Rank (Messer, 2001). Formulation and problem focus, the centrality of affective experience, technical competence, and the timely and apt use of intervention are all areas that are integral to current practice now (Summers & Barber, 2010).

All in a day's work: hating your patients

Main citation

Winnicott, D. W. (1949). Hate in the counter-transference. *The International Journal of Psychoanalysis*, 30, 69–74.

Background

In the 1940s, two schools of practice arose in psychodynamic psychotherapy—classical drive theory, led by Freud's daughter, Anna (Freud, 1963), and object relations, a system focusing on the cognitive-affective representations of interpersonal relationships, led by Melanie Klein (Klein, 1952). Object relations is an unfortunately mechanistic term, as objects refer to mental stand-ins for important people in a person's life, and relations are the emotional bonds and boundaries between self and others. We use these representations, derived from early encounters and expectations, to shape present relating. Tensions were high between these two groups, each claiming the legacy of Freud. Donald Winnicott's perspective, while largely derived from object relations, represented the 'middle group', which creatively straddled both schools and attempted to incorporate the considerable strengths of each.

Methods

Initially a paediatrician, Winnicott was known for his playful writing style. He took up a serious topic in this paper—lower-functioning patients[1] that make therapy difficult by bringing up feelings in the therapist, or countertransference. The traditional view was that the therapist should use personal analysis and supervision to be objective and motivation-free regarding patients, and countertransference was a harmful contagion or misstep on the part of the therapist. Winnicott, in daring to work with these unanalysable individuals, confronted his strong negative feelings of frustration and, indeed, found them integral to the treatment.

Results

Winnicott assumed negative countertransference is a normative reaction to patients' sometimes exasperating behaviour. He compared this to the relationship between infants and caregivers. Caregivers must inevitably feel frustration at the mercurial needs and moods of their infants, who are allowed to be implacably demanding due to their development. However, as infants mature into children, they are slowly made aware of the consequences of their desires and behaviours for those around them, and given the opportunity to take responsibility for the negative feelings they engender. Until that point, caregivers must contain their reactions and, in unveiling them, must be supportive even when they are the targets of their child's thoughtlessness. This same process is enacted in the therapy, as the patient's symptoms are often vexing arrests in development. Ignoring the inevitability of negative countertransference in the therapy is unhelpful, as it leads to unconsidered action on the part of the therapist, including reactions as minor as looking forward to the end of the session, and as great as deciding to terminate the treatment. Avoidance of the negative countertransference may also perpetuate the symptom, as the patient is never exposed to the impact of his or her behaviour. Therapists must be willing to offer their uncomfortable reaction to the patient at an opportune time to facilitate the patient's growth.

> [Therapy] is incomplete if even towards the end it has not been possible for the analyst to tell the patient what he, the analyst, did unbeknown for the patient whilst he was ill, in the early stages. Until the interpretation is made the patient is kept to some extent in the position of the infant, one who cannot understand what he owes to his mother. (Winnicott, 1949, p. 74)

Winnicott, D. W. (1949). Hate in the counter-transference.
The International Journal of Psychoanalysis, 30, 69–74.

Conclusions and critique

Hate in the Countertransference was a bellwether of change in the psychodynamic community. Prior to this, therapy was expected to be a sterile process, and any countertransference

---

[1] Using the terminology of the time, he labelled these individuals 'psychotics', meaning those who had extreme difficulty in interpersonal relationships and were unlikely to do well in traditional psychoanalysis.

about the patient was blamed on the therapist for contaminating the therapy with his or her reactions. Winnicott expressed the secret that most therapists held—namely, that they had feelings for their patients. He suggested it was appropriate to have such feelings, leading to a greater consideration of the therapist as a person in the therapeutic encounter and the reciprocal nature of the therapy relationship. More than that, bringing those feelings into the treatment was therapeutically and developmentally advantageous. Discussion of countertransference, its management, and its use is now found in all treatment orientations to assist patients, avoid therapeutic failures, and prevent ethical boundary violations.

To thine patient's self

Main citation

Kohut, H. & Wolf, E.S. (1978). The disorders of the self and their treatment: an outline. *The International Journal of Psychoanalysis*, 59, 413–425.

Background

Originality in psychodynamic therapy was a casualty in the stalemate brokered between practitioners of classical drive theory and of object relations, as each group competed to be most adherent to the legacy of Freud. Outside the psychodynamic community, new approaches to treatment, like client-centred and cognitive behavioural therapies, were mushrooming, but these developments were not taken seriously by analysts. Heinz Kohut created a method that was perpendicular to existing dynamic therapies and responded to the emptiness experienced by many in the post-war materialism of the 1950s, and that truly came of age in the excess of the 1970s. In Kohut's experience, traditional psychodynamic approaches were deemed by certain patients, specifically those with fragile self-esteem, as unnecessarily withholding, challenging, and shaming, and so were only nominally successful.

Methods

Kohut proposed a new structure of the mind—the self—which is a cascading series of related experiences, expectations, and fantasies. In development, the self moves toward cohesion and requires empathic nurturance in order to congeal and sustain itself later in adult life. Early caregivers serve self-object functions; that is, they hold together and bolster the transient experience of self. Examples of self-object functions are mirroring, which allows a person to feel verified and esteemed, and idealizing, which allows for belonging, soothing, and reflected accomplishments. Empathy is the primary vehicle through which these self-object functions are accomplished. In healthy development, the self is provided empathy, becomes cohesive, and is less reliant on others for those functions. In the absence of empathy in early life, the individual repeatedly demands this function from others later on, leading to acting out behaviours, grandiose fantasies, and withdrawal when not forthcoming.

Results

Kohut and Ernest Wolf first suggested that self-psychological processes occur in everyone and result in both adjustment and psychopathology. Healthier individuals are not crushed in failure, nor do they get carried away by success, even though the self is implicated in these experiences. Other individuals, whose early attempts at mirroring and idealizing are rebuffed, have lasting damage to the self-structure that is either worn outwardly or is compensated for through defensive reactions. Disorders of the self are not just restricted to narcissism, but are the basis of many types of symptoms such as forgetfulness, anxiety, impulsivity, and depression. In terms of technique, withholding and interpretation frustrate and shame the person, so empathy is applied instead. Kohut and Wolf thought that when empathic responding is shown to the patient

> who demands praise, despite the availability of external responses, [who] must continue to 'fish for compliments' because the hopeless need of the unmirrored child in him remains unassuaged [and who rages because] he cannot assert his demands effectively, then the old needs will slowly begin to make their appearance more openly as the patient becomes more empathic with himself. (Kohut & Wolf, 1978, p. 423)

Kohut, H., & Wolf, E. S. (1978). The disorders of the self and their treatment: An outline. *The International Journal of Psychoanalysis, 59*(4), 413–425.

Empathy allows the therapist simultaneously to know and provide for the needs of the patient and present them back to the patient in a tolerable and edifying way for the self.

Conclusions and critique

Self-psychology broke up the hegemony of classical theory and object relations and allowed for new ideas to enter into mainstream dynamic therapy. It threw off the required persona of the abstinent and withholding therapist. Empathy was the pre-eminent therapeutic tool, and the most accurate and useful way to gain knowledge about the patient. Psychodynamic treatment of patients with difficult conditions like narcissistic personality disorder was now possible because empathy permitted a foothold for the therapist into the otherwise distasteful psyche of these persons. Lastly, self-psychology invited the concept of multiple conflicting self-states, as the self is made up of various ways of being and experiencing based on the context at hand.

A critique of self-psychology was that the self was never clearly defined, so the approach could be applied generically to many forms of treatment. Additionally, self-psychology overly distinguished itself from the mainstream of psychodynamic thinking by not acknowledging its similarities to other psychodynamic theorists and practitioners, nor its convergence with the work of another expert in empathy, Carl Rogers, who believed that showing conditions of worth to individuals allowed them to become aware of and reach their potentials. Opportunities for greater development and extension of self-psychology might have occurred but were missed.

A therapy of her own: a feminist perspective

Main citation

Chodorow, N. J. (1974). Family structure and feminine personality. In: *Feminism and Psychoanalytic Theory*, ed. M. Z. Zimbalist and L. Lamphere. Redwood City, CA: Stanford; pp. 45–65.

Background

Even though psychodynamic psychotherapy was shaped by many strong women theorists and practitioners, it retained an assumption of the dominance of men. The crux of development was thought to be the dawning of awareness of sex differences (noticing differences in external genitalia) and the psychological consequences of that knowledge (anxiety over the imagined loss and meaning of external genitalia). Melanie Klein, Karen Horney, and Helene Deutsch, among others, all wrote about the experience of women from a psychoanalytical perspective; however, as insiders to dynamic therapy, their thinking largely agreed with the classical lines that had been drawn. Coming from a feminist sociological perspective, Nancy Chodorow was free from the pressures to conform and was the first to offer an enduring critique of dynamic therapy and its treatment of women.

Methods

Chodorow used feminist inquiry, models of social oppression, and anthropological data on women and families to construct her argument for the psychology of women. She started with two premises that she saw as universal across cultures: women perform most of the childcare, and they share unique relationships with their daughters and their sons. Mothers hold a stronger identification with their daughters due to their similarity and to the woman's own memories of caregiving from her mother. Daughters, in looking toward their mothers and other female caregivers, see femininity and relationships as positive and directly rewarding. Based on this experience, women develop a deep, personal, feminine identification and an uncomplicated relationship with dependency. Boys, on the other hand, are seen by their women caregivers as separate and different, and, at every chance, boys' autonomy is encouraged in fulfilment of societal expectations. Fathers and other men are not traditionally present in the household and therefore do not provide immediate objects for identification. Instead, in the boy's identity formation, he must rely on his fantasy of what it means to be a male, which is often a rejection of the femininity he sees around him and of the dependency he experiences in his everyday life during boyhood.

Results

What follows from these premises is the development of the gendered personality. Women, due to their early unbroken attachment to the female caregivers in their life, remain more motivated by connectedness. Their relationship to female role models in early life facilitates the acceptance of this identity. Unique experiences arise within the female life cycle that might bring women to therapy: separating from mothers, family, and significant others; concerns about mothering; and having to occupy a lesser status in society.

For men, autonomy and separateness are thrust on them at an early age regardless of their readiness. The masculine identity foundationally consists of a counterphobic avoidance of dependency and, therefore, is easily threatened by the incursion of attachment needs. Traditional psychodynamic therapy privileged these stereotypically male attributes: the autonomy of the patient was frequently the explicit goal and dependency was viewed as regressive.

Gender identity development affects the way that women and men later interact. As Chodorow described, 'the structural situation of child-rearing, reinforced by female and male role training, produces these [psychodynamic] differences, which are replicated and reproduced in the sexual sociology of adult life' (Chodorow, 1974, p. 46). Men are often more concerned about dominance and appearing without vulnerability. Women, being concerned about the well-being of others, are often content to give men that experience, or at least that illusion. As a consequence, the different intrapsychic organizations cultivated in women and men reinforce gender oppression and disparagement of the traditional roles of women.

Conclusions and critique

As a sociologist, Chodorow initially developed her intervention to be applied society-wide, advocating for a new social structure in which there is greater gender equity and men share more in childcare. Greater balance in gender roles would reduce the pressures forcing girls and boys toward specific intrapsychic organizations. The impact of her work on the practice of psychodynamic therapy has been in the consideration of women's psychology and in challenging the gender-stereotyped assumptions that dynamic therapy has used to treat patients (preoccupation with external genitalia; focus on autonomy and independence). Chodorow's initial focus did not include other identities besides gender and did not account for the heterogeneity of women's experiences. Subsequent explorations of race, sexuality, religion, social class, immigration status, and ability status, as well as more recent reflections on non-binary gender, among others, have been inspired by her attempt to incorporate diversity into dynamic therapy (Tummala-Narra, 2013).

The developmental tilt

Main citation

Mitchell, S.A. (1984). Object relations theories and the developmental tilt. *Contemporary Psychoanalysis*, 20, 473–499.

Background

Many object relations thinkers and practitioners viewed their model as an outgrowth or extension of drive theory, believing that development began with attachment and relational needs and matured to the management of drives and societal expectations. Distortions in object relations happen earlier in development and therefore cause dysfunctions that are more primitive and harder to treat, whereas conflicts between instinctual drives and social acceptability become salient slightly later and lead to less complicated neuroses. This precarious balance between the two approaches, which Stephen Mitchell styled the 'developmental tilt', allowed for continued loyalty to classical psychodynamic therapy along with a commitment to understanding and working with attachment problems. However, postmodern thinking called into question this theoretical manoeuvring because it privileged one tradition over another and contradicted the immediacy and importance of current relationships.

Methods

Outlining the problems with the developmental tilt, Mitchell suggested it minimizes the relational nature of life to the first few months and years, and treats object relations as a cursory step toward the more sophisticated problems of conflict. It denies that contemporary relationships are in themselves important, including the therapeutic relationship. Attachment behaviours in a person are seen as regressive, resulting from earlier experiences, and as passive, denying the person's present needs and contributions to the encounter. When an individual exhibits interpersonal needs in a current relationship, this is attributed to a persisting deficit in the individual, and not seen as an opportunity for the negotiation of that need between the two persons.

Results

Mitchell's solution to the developmental tilt was to abandon drive theory altogether. He posited a new relational model where the individual exists in an interpersonal matrix with numerous relationships to self and others. The primary motive of the individual is relatedness, and the negotiation of interpersonal connection is ongoing throughout the lifespan. Early experiences alter the person's perceptions and motivations about relationships, and distress occurs when the individual engages in relationships without knowledge of these starting values and loses the potential for full and authentic engagement with others. The therapist helps the patient to understand the past, but even more importantly, represents a novel object who stretches the patient in a new, voluntary, and negotiated experience. Mitchell asks us 'to put more emphasis on what is new in the analytic relationship. The past is still important, but as a vehicle for understanding the meaning of the present relationship with the analyst, and it is in the working through of that relationship that cure resides' (Mitchell, 1984, p. 478).

Conclusions and critique

Mitchell's paper ushered in a new school of thought and practice—the relational model. The encounter between the therapist and patient is primary, and therapist disclosure and authenticity are new tools to use to deepen the relationship. The therapeutic relationship is the goal of treatment, not just a medium used to understand earlier experiences. Major topics of study that have come out of the relational model include alliance rupture and resolution, the inevitable breakdown and repair of the bond between therapist and patient that can be restorative practice for relationships (Saffra et al., 2011), and intersubjectivity, the experience created and shared between two individuals (Benjamin, 1998). The relational approach, however, has been criticized for its ephemeral nature. Having a relationship is the symptom, goal, task, and outcome of treatment, which makes the treatment less pragmatic, especially for patients in distress.

Envelope please …

Main citation

Leichsenring, F., Rabung, S., & Leibing, E. (2004). The efficacy of short-term psychodynamic psychotherapy in specific psychiatric disorder: a meta-analysis. *Archives of General Psychiatry*, 61, 1208–1216.

Background

Dynamic therapy works to reduce symptoms, and voluminous evidence for its outcomes has been amassed in the clinical literature. Periodically, there arises a challenge to this supposition, most recently whether psychodynamic therapy meets criteria for an 'empirically supported' designation for specific disorders. Current positivist paradigms of science prioritize the randomized clinical trial and discount much of the constructivist and qualitative forms of study for which psychodynamic therapy has greater affinity. In this context, Falk Leichsenring and colleagues sought to spotlight the considerable quantitative evidence already in existence for dynamic therapy.

Methods

Leichsenring and co-workers used the research technique of meta-analysis to distil the overall effect of psychodynamic therapy across a number of studies. They reviewed 141 studies of dynamic therapy versus control conditions (no treatment, wait list) or versus other active treatments (medication, cognitive behavioural therapy) and selected 17 that satisfied several stringent criteria, including recent publication, use of manualized treatments (systematic procedures of how and when to employ dynamic principles and techniques) with trained therapists, targeting of specific disorders, and administration of reliable and valid assessments. The meta-analysis represented data from over 1,600 participants with a wide array of presenting problems.

Results

Leichsenring and colleagues made two major comparisons: first, whether the average patient in dynamic therapy changed more than the average patient in a control treatment, which they hypothesized would be true; and second, whether the average dynamic-therapy patient changed more than the average patient in an active treatment, for which they did not predict a difference given that both types of treatments were expected to work. On symptoms, patients in psychodynamic therapy performed better than patients in control conditions 88% of the time (a large effect size) and better than patients in active conditions 52% of time (a negligible effect size, essentially a coin toss). These values were similar for other outcome measures like social functioning and at follow-up.

Conclusions and critique

Such is the contentious environment surrounding psychotherapy efficacy that criticism of this article by detractors of psychodynamic treatment was immediate and reflexive. Studies included in the meta-analysis were diverse, and so it is difficult to draw conclusions about efficacy for any one specific problem. However, Leichsenring and co-authors' findings converge with a substantial body of evidence for dynamic therapy in the literature and in other meta-analytical research consistently upholding these results (Barber et al., 2013). Several forms of dynamic treatment have achieved an empirically supported designation. With current funding trends, it is becoming less likely that large quantitative studies like those found in Leichsenring and colleagues' meta-analysis will be conducted. Novel ways of documenting outcomes will have to be found, perhaps in research on the moderators and mechanisms of treatment. In addition, emphasis has shifted toward evidence-based practices, in which multiple types of evidence (including the randomized clinical trial, patient characteristics and preferences, clinical opinion, and many other types of extant evidence) will become increasingly important.

Conclusion

Psychodynamic practice has evolved over the past 125 years. New theories and applications have been developed to help a wider range of individuals with diverse problems and experiences. Forces impinging on psychodynamic therapy from outside, like accountability to show outcomes and the need to become more inclusive, have been accommodated, and many innovations developed inside from the thinking of skilled practitioners and researchers.

However, the field of dynamic therapy has continued challenges, often hinted at by the authors of these landmark papers. First is the variable emphasis on behaviour change. Insight, attainment of developmental needs, or personality change are sometimes the stated goals of treatment. However, the translation of these mechanisms into behaviour and interpersonal patterns is inexact. Psychodynamic therapists are sometimes ill-equipped to handle the question from patients, 'I know what I am doing, but how do I change it?' Worse, it can be interpreted as resistance rather than an honest request for help. Dynamic therapy needs to develop ways within and outside the current frame of therapy to answer this question satisfactorily.

Training and competence are areas for increased attention in psychodynamic psychotherapy. Assuring technical skill is important not only for the outcome of patients but also for teaching the next generation of psychodynamic practitioners. We must observe empirical treatment outcomes and, importantly, listen to practicing therapists in order to know what interventions work, when, and for whom. Indoctrination needs to be avoided, as the history of dynamic therapy shows that growth can be inhibited when conformity is expected. Competence is multifaceted, incorporating timing, accuracy, interpersonal skill, and patient characteristics. It cannot be determined by theory alone.

Neurobiological approaches are rapidly advancing as ways to understand social behaviours and affects. Psychodynamic therapy must, with some humility, acknowledge the undeniable influence of neurobiology on individuals. However, it should also not give up its ambitious attempts to explain our psychology. Even as somatic interventions are increasingly effective, meaning-making, relationships, and symbolism are still valuable and irreducible elements of the human experience.

Finally, inclusion of diversity is occurring in psychodynamic psychotherapy, and dynamic therapy's focus on relationships, identity, and interpersonal conflict make it well-suited to address issues of multiculturalism (Tummala-Narra, 2013). However, rigid adherence to obsolete ways of thinking and previous misuses of psychodynamic treatment in minority populations slow this process. Modern dynamic psychotherapy must justify how it is useful and relevant for today's society and its pluralistic constituents. Such work is critical to the vitality of psychodynamic therapy and to inspire the next generation of landmark thinkers and practitioners.

References

Barber, J. P., Muran, J. C., McCarthy, K. S., & Keefe, J. R. (2013). Research on psychodynamic therapies. In: *Handbook of Psychotherapy and Behavior Change*, 6th edn, ed. M. J. Lambert. New York: Wiley; pp. 443–494.

Benjamin, J. (1998). Recognition and destruction: an outline of intersubjectivity. In: *Like Subjects, Love Objects: Essays on Recognition and Sexual Difference*. New Haven: Yale University Press; pp. 27–48.

Breuer, J. & Freud, S. (1893–1895). Studies on hysteria. In: *The Standard Edition of the Complete Psychological Works of Sigmund Freud*, Volume *II* (1893–1895), ed. and trans. J. Strachey (1955). London: Hogarth.

Chodorow, N. J. (1974). Family structure and feminine personality. In: *Feminism and Psychoanalytic Theory*, ed. M. Z. Zimbalist & L. Lamphere. Redwood City, CA: Stanford; pp. 45–65.

Ferenczi, S. & Rank, O. (1925). *The Development of Psycho-Analysis*, trans. C. Newton. New York: Nervous and Mental Disease Publishing Company.

Freud, A. (1963). The concept of developmental lines. *The Psychoanalytic Study of the Child*, **18**, 245–265.

Freud, S. (1911–1915). Papers on technique. In: *The Standard Edition of the Complete Psychological Works of Sigmund Freud, Volume* XII *(1911–1913)*, ed. and trans. J. Strachey (1955). London: Hogarth; pp. 83–171.

Gay, P. (2006). *Freud: A Life for Our Time*. New York: Norton.

Klein, M. (1952). The origins of transference. *The International Journal of Psychoanalysis*, **33**(4), 433–438.

Kohut, H. & Wolf, E. S. (1978). The disorders of the self and their treatment: an outline. *The International Journal of Psychoanalysis*, **59**, 413–425.

Leichsenring, F., Rabung, S., & Leibing, E. (2004). The efficacy of short-term psychodynamic psychotherapy in specific psychiatric disorder: a meta-analysis. *Archives of General Psychiatry*, **61**, 1208–1216.

Messer, S. B. (2001). What makes brief psychodynamic therapy time efficient. *Clinical Psychology: Science and Practice*, **8**(1), 5–22.

Mitchell, S. A. (1984). Object relations theories and the developmental tilt. *Contemporary Psychoanalysis*, **20**, 473–499.

Redmond, J. & Shulman, M. (2008). Access to psychoanalytic ideas in American undergraduate institutions. *Journal of the American Psychoanalytic Association*, **56**, 391–408.

Safran, J. D., Muran, J. C., & Eubanks-Carter, C. (2011). Repairing alliance ruptures. *Psychotherapy*, **48**(1), 80–87.

Summers, R. F. & Barber, J. P. (2010). *Psychodynamic Therapy: A Guide to Evidence-Based Practice.* New York: Guilford.

Tummala-Narra, U. (2013). Psychoanalytic applications in a diverse society. *Psychoanalytic Psychology*, **30**(3), 471–487.

Winnicott, D. W. (1949). Hate in the counter-transference. *The International Journal of Psychoanalysis*, **30**, 69–74.

Chapter 12

Cognitive behavioural therapy

Keith S. Dobson

Introduction

This chapter provides a selection of important historical articles in the development of the field of cognitive behaviour therapy (CBT). CBT emerged in the mid to late 1970s, but has since developed as the dominant contemporary model in psychotherapy. Recent articles have referred to CBT as the 'gold standard' for the treatment of a range of mental disorders (David et al., 2018; Otte, 2011), and a series of meta-analyses and reviews of meta-analyses (cf. Butler et al., 2006; Cuijpers et al., 2016) continue to reinforce the strong evidence in favour of the efficacy of CBT.

While there is global positive evidence for the efficacy of CBT, this evidence has only emerged over time. Further, although CBT is often referred to as a single psychotherapy model, it has been widely recognized that in fact its history can be distinguished by three predominant phases (Dozois et al., 2019). The first of these was the emergence of cognitive models (as described in Chapter 6) and techniques as an adjunct to what was then the more typical behaviour therapy. Indeed, some of the earliest texts in the field referred to 'cognitive behaviour modification' (Meichenbaum, 1977) or explicitly discussed the incremental value of considering thoughts in the context of behavioural change (Mahoney, 1974). These early approaches also were highlighted by a continual focus on logical empiricism and an emphasis on behavioural change as the primary index of treatment outcome.

The second phase of CBT can be distinguished as fully fledged cognitive models and treatments for various forms of psychopathology. These approaches placed cognitive processing as a critical construct in human adaptation. They often made reference to ancient philosophy: one often-quoted reference, for example, is the Greek Stoic Epictetus ('People are not disturbed by things, but by the view they take of them'). Some of the seminal articles in CBT featured in this chapter clearly position either general beliefs or situational appraisals as critical to the emotional and behavioural disturbances that humans can experience. The treatment models based on these assumptions characteristically suggest that the key to treatment is to identify and remediate dysfunctional thinking through techniques such as 'cognitive restructuring' or 'cognitive therapy'.

The third phase of CBT has taken some exception to what is sometimes viewed as an overly mechanistic approach adopted in the second phase of CBT development. It has recognized that all cognition and experience needs more broadly to be considered in its context. From this perspective, not all negative cognition needs to be remediated, since sometimes bad things do happen. As such, these approaches have adopted aspects of Eastern philosophy and incorporated elements of acceptance and commitment as principles that might, in some circumstances, override the need for cognitive and/or behavioural change. For example, the Chinese proverb 'Tension is who you think you should be; relaxation is who you are' enjoins the listener to strive less and accept one's current position in life more. As further described here, these approaches incorporate a variety of methods in which the therapeutic change process is more a cognitive shift or emotional change than enactment of change.

These three phases were not chronologically sequential, and as the articles in this chapter demonstrate by their dates, there has been considerable dialogue and cross-fertilization amongst the various approaches within the overall field of CBT. In some respects, the flexibility and dynamism of the field is itself a reflection of human adaptability. The field now encompasses a fairly wide range of concepts, constructs, and methods, and in some cases unique treatment components exist for specific disorders or applications. As a result, it has become increasingly difficult to find central or essential elements of all of the CBT approaches.

In selecting the articles for this particular chapter, the author chose to emphasize primary research articles, as opposed to significant chapters, theoretical descriptions, or case reports. As much as possible, these articles were the earliest to represent a particular development, and they have been selected because of their seminal influence either on the field at large or the treatment of a particular set of disorders.

Origins: Cognitive therapy of major depression

Main citation

Rush, A. J., Beck, A. T., Kovacs, M., & Hollon, S. (1977). Comparative efficacy of cognitive therapy and pharmacotherapy in the treatment of depressed outpatients. *Cognitive Therapy and Research*, 1, 17–37.

Background

This is perhaps the earliest and most fundamental article to precipitate the emergence of the field of cognitive behaviour therapy. It consists of a randomized clinical trial that compared what was referred to as cognitive therapy (a specific version of CBT) to what was then state-of-the-art pharmacotherapy in the treatment of patients with major depression. Its importance in the field is twofold. First, it represents one of the first direct head-to-head comparisons between a psychotherapy and drug therapy for a recognized mental disorder. Secondly, the results of the trial indicated that the psychotherapy led to significantly greater improvement than the drug therapy on several outcome measures, and with a significantly lower dropout rate than for the drug treatment. When this article emerged, in the very first issue of a new journal dedicated to CBT, there was considerable response in the psychiatric community, which further reinforced the importance of this clinical trial.

Methods

This study was a randomized clinical trial of 41 depressed outpatients who were determined to be at least moderately depressed, and able and willing to be randomized to either treatment condition. Participants were given either a maximum of 20 cognitive therapy sessions over a 12-week period or a maximum dose of 250 mg per day of imipramine for a maximum of 12 weeks. Patients were assessed at baseline, end of treatment, and three and six months following the conclusion of treatment, using a combination of self-report and interview-based severity outcomes. Relatively novel features of this trial were that the psychotherapists were required to use a treatment manual (the precursor to the Beck et al. 1979 book) and that the pharmacotherapists were required to follow a predetermined but flexible dosing schedule to maximize patient outcome.

Results

Dropouts varied between the two treatments. Nineteen out of twenty cognitive-therapy patients finished the trial, compared to only 14 out of 22 patients treated with pharmacotherapy. The essential result of this trial was that patients who completed a trial of either cognitive therapy or pharmacotherapy benefitted, as indicated by both lower depression ($p < 0.001$) and anxiety ($p < 0.001$ for cognitive therapy and $p < 0.01$ for pharmacotherapy) outcome measures. When only the patients who completed the trial were considered, there was no difference between treatments (average Hamilton Rating Scale for Depression scores of 5.80 and 9.29, respectively). However, when the entire sample was considered (completers plus dropouts), the results clearly favoured the participants who had received cognitive therapy. When considered in terms of amount of improvement, patients treated with cognitive therapy (both those who completed the study and those who entered the treatment) fared better than patients treated with medications, both in the short term and at each of the two follow-up periods. Finally, patients treated with pharmacotherapy were more likely to return to therapy if they successfully completed treatment.

Conclusions and critique

This study was truly revolutionary in its intent, and it caused a major response in both the fields of psychotherapy (favourable) and psychiatry (unfavourable) when it emerged. Some argued that the study was biased against the pharmacotherapy condition, in that providers were limited to one medication, had to engage in a tapering of medications before the end of the trial, that there was no placebo control condition, and that the study group was comprised of adherents to the newly emerging cognitive therapy model. In contrast, the authors of the article noted the randomization of patients to treatment, the use of what was then the dominant antidepressant medication in the field, the blind assessment of patients, and a number of statistical analyses that are today considered essential features of randomized trials (for example, analysing both completers and what are now called intent-to-treat patients).

This article received so much attention that the National Institute of Mental Health in the United States supported and funded the largest direct comparison between psychotherapies and pharmacotherapy to date (Elkin et al, 1989). The Treatments of Depression Collaboration Research Program (TDCRP) contrasted cognitive therapy, pharmacotherapy, and interpersonal therapy for the outpatient treatment of depression in three different cities. It found no overall significant differences among the treatments in depression outcome, although these results were complicated by differential group dropout and site differences in outcomes. In any event, the positive results of the Rush et al. (1977) trial, combined with the publication of the Beck et al. (1979) treatment manual, quickly catapulted cognitive therapy to a dominant position in the treatment of depression, which is a position that it still enjoys.

Cognitive behavioural therapy for panic disorder

Main citation

Clark, D. M., Salkovskis, P. M., Hackmann, A., Middleton, H., Anastaasiades, P., & Gelder, M. (1994). A comparison of cognitive therapy, applied relaxation and imipramine in the treatment of panic disorder. *British Journal of Psychiatry*, 164, 759–769.

Background

Although depression may have been the initial condition to develop and test cognitive models of psychopathology and therapy, the anxiety disorders soon followed. In part, this was a logical extension of the earlier work, as depression and anxiety are highly comorbid, and as some of the belief systems and processes that underpin both conditions are similar (e.g. perfectionism, self-denigration, worry and rumination). Clark's (1986) highly influential paper described a cognitive model of panic disorder which considered catastrophic interpretations of bodily sensations as a pivotal aspect for the development and maintenance of panic. This model clearly implied that exposure to anxiety-related symptoms, in a manner that enabled reinterpretation and decatastrophization of internal sensations and panic triggers, could be an effective treatment for panic disorder. The article summarized some early results from case studies and open trials, but it remained until the current randomized trial to provide more definitive results about the cognitive model of panic.

Methods

This was a randomized clinical trial of 64 adult patients with a primary diagnosis of panic disorder (with or without agoraphobia), who had a current episode of at least six months' duration, and who had experienced at least three panic attacks in the previous three weeks. Patients with a current depressive disorder and several other diagnoses (e.g. schizophrenia, epilepsy) were excluded, and patients had to be willing to accept assignment to any of the four treatment conditions (cognitive therapy, applied relaxation training, imipramine, wait list; $n = 16$ per group). Outcomes were assessed comprehensively both pre-test and post-test, and at 3, 6, and 15 months.

Results

The results of this trial are complex, in part as there were four treatment conditions, multiple outcome measures, and varied assessment periods for the treatment conditions (for example, the wait list only lasted three months, and then concluded). A primary outcome was that at the post-test point, all of the active treatments were significantly better than the wait-list condition on a panic/anxiety composite score. By the time of the three-month follow-up, the patients treated with cognitive therapy had superior outcomes to the other two treatment groups ($p < 0.01$) on the panic/anxiety composite score, but not on a measure of depression. The patients treated with medications continued to improve over time and, by the six-month assessment, the pharmacotherapy and cognitive therapy groups had the same panic/anxiety composite score, and both were superior to the applied relaxation group. Results on other outcomes favoured the cognitive therapy group: compared to other groups, they had a higher percentage of patients who were panic-free at the final follow-up (85%, versus 47% for applied relaxation and 60% for medications). Further, the cognitive therapy group had a higher percentage of patients who achieved what was defined as 'high end-state functioning' (70%, as opposed to 32% for the relaxation group and 45% for the pharmacotherapy group), and lower relapse rates (5%, as opposed to 26% and 40%, respectively).

Conclusions and critique

The authors of this important study concluded that 'cognitive therapy was the most consistently superior treatment, followed by imipramine' (Clark et al., 1994, p. 767). These results were especially compelling at the final follow-up, and were taken as evidence in support of the cognitive model of panic disorder and cognitive therapy for that condition. The study had several limitations. These included the fact that their relaxation group actually received a modified version, to be more consistent in format with the other treatments. They only used medication to treat patients in the pharmacotherapy condition, which is not how many psychiatrists would approach the problem. Also, patients in any of the treatment conditions were allowed to continue with medications they were taking at the start of the trials—a potential confounder to some of the study results. In any event, this research study clearly identified a CBT approach as an effective treatment for panic disorder, and propelled it to a dominant position for both this disorder and anxiety disorders more generally. The CBT approach to panic disorder remains one of the treatments with the best short- and long-term results for this disorder, and is recommended as a first-line treatment in many countries.

Uncharted territory: Cognitive behaviour therapy for eating disorders

Main citation

Fairburn, C. G., Kirk, J., O'Connor, M., & Cooper, P. J. (1986). A comparison of two psychological treatments for bulimia nervosa. *Behavior Research and Therapy*, 24, 629–643.

Background

By the early 1980s, several clinical trials had emerged that contrasted cognitive behaviour therapies with either other active treatments (including psychological treatments and pharmacotherapies) or placebo control conditions. For the most part, these trials focused on anxiety disorders and depression, primarily in adults, and with results that were generally favourable for CBT. Not surprisingly in this context, theorists and researchers began to consider and then examine the boundary conditions of CBT, with disorders that had not been previously treated. One such disorder was bulimia nervosa. In this study, Christopher Fairburn and colleagues built on *a prior* treatment manual, and then conducted a randomized trial of patients who met diagnostic criteria for this condition, comparing CBT to a short-term focal psychotherapy that was specifically tailored for patients with bulimia nervosa. It was argued by the study's authors that this comparison provided a relatively strict assessment of the efficacy of CBT, as it was contrasted with another active treatment.

Methods

This was a randomized clinical trial of adult females who met diagnostic criteria for bulimia nervosa, had an initial weight of at least 80% of their population mean weight, but who did not have other major psychiatric disorders, current alcohol or drug dependence, need for hospitalization, or other ongoing treatment. From an initial group of 46 referred patients, 24 patients met criteria and were randomized to one of the two active treatment conditions, treated for up to 18 weeks, and then followed for 12 months (two patients dropped out, leaving 11 patients in each condition). Outcomes were assessed comprehensively, including number of bulimic episodes, number of episodes of vomiting, weight, and a large number of self-report measures reflecting mental health status and psychopathology.

Results

Patients who were assigned to both of the two active treatments in the study were described as being 'improved substantially' by the authors. For example, the frequency of bulimic episodes and self-induced vomiting decreased significantly with both treatments ($p < 0.005$), and this improvement was maintained during the follow-up. This said, the patients in the CBT group had superior outcomes than the comparison treatment with respect to a global clinical score and on an eating disorder questionnaire at the post-test and follow-up assessment points. Further, 10 out of 11 of the patients treated with CBT rated themselves as having either no eating problem or having minor problems that did not warrant further care, compared to only 6 out of 11 of the participants in the comparison group.

Conclusions and critique

This study was the first randomized clinical trial of a CBT treatment manual for bulimia nervosa, and it established that this treatment could be effective with this difficult clinical problem. This said, there were several qualifications to the study. For example, the referral methodology meant that the patients were not typical of those in clinical care. It was also noted by the authors that since both groups of patients received a psychological treatment, it was impossible to fully differentiate which elements of the treatments were similar and which were distinguishing. Indeed, this issue of common factors in psychotherapy has been repeatedly raised as a concern in studies that have tried to demonstrate the unique elements of CBT that help to explain its efficacy. It has been noted that studies that use placebo conditions or sham psychotherapy can help to identify unique features of treatments that work, but this feature was not employed in the current study. It can also be questioned whether a 12-month follow-up period was adequate for a condition such as bulimia nervosa, since it often manifests with long-term difficulties. Finally, similar to a large number of other psychotherapy trials, this study had a relatively small sample size, and so it is possible that the lack of difference between the two treatment conditions seen on many outcomes was the result of inadequate statistical power, as opposed to true outcome equivalence between the two treatments. Nonetheless, this study was notable for its innovative application of CBT to a notoriously difficult condition to treat. The model has become one of the key evidence-based treatments for bulimia nervosa and has been expanded into an enhanced model for eating disorders; it is now available in a web-based format as well.

Age is not a barrier: Cognitive behaviour therapy in children and youth

Main citation

Kendall, P. C. (1984). Treating anxiety disorders in children: results of a randomized clinical trial. *Journal of Consulting and Clinical Psychology*, 62, 100–110.

Background

As previously noted, the earliest applications of cognitive behaviour therapies were for depression and anxiety disorders in adults. This work has generated an enormous body of data that supports the CBT model in these cases, and also documents that these treatments have considerable efficacy. It was perhaps inevitable that CBT would also be applied to children who suffer from anxiety, as this work would be a natural extension of the adult work, and as many children who suffer from anxiety normally go on to experience adult anxiety problems. At the same time, arguments had been made about whether or not children could use the skills associated with CBT, as their cognitive and self-regulation skills are not as developed as those typically seen in adults. Although other CBT models had emerged for specific skills with children (for example, teaching them how to use self-talk to learn new skills), this article presents the first randomized clinical trial that investigated the efficacy of cognitive behaviour therapy in children with anxiety disorders.

Methods

This randomized clinical trial contrasted a manualized treatment for anxiety disorders entitled the Coping Cat Program. The 47 participants in the study had a primary anxiety disorder, although several specific diagnoses were permitted (overanxious disorder, $n = 30$; separation anxiety disorder, $n = 8$; avoidant disorder, $n = 9$). Participants were randomly assigned either to receive the Coping Cat CBT approach ($n = 27$) or to enter a wait-list control condition ($n = 20$). The therapists were graduate students who were trained by the principal investigator and who had an allegiance to the Coping Cat treatment model. Outcomes were assessed comprehensively, but with a focus on childhood anxiety and depression, negative self-statements, and parental report of child behaviour and anxiety. The treatment lasted for approximately 16 weeks, which was also the length of time for the wait-list control pre- and post-test assessment, and a follow-up assessment was conducted approximately one year after treatment for those participants who were available.

Results

The results supported the efficacy of the Coping Cat program relative to a wait-list control condition across almost all of the outcome measures. These outcomes included self-reported anxiety, parental reports of anxiety, depression, general fears, improved coping ability, and anxious self-talk. For example, scores on the Revised Children's Manifest Anxiety Scales fell from 54.82 to 41.43 from pre-test to post-test in the treated group, but were essentially unchanged in the control group. When assessed in terms of clinical significance, 60% of the treated children had scores in the normal range of functioning, and 64% of the treated cases no longer qualified for an anxiety diagnosis (compared to only 5% in the control group). The one-year follow-up data revealed that self-reported anxiety remained at a low level, as did the assessments from parents and teachers.

Conclusions and critique

This was a well conducted trial of CBT for anxious children relative to a wait-list condition. It should be noted that comparing any given treatment to a wait list is a relatively weak comparison, but that the magnitude and stability of results for the CBT condition in the current trial provided strong evidence for the efficacy of CBT. Further, the fact that a variety of informants (the patients themselves, parents, and teachers) all provided convergent results strengthened the conclusion that the treatment was effective.

Limitations of the study included the fact that the sample sizes were relatively small, which precluded subgroup analyses or the investigation of the mediators of treatment outcomes. The use of a relatively weak comparison, and one that did not include active treatment ingredients, precluded the ability to study non-specific treatment factors. Third, although the treatment was focused on work with children, parents were involved during the treatment, which means that the treatment results cannot be directly and conclusively attributed to the work with the children. The two arms of the study had different lengths, as the treatment lasted approximately 16 weeks, whereas the wait-list control condition only lasted eight weeks. Although it was argued that this was an ethical consideration, these different study links open the possibility that the time to treat was a significant factor in the outcomes that were observed.

Notwithstanding these considerations, this study represented a groundbreaking extension of the work in anxious adults and tested the extent to which these approaches could also be effective in children. The results of this trial significantly advanced the care and treatment of childhood anxiety disorders. Indeed, the Coping Cat has become one of the validated programmes for anxiety in youth, and it has been extended in terms of delivery mechanisms (it is now web-based) and the diagnostic groups for which is has been validated (e.g. mixed anxiety and depression).

Treating the untreatable: The emergence of dialectical behaviour therapy

Main citation

Linehan, M. M., Armstrong, H. E., Suarez, A., Allmon, D., & Heard, H. L. (1991). Cognitive-behavioral treatment of chronically parasuicidal borderline patients. *Archives of General Psychiatry*, 48, 1060–1064.

Background

Despite other early successes with cognitive behaviour therapy, certain conditions such as psychosis and personality disorders were generally believed to be too difficult to treat successfully with this treatment model. This relatively brief paper is generally credited with debunking this belief. In it, the approach that had recently been identified as dialectical behaviour therapy (DBT) (Linehan, 1991) was used in a randomized clinical trial to treat patients who had chronic parasuicidal behaviour and who met the criteria for borderline personality disorder. This study represents the first efficacy trial of DBT and provided preliminary but compelling evidence that what was seen to be a largely untreatable condition could in fact receive benefit from CBT.

Methods

This was a randomized clinical trial of 44 women, half of whom received up to one year of DBT and half of whom received treatment as usual, as it was determined that a no treatment or placebo control condition would not be ethically justifiable. DBT was offered as a manualized treatment, and outcomes were comprehensively assessed throughout the 12 months of the trial, including the use of self-report questionnaires and other behavioural outcomes. Analyses consisted of both parametric and non-parametric tests, as some of the variables failed to meet statistical assumptions.

Results

Outcomes generally favoured patients who received DBT as compared to those in the usual care, particularly in the latter half of the year of the study. For example, the results showed that patients who received DBT had fewer instances of parasuicidal behaviour, were more likely to stay in treatment, and had fewer days of inpatient care than the group of patients who received treatment as usual. In contrast, it is notable that the relatively large number of questionnaires that were administered failed to show group differences (although this result may have been the result of a relatively small sample size and inadequate statistical power).

Conclusions and critique

As noted earlier, this paper constituted a major development in the field of cognitive behaviour therapy, as it presented an efficacy study for what had previously been considered to be a largely untreatable clinical problem. Also, the model incorporated novel concepts such as the use of dialectical reasoning and validation before change, coupled with methods such as treatment teams, to transform the field of CBT. Patients with personality disorders are often considered to be highly challenging, and borderline personality disorder in particular is seen as a difficult condition to treat. The success of DBT with this patient population was remarkable.

One of the important results of this particular trial was the reduced number of inpatient days for patients who received DBT relative to treatment as usual, since this outcome had direct implications for patient care, quality of life, and the costs of treatment. As a consequence, this paper was widely read and had major impact on the development and dissemination of DBT. This being stated, the study did have several limitations. The sample was relatively small and limited to females. The therapists were experienced in DBT and the study was conducted by advocates of the approach. The generalizability of the results to other types of personality disorder was uncertain. Finally, some of the statistical analyses were constrained by the sample size, rendering some of the conclusions tentative and in need of replication.

Acceptance and commitment therapy: Behaviour-analytical cognitive behaviour therapy

Main citation

Hayes, S. C., & Wilson, K. G. (1994). Acceptance and commitment therapy: Altering the verbal support for experiential avoidance. *The Behavior Analyst*, 17, 289–303.

Background

One of the historical origins of the development of CBT is from behaviour therapy. In fact, treatment methods such as setting goals, examining behavioural skills, conducting experiential exercises to maximize goal-oriented behaviour, and examination of situations that facilitate or hinder goal-directed behaviour are all parts of the history of CBT. Within this context, however, a particular approach that has been entitled 'acceptance and commitment therapy' (Hayes et al., 1999) emerged. This approach had been written about extensively before this specific publication, and the authors had published theoretical arguments about the need for a contextual approach to rule governed behaviour change. Thus, they emphasized the important role of language and other private events that determine the meaning associated with various behaviours, and how modification of these meanings can lead to effective behaviour change. Further, they noted that changes in meaning can encourage patients to accept negative circumstances and/or emotional experiences, but nonetheless identify goals that are consistent with their values and purposes, and then commit to enacting behaviour change to fulfil those goals.

Methods

This paper summarizes the key elements of relational frame theory, which is the model that underpins acceptance and commitment therapy (ACT). The paper notes that the goals of ACT are to reduce emotional avoidance, manage responses to cognitive content, and improve the ability to make and meet behavioural commitments. While this paper does not present efficacy data, case materials are presented, including general descriptions of ACT methods as well as transcripts of specific therapist–client interactions, so that the reader can appreciate both the theoretical approach and the application of ACT.

Results

This article really has no conclusion. It is a theoretical and case-driven description of relational frame theory and ACT. The article does include a brief description of outcome and process data on ACT, although it acknowledges that 'the outcome data are still limited' (p. 301). Indeed, whilst some process research is cited, the major outcome reference is an unpublished dissertation (Zettle, 1984), which significantly predates the formalization of the model and ACT approach to psychotherapy.

Conclusions and critique

ACT (and related mindfulness-based approaches) has had an enormous impact on the field of CBT in general. It is a model that, in some respects, challenges the need to examine and modify negative thinking on the part of patients who experience various disorders, and is thus outside of the main corpus of CBT theory and research. At the same time, ACT relies heavily on the meanings that people attach to their experiences, the way that they find value in life (which is, by the way, another CBT perspective driven by core beliefs and attitudes), and the commitment to behaviour change that is consistent with personal values and goals. Thus, while the ACT approach has sometimes been referred to as a 'third wave' of CBT, at least from the perspective of the current author it can be nicely framed within the general principles associated with the overall field of CBT. Undoubtedly, randomized clinical trials that have compared the efficacy of ACT to other existing models of treatment and to wait-list or placebo conditions (A-Tjak et al., 2015) have since significantly enhanced the status of the approach.

Conclusion

The field of CBT has grown dramatically since its first efforts to incorporate cognitive elements into what were predominantly behaviour-change strategies. Beginning in the 1970s, these efforts emerged as a fully developed set of models, and then, in the 1980s, expanded into a broad set of applications through theoretical advances, field trials, and randomized trials. These applications were widely applied to depression, anxiety disorders, eating disorders, and personality disorders. By the end of the 1980s, a variety of models had emerged, with both a strong conceptual framework and evidence base. Even so, innovations in the field of CBT demanded that the model expand during the 1990s to incorporate some of what are now occasionally referred to as 'third wave' elements (that is, aspects of acceptance, mindfulness, and dialectical principles).

One of the hallmark principles of the field of CBT has been its emphasis on the evaluation of therapeutic developments. This evaluation process was relatively easy when specific disorders were targeted for change, but has become somewhat more complex as psychological processes have emerged as the focus of intervention (e.g. acceptance). Nonetheless, many of the technologies associated with CBT have an evidence base to support them, and it is for this reason that they have been promoted within the field of psychotherapy and health care more broadly.

CBT continues to evolve (Dobson & Dozois, 2019); several recent directions will likely continue into the future. These include testing the limits of various models (e.g. different diagnostic applications, age ranges). The development and validation of transdiagnostic processes and therapeutic procedures continues to be a focus of research and development. The development, evaluation, and delivery of optimal strategies to provide access to CBT to the millions of people who could benefit is an ongoing concern. Both public and private groups are examining the use of internet, smartphone, and other technological strategies to appropriate target problems. There has been the genesis of CBT models to prevent disorders and promote health, and not simply treat disorders once they emerge. There has also been an explosion of application of CBT models and methods into diverse cultures and subcultural groups.

From a global perspective, it can now be argued that there have been four large movements in the overall field of psychotherapy. The first was the development of psychoanalysis and psychoanalytical approaches. This model was juxtaposed with behaviourism and behavioural therapy, as well as the humanistic approaches that emerged in the period following the Second World War. Recent years, however, have witnessed the evolution of the large set of therapies that fall under the rubric of cognitive behaviour therapies. This chapter has tried to capture some of that development, through the exposure of landmark empirical papers in a diverse set of domains. Even the act of including these articles and authors is open to criticism, though, as their selection perforce meant the omission of other innumerable developments and key figures.

References

A-Tjak, J., Davis, M. L., Morina, N., Powers, M., Smits, J, & Emmelkamp, P. (2015). A meta-analysis of the efficacy of acceptance and commitment therapy for clinically relevant mental and physical health problems. *Psychotherapy and Psychosomatics*, **84**. 30–36. doi:10.1159/000365764

Beck, A. T., Rush, A. J., Shaw, B. F., & Emery, G. (1979). *Cognitive Therapy of Depression*. New York: Guilford Press.

Butler, A. C., Chapman, J. E., Forman, E. M., & Beck, A. T. (2006). The empirical status of cognitive behavioral therapy: a review of meta-analyses. *Clinical Psychology Review*, **26**, 17–31.

Clark, D. M. (1986). A cognitive approach to panic. *Behaviour Research and Therapy*, **24**(3), 461–470.

Cuijpers, P., Cristea, I. A., Karyotaki, E., Reijnders, M., & Huibers, M. J. (2016). How effective are cognitive behavior therapies for major depression and anxiety disorders? A meta-analytic update of the evidence. *World Psychiatry*, **15**(3), 245–258. doi:10.1002/wps.20346

David, D., Christia, I., & Hoffman, S. G. (2018). Why cognitive behavioral therapy is the current gold standard of psychotherapy. *Frontiers in Psychiatry*.

Dobson, K. S., & Dozois, D. J. A. (Eds) (2019). *Handbook of the Cognitive-Behavioral Therapies*, 4th edn, New York: Guilford Press.

Dozois, D. J. A., Dobson, K. S., & Rnic, K. (2019). Historical and philosophical bases of the cognitive-behavioral therapies. In: *Handbook of the Cognitive-Behavioral Therapies*, 4th edn, ed. K. S. Dobson & D. J. A. Dozois. New York: Guilford Press; pp. 3–31.

Elkin, I., et al. (1989). National Institute of Mental Health Treatment of Depression Collaborative Research Program. General effectiveness of treatments. *Archives of General Psychiatry*, **46**(11), 971–982.

Hayes, S. C., Strosahl, K., & Wilson, K. D. (1999). *Acceptance and Commitment Therapy: The Process and Practice of Mindful Change*. New York: Guilford Press.

Linehan, M. M. (1991). *Cognitive-Behavioral Treatment for Borderline Personality Disorder: The Dialectics of Effective Treatment*. New York: Guilford Press.

Mahoney, M. J. (1974). *Cognition and Behavior Modification*. Cambridge, Mass.: Ballinger.

Meichenbaum, D. (1977). *Cognitive Behavior Modification*. New York: Plenum.

Otte, C. (2011). Cognitive behavioral therapy in anxiety disorders: current state of the evidence. *Dialogues in Clinical Neuroscience*, **13**(4), 413–421.

Zettle, R. D. (1984). *Cognitive therapy of depression: a conceptual and empirical analysis of component and process issues*. Unpublished doctoral dissertation, University of North Carolina at Greensboro.

Chapter 13

Third-wave psychotherapies

Amanda A. Uliaszek, Nadia Al-Dajani, Amanda Ferguson, and Zindel V. Segal

Introduction

While cognitive and behaviour therapies were firmly entrenched in the psychotherapy landscape of the late 1980s and 1990s, there were clear indications that these approaches were in need of refinement. A number of studies and reviews (Keller & Boland, 1998; Linehan, 1993; Safran et al., 1988; Shea et al., 1992; Wierzbicki & Pekarik, 1993) noted that these models were failing to reach traditionally disenfranchised, comorbidly diagnosed, or treatment-resistant populations and, additionally, that few studies examined the mechanisms of action through which symptoms improved, thereby shedding little light on the linkage between psychopathology and psychotherapeutic interventions. In response to these concerns, a number of therapeutic modalities were developed in the mid to late 1990s that featured, at their core, skills in mindfulness, contextual analysis, valued action, and behavioural activation. Steven Hayes (2004) coined the term 'third wave' as a way of distinguishing these interventions from their largely cognitive (second wave) and behavioural (first wave) progenitors, and defined them as drawing from the 'less empirical wings of clinical intervention and analysis, emphasizing such processes as acceptance, mindfulness, cognitive defusion, dialectics, values, spirituality, and relationship. Their methods were often more experiential than didactic; their underlying philosophies more contextualistic than mechanistic' (Hayes, 2004, p. 640).

Here we focus on mindfulness-based stress reduction (MBSR), mindfulness-based cognitive therapy (MBCT), behavioural activation (BA), dialectical behaviour therapy (DBT), and acceptance and commitment therapy (ACT). We have chosen to highlight books and papers that not only demonstrate the efficacy of each approach, but also address three important themes that were influential in garnering support for the third-wave movement. The first theme involves the willingness to target traditionally difficult-to-treat and/or underserved populations. The authors of these books and papers noted that, while evidence-based treatments existed for a particular disorder, these treatments often fell short in their ability to impact those that suffer more severely. This is seen in the work of Willem Kuyken and colleagues (2015), who addressed depressive relapse prophylaxis in recurrent depression. Marsha Linehan (1993) and Patricia Bach and Steven Hayes (2002) focused on populations that were often thought to be non-responsive to psychotherapy, those with borderline personality disorder and those with positive psychotic symptoms. Finally, Jon Kabat-Zinn (1990) focused on those with chronic pain and medical illness—problems where first-line defences included medication and surgeries that often were ineffective or caused greater long-term problems (e.g. opioid dependence).

Secondly, these papers all demonstrate a fundamental shift away from traditional cognitive behavioural approaches. By the 1990s, the majority of evidence-based practice emphasized specific cognitive techniques aimed at distracting from unpleasant experiences or symptoms. Third-wave therapies, in contrast, seek to de-emphasize the importance of such cognitions and reduce avoidance tactics that could well serve to increase unpleasant experiences over time. Instead, patients are encouraged to develop metacognitive skills that support them in observing their thoughts as mental events without getting wrapped up in their content. This ability to defuse or decentre from thinking leaves room for people to consider adaptive behaviours, in turn decreasing symptomatology.

Finally, third-wave therapies place a greater emphasis on understanding and testing underlying theory and treatment mechanisms. For example, Neil Jacobson and colleagues (1996) undertook a component analysis of cognitive behavioural therapy for depression in order to examine the theory that a change in cognition is a necessary and sufficient condition for a reduction in depressive symptoms. In demonstrating that behavioural techniques alone resulted in a change in attributional style and that this predicted treated outcome, that paper highlighted the importance of mechanistic research in refining and streamlining therapeutic techniques. Richard Davidson and colleagues (2003) went a step further by examining the specific neurological and immunological mechanisms that explain the effect of mindfulness on emotion regulation. These studies were exciting and important steps forward in spurring the field to consider the role of contextual and acceptance-based approaches in the larger field of psychological treatment.

Mindfulness-based stress reduction: a self-help guide for physical and psychological pain

Main citation

Kabat-Zinn, J. (1990). *Full Catastrophe Living: Using the Wisdom of Your Body and Mind to Face Stress, Pain, and Illness*. New York: Delacorte.

Background

After being introduced to Zen Buddhism in the 1970s, Kabat-Zinn combined these practices with his knowledge of behavioural health to create the Stress Reduction and Relaxation Program, now known as MBSR. This clinic accepted patients with a diverse range of medical problems and offered a treatment that featured intensive training in meditation and yoga practice. The book *Full Catastrophe Living* offers a compelling rationale for the components of the eight-week MBSR programme and, more broadly, provides a template for how third-wave treatments can integrate traditional therapy elements with contemplative practices in supporting patients' search for greater wellness.

Methods

Those afflicted by chronic illnesses, medical problems, and stress may concentrate too intensely on the avoidance of unpleasant aspects of mood or physical sensations, or may live on 'automatic pilot', unaware of the present moment. Kabat-Zinn suggested that by listening to the body and mind, we can begin to trust our actual experience in the world. This 'way of mindfulness' includes seven interconnected attitudinal factors that make up its major pillars: non-judging (a stance of impartial witness to experience), patience (letting things unfold in their own time), beginner's mind (attitude of seeing everything as if for the first time), trust (in yourself, your experience, and intuition), non-striving (a focus on the process not the goal), acceptance (seeing things as they actually are), and letting go (non-attachment). Through the cultivation of these intentions, people begin to relate to their thoughts, bodily sensations, and feelings in new and more deliberate ways. Different mindfulness practices are introduced (e.g. mindful eating, sitting and walking meditation, the body scan, yoga), with emphasis on how each can be used to cultivate a state of present moment awareness and integrated into daily-life activities. A detailed eight-week practice schedule is provided, allowing the reader to follow the MBSR programme.

Results

MBSR may be helpful for anyone experiencing chronic pain, illness, or health obstacles. This might include chronic back pain, fibromyalgia, heart disease, or cancer. Seventy-two percent of MBSR patients with chronic pain reported a 33% reduction, while 61% achieved at least a 50% reduction in ratings of pain intensity. Patients also reported taking less analgesic medication and being more physically active, and 55% reported a reduction in negative mood states. Furthermore, longitudinal follow-up of clinic patients ($n = 400$) has shown that over 90% maintain some form of meditation practice for up to four years after treatment.

Conclusions and critique

'Facing the full catastrophe' means finding and coming to terms with our humanity. By learning about the mind and body through meditation, one can begin to see connection and relatedness where it was not seen before (e.g. the connection between the experience of physical pain and the feeling of frustration or fear), and begin to put space between the content of an event and the actual experience in the moment. For treatment providers, MBSR represents an experience-based intervention with reliable outcomes. Instead of describing symptoms as problems and discussing how to get rid of them, MBSR encourages tuning in to the actual experience of the symptoms as they are present in the mind and body. MBSR invites the patient to get out of 'doing mode' and move toward simply being by allowing body and mind to come to rest in the moment, even in the context of persistent thoughts and physical pain. Since *Full Catastrophe Living* was published, the methods described by Kabat-Zinn have been widely adopted by psychological treatment providers. The book itself offers a largely anecdotal account of MBSR, but it was an important conceptual advance; the subsequent research it has engendered has provided considerable empirical support for its health benefits (for a review, see Grossman et al., 2004). One such paper is described next.

Neurological and immunological functioning after mindfulness meditation training

Main citation

Davidson, R. J., et al. (2003). Alterations in brain and immune function produced by mindfulness meditation. *Psychosomatic Medicine*, 65, 564–570.

Background

Twenty years ago, there was promising case evidence that teaching individuals mindfulness and other meditative practices might have important health benefits. However, the actual evidence base for this work was founded largely on self-report, with little research on the biological correlates of meditative practice or data on changes over time. One source of credibility for mindfulness training as a self-regulation strategy would be evidence of the engagement of biological mechanisms during the intervention. The present paper sought to evaluate change in neural and immune biomarkers in individuals participating in an MBSR programme and was one of the first to use a pre/post design to assess the effects of training in mindfulness meditation.

Methods

Participants were employees of a biotechnology corporation who were randomly assigned to a meditation group ($n = 25$) or wait-list control group ($n = 16$). The meditation group was modelled on MBSR and training consisted of eight weekly group sessions and one-hour daily home practice. Measures of brain electrical activity in response to aneutral, positive, and negative mood induction were recorded at three time points: before random assignment to each of the two groups (Time 1), immediately after the eight-week intervention (or equivalent time on wait list; Time 2), and four months after the training period ended (Time 3). Participants in both groups were vaccinated with influenza vaccine at the end of the eight-week period. Immune function was assessed by examining antibody titres from blood draws obtained at 3–5 weeks and 8–9 weeks post-vaccination.

Results

Based on previous findings linking asymmetric anterior activation to positive affect, specific changes in four anterior electrode sites (F3/4, FC7/8, T3/4, and C3/4 in the International 10/20 system) were examined. At both Time 2 and Time 3, meditators showed significantly greater left-sided activation at C3/4 compared to the wait-list group ($p < 0.05$ for each) during baseline periods. Following a positive mood induction, meditators showed a significant increase in left-sided anterior temporal activation from Time 1 to Time 2 ($p < 0.05$), whereas controls showed no change. Following a negative mood induction, participants in the meditation group demonstrated a significant increase in left-sided activation (C3/C4) from Time 1 to Time 2 ($p < 0.05$) and at Time 3 ($p < 0.05$), and significantly greater activation in this region compared with those in the control group (for Time 2: $p < 0.05$; for Time 3: $p < 0.01$)

In response to the influenza vaccine, meditators displayed a significantly greater rise in antibody titres from the first to the second blood draw compared with the controls [$t(33) = 2.05$, $p < 0.05$]. Among subjects in the meditation group, those who showed a greater increase in left-sided activation from Time 1 to Time 2 displayed a larger rise in antibody titres ($r = 0.53$, $p < 0.05$), while there was no significant relation between these variables for subjects in the control group ($r = 0.26$).

Conclusions and critique

These results demonstrated that an MBSR-based programme could produce significant changes in brain and immune function, while providing clues to possible biological mechanisms underpinning the benefits of mindfulness-based interventions as they pertain to ongoing regulation of illness/stress processes. For example, this study was the first of its kind to demonstrate anterior activation asymmetry as a function of meditation training; a neurological pattern related to dispositional affect. Research interest in the biological markers of mindfulness and meditation has soared following this publication. An increase in the use of sophisticated imaging techniques has since allowed for more detailed and nuanced understanding on such topics: for example, that mindfulness meditation increases grey-matter density (e.g. Holzel et al., 2011) and enhances prefrontal cortical regulation of affect (e.g. Creswell et al., 2007).

An important limitation of this study is its relatively small sample size and associated lack of statistical power, as well as the fact that participants were relatively healthy and were not chosen for elevated levels of symptoms. Although many hypothesized effects were in the predicted direction, a lack of power limits the strength of the inferences that can be drawn from the results. Nonetheless, the design and methods of the study represented an important step toward further delineating the biological mechanisms of change associated with the practice of mindfulness meditation.

Mindfulness-based cognitive therapy: a prophylactic treatment for recurrent depression

Main citation

Kuyken, W., et al. (2015). Effectiveness and cost-effectiveness of mindfulness-based cognitive therapy compared with maintenance antidepressant treatment in the prevention of depressive relapse or recurrence (PREVENT): a randomised controlled trial. *The Lancet*, 386, 63–73.

Background

Major depressive disorder frequently has a recurrent course; thus, comprehensive treatment should address both acute symptoms and prevention of future episodes. While maintenance antidepressant pharmacotherapy is the standard of care for prevention of depressive relapse, psychological therapies that teach skills to be employed during remission have also generated positive prevention outcomes. MBCT is an eight-week group intervention that integrates the practice of mindfulness meditation with the tools of cognitive therapy. Derived from MBSR, it was designed to teach people with recurrent depression the skills to stay well in the long term. An early review of MBCT studies demonstrated its efficacy in comparison to usual care, which was an important step in justifying the use of meditative practices in mood disorder populations (Piet & Hougaard, 2011). However, these data had little effect on front-line practice patterns because most patients treated for depression receive antidepressant medication. The next step in testing MBCT's suitability for widespread adoption lay in comparing it to antidepressant medication. It was in this context that Kuyken and colleagues set out to examine the two-year efficacy of MBCT in patients who had initially been treated to remission with antidepressant medication.

Methods

Participants in this trial were on a maintenance dose of any antidepressant medication and had a diagnosis of recurrent major depressive disorder, in full or partial remission, with three or more previous major depressive episodes ($n = 424$). They were randomized to either MBCT-TS (taper support: they were provided with support to taper or discontinue their antidepressant treatment) or to maintenance antidepressant medication, and then entered a two-year clinical follow-up. Assessments were conducted at six time points: baseline (before randomization), one month after the end of the eight-week MBCT-TS programme (or the equivalent time in the maintenance antidepressant group), and at 9, 12, 18, and 24 months post randomization. The primary outcome measure was time to relapse or recurrence of depression (i.e. defined as an episode meeting DSM-IV criteria for a major depressive episode) using a Cox regression proportional hazards model. Analysis was intention to treat. Secondary outcome measures included total health and social care cost per participant.

Results

Rates of relapse were similar across both groups: 94 (44%) of 212 patients in the MBCT-TS group relapsing compared with 100 (47%) of 212 in the maintenance antidepressant group. There was no difference on the primary outcome of time to relapse (hazard ratio = 0.89). Total health and social care cost per participant did not differ significantly across the two groups (mean difference £124, 95% CI –749.98 to 972.57, $p = 0.80$), nor did productivity losses and out-of-pocket expenditures.

Conclusions and critique

Kuyken et al. (2015) found that MBCT with support to taper antidepressant medication was as effective as maintenance antidepressant medication in preventing depressive relapse, offering a viable alternative to interminable maintenance medication. Side-effect burden, pregnancy/breastfeeding concerns, or tachyphylaxis can often lead to the unsupervised discontinuation of antidepressants and can increase the risk of relapse/recurrence. The data generated by Kuyken et al. (2015) suggest that MBCT can be an equally effective prevention option. While the findings from this study address the efficacy of MBCT as a multi-component treatment package, it is not possible to discern which particular elements of MBCT (mindfulness meditation, yoga, compassion, or psychoeducation) contributed most to the outcomes observed. This is an important question to answer because the therapeutic components featured in MBCT are also prominent in other third-wave therapies. Perhaps the findings of Kuyken et al. will allow the field to shift its focus towards more mechanism-based studies which can help isolate the active ingredients of change in third-wave therapies and inform the design of more efficient interventions.

Behavioural activation as an active treatment for depression

Main citation

Jacobson, N. S., Dobson, K. S., Traux, P. A., Addis, M. E., & Koerner, K. (1996). A component analysis of cognitive-behavioral treatment for depression. *Journal of Consulting and Clinical Psychology*, 64, 295–304.

Background

By the mid-1990s, the efficacy of cognitive behavioural therapy (CBT) for treating depression had been investigated in numerous studies, with many purporting that CBT was more effective than behaviour therapies and wait-list control conditions and as effective as antidepressant medication (see Dobson, 1989). Others identified that CBT had sustained prevention effects that were on par with interpersonal psychotherapy and pharmacotherapy (Shea et al., 1992). Like many psychological interventions, CBT featured many therapeutic elements, including behavioural strategies, cognitive change strategies, psychoeducation, and homework, yet no one had investigated which components made CBT effective. Jacobson et al. (1996) identified two potential mechanisms of change in CBT: behavioural activation (BA), which includes increased frequency of engaging in reinforcing tasks and events, and coping skills, which includes learning how to cope with negative thinking styles more effectively. They then designed a dismantling study to gauge the impact of behavioural versus cognitive strategies across three components of CBT: (1) BA; (2) BA plus coping with automatic thoughts (AT); and (3) BA, AT, plus schema change (CBT) (i.e. the entire CBT 'package').

Methods

Participants were diagnosed with major depressive disorder (*n* = 152) and scored at least 20 on the Beck Depression Inventory and 14 on the Hamilton Rating Scale for Depression. Participants were then randomized to BA, AT, or the CBT conditions. Assessments were completed pre-treatment, post-treatment, and at six-month follow-up. Mechanism variables were assessed through self-report questionnaires, pre- and post-treatment. Analyses of covariance, with baseline symptom measures as covariates, were used to compare the efficacy of the treatment conditions.

Results

No differences in depression severity or recovery from major depressive disorder were obtained between any of the treatment conditions, post-treatment or at six-month follow-up. In addition, there were no differences in relapse rates, mechanisms, and long-term functioning across treatments at six-month follow-up. Interestingly, cognitive schema change in the BA condition was related to better outcomes later in treatment, whereas early BA change was associated with better outcomes later in treatment in the CBT condition.

Conclusions and critique

The authors were unable to identify any differences between groups on depression, relapse rates, or long-term functioning. This is unlikely due to lack of power in their analyses, as scores on outcome measures across treatment components were comparable. Contrary to the study hypotheses, changes in attributional styles (a cognitive variable) were related to reduced depression severity only in BA and not in CBT, suggesting that BA might be as effective in changing thinking styles as a cognitive intervention. A broader implication is that BA may be a more cost-effective option for treating depression; the authors suggest that paraprofessionals could be trained in larger numbers than CBT therapists and for less cost, in this way increasing access to depression care.

One critique is that the division of the elements of CBT was somewhat artificial. For example, the AT condition they created is not representative of CBT practice in the community. The fact that this artificial condition preformed as well as the full CBT package and BA suggests that the overall level of treatment efficacy across conditions may have been low. The lack of a placebo condition or no-treatment control makes it hard to rule out the latter as an interpretive confound for these findings.

Dialectical behaviour therapy for borderline personality disorder and suicidality

Main citation

Linehan, M. M. (1993). *Cognitive-Behavioral Treatment of Borderline Personality Disorder.* New York: Guilford Press.

Background

During the 1980s, interest in borderline personality disorder (BPD) was increasing for two reasons: individuals with BPD represented a disproportionate number of both inpatients and outpatients in psychiatric settings, and also available treatment modalities were inadequate, leading many to label those with BPD as 'treatment-resistant'. In addition, the most distinguishing features of those with BPD—non-suicidal self-injury and suicidal behaviour—were often ignored as important treatment targets. Linehan adapted cognitive behavioural therapy to specifically target the BPD population by focusing on: (1) acceptance and validation of behaviour; (2) addressing therapy-interfering behaviour; (3) using the therapeutic alliance to strengthen patient engagement; and (4) balancing the emphases on acceptance and change in evaluating therapeutic outcomes. This book represents the hallmark DBT text, providing both an aetiological theory of BPD and an underlying theory of DBT, as well as a detailed description of how to perform the intervention.

Methods

A primary focus of DBT was to reconceptualize and destigmatize BPD as a disorder through a theoretically sound aetiological model and a reduction in pejorative language. Linehan's biosocial theory posits that BPD is primarily a disorder of emotion dysregulation and that other marked symptoms are secondary manifestations of this dysregulation. Using a stress-diathesis framework, the biosocial theory posits that individuals with BPD possess a biological temperament (diathesis) that predisposes them towards emotional lability/reactivity. When this person is placed in an environment (stress) where their behaviour is systematically invalidated, they will be prone to exhibit emotion dysregulation which typically manifests as the behavioural, interpersonal, and self-focused symptoms characteristic of BPD.

Results

DBT is a one-year treatment that is based on the premise of dialectics (i.e. finding the synthesis between two seemingly opposing factors), with the major dialectic in treatment being that of acceptance and change. This treatment has four main components: (1) weekly individual therapy; (2) weekly group therapy; (3) 24-hour phone coaching; and (4) weekly consultation team for the therapist. Individual therapy consists of identifying problematic behaviours based on the DBT hierarchy: life-threatening behaviours, therapy-interfering behaviours (e.g. not coming to session), and behaviours that interfere with quality of life. A behavioural treatment is then implemented that identifies which factors reinforce the problematic behaviours and which alternative behaviours could be implemented. Group therapy is a skills-based treatment that focuses on teaching skills in four areas: mindfulness, distress tolerance, emotion regulation, and interpersonal effectiveness. Mindfulness skills are considered to be a 'core skill' in DBT, as they are necessary in enhancing the effectiveness of other skills. Indeed, each DBT group begins with a mindfulness exercise, illustrating its importance in this treatment. Phone coaching includes coaching calls made by the patient to the therapist when the patient needs the therapist to assist in 'in the moment' skill usage. Many of these interventions are based on a resilience model, where the emphasis lies in building self-regulatory capacities within treatment that the patient can rely on once treatment has ended.

Conclusions and critique

It is posited that DBT for BPD is more effective than cognitive interventions as it introduces several new elements, specifically mindfulness and validation, meant to target the specific symptoms of BPD. For individuals with BPD who are hypothesized to be sensitive to forms of invalidation, it is believed that a treatment that only focuses on change (like CBT) is likely to result in high dropout rates. In addition, DBT places life-threatening behaviours as primary treatment targets. Further, DBT introduces phone coaching as a necessary treatment component in that additional support outside of treatment is needed for safety, treatment retention, and skills generalization. Since the publication of this book, numerous studies have illustrated the effectiveness of DBT with respect to treatment retention (e.g. Linehan et al., 1999). Most recently, researchers have been examining the effectiveness of DBT in other populations that are difficult to treat, including those with eating disorders and substance use disorders (Dimeff & Linehan, 2008; Wisniewski & Kelly, 2003).

Acceptance and commitment therapy for psychosis

Main citation

Bach, P., & Hayes, S. C. (2002). The use of acceptance and commitment therapy to prevent the rehospitalization of psychotic patients: a randomized controlled trial. *Journal of Consulting and Clinical Psychology*, 70, 1129–1139.

Background

Historically, psychosocial interventions aimed at reducing hallucinations and delusions employed strategies that included challenging beliefs, distraction, reality testing, and improving perceived control (Alford & Beck, 1994; Haddock et al., 1998; Himadi & Kaiser, 1991). However, the use of avoidance and suppression as strategies to cope with hallucinations and delusions might unintentionally increase the frequency of such thoughts (Salkovskis & Campbell, 1994; Wegner et al., 1987) and reduce conscious control over co-occurring overt behaviours (Bargh & Chartrand, 1999). ACT (Hayes et al., 1999) is a therapy in which patients are taught to accept difficult thoughts and feelings, to 'just notice' these states without any attempt to alter them, and to focus on managing and controlling overt behaviours. In ACT, it is believed that active avoidance and suppression of thoughts, feelings, and bodily sensations leads to maladaptive behaviours (Hayes et al., 1996). It was originally developed in the early 1980s as a way to combine cognitive and behavioural techniques for a range of emotional difficulties. The objective of this study was to examine if a brief version of ACT would lead to reduced believability of positive psychotic symptoms and if, consequently, this would lead to reduced rates of rehospitalization.

Methods

Inpatients experiencing auditory hallucinations or delusions at admission and who would receive follow-up outpatient care were recruited for this study (n = 80). The majority of patients had schizophrenia (n = 43), schizoaffective disorder (n = 19), or a mood disorder with psychotic features (n = 12). Patients were randomly assigned to receive treatment as usual (TAU) or brief ACT plus TAU (labelled ACT henceforth). TAU consisted of medication, three or four weekly psychoeducational groups, and potential weekly individual psychotherapy if hospitalized for more than a few days. Rehospitalization data was collected during a four-month follow-up period using public hospital records. Participants also reported on the frequency of psychotic symptoms, the level of distress associated with these symptoms, medication compliance, and the believability of these symptoms. A series of analyses of variance or covariance (with baseline measures as covariates) were conducted.

Results

Individuals in the ACT condition stayed out of hospital an average of 22 days longer than individuals in the TAU condition during the four-month follow-up (a significant difference) and were rehospitalized at a significantly lower rate. Enhanced medication compliance and reduced symptom frequency were not found to significantly differ between groups. In fact, individuals in the ACT condition reported significantly higher symptom frequency at the follow-up assessment time point in comparison to those in the TAU condition. The authors suggest that this might be related to acceptance and acknowledgement of symptoms. In support of this hypothesis, 36% of individuals in the ACT condition who denied symptoms were rehospitalized, whereas only 9.5% of those in ACT who acknowledged symptoms were rehospitalized. This pattern of results was not observed for individuals in the TAU condition. Further, significant differences in distress levels associated with symptoms were not observed between the conditions. As predicted however, individuals in the ACT condition reported significantly reduced believability in psychotic symptoms in comparison to individuals in the TAU condition.

Conclusions and critique

This paper supported a brief ACT intervention as efficacious in reducing rehospitalization in patients with psychotic symptoms. Participants in the ACT condition were also more likely to report symptoms and, if they did, they were three times less likely to be rehospitalized in comparison to individuals in the TAU condition. Reduced rates of rehospitalization could not be due to increased medication compliance, reduced levels of distress, or lower symptom frequency; instead, reduced believability and increased acceptance of symptoms were associated with positive outcomes. More broadly, this paper's findings suggest that, while cognitive modification did not occur, mindfulness and acceptance techniques resulted in reduced distress when symptoms were present, thereby lowering rates of rehospitalization in this population.

Conclusion

Third-wave therapies have gained prominence over the past three decades as a response to the perceived insufficiencies of cognitive and behavioural therapies to fully address the needs of underserved patients and/or populations that are difficult to treat, and to the deleterious effects of challenging and disputational techniques utilized to modify cognitive content. MBSR, MBCT, BA, ACT, and DBT all shifted the focus from the second-wave tradition of challenging and changing automatic thoughts to a relationship with thinking that emphasized decentring of metacognitive observing of thoughts without addressing their content. Within these therapies, the introduction of strategies such as present moment awareness, reduced experiential avoidance, contextual analysis, and behavioural activation toward valued action has augmented the armamentarium of front-line clinicians. The integration of these tenets into existing treatment (e.g. MBCT, DBT) or as new standalone treatment approaches (e.g. MBSR, ACT) has provided exciting and fruitful avenues not only for the alleviation of myriad symptoms for thousands of patients but also for new research areas exploring the efficacy and effectiveness of these treatments, as well as their purported mechanisms. As this research literature continues to grow, new insights will likely emerge regarding the types of patients and conditions for whom third-wave therapies are optimally suited.

References

Alford, B. A., & Beck, A. T. (1994). Cognitive therapy of delusional beliefs. *Behaviour Research and Therapy*, 32(3), 369–308.

Bach, P., & Hayes, S. C. (2002). The use of acceptance and commitment therapy to prevent the rehospitalization of psychotic patients: a randomized controlled trial. *Journal of Consulting and Clinical Psychology*, **70**(5), 1129–1139.

Bargh, J. A., & Chartrand, T. L. (1999). The unbearable automaticity of being. *American Psychologist*, 54(7), 462–479.

Creswell, J. D., Way, B. M., Eisenberger, N. I., & Lieberman, M. D. (2007). Neural correlates of dispositional mindfulness during affect labeling. *Psychosomatic Medicine*, **69**(6), 560–565.

Davidson, R. J., et al. (2003). Alterations in brain and immune function produced by mindfulness meditation. *Psychosomatic Medicine*, **65**(4), 564–570.

Dimeff, L. A., & Linehan, M. M. (2008). Dialectical behavior therapy for substance abusers. *Addiction Science and Clinical Practice*, **4**(2), 39–47.

Dobson, K. S. (1989). A meta-analysis of the efficacy of cognitive therapy for depression. *Journal of Consulting and Clinical Psychology*, 57(3), 414–419.

Grossman, P., Niemann, L., Schmidt, S., & Walach, H., 2004. Mindfulness-based stress reduction and health benefits. *Journal of Psychosomatic Research, 57*, pp.35–43.

Haddock, G., Slade, P. D., Bentall, R. P., Reid, D., & Faragher, E. B. (1998). A comparison of the long-term effectiveness of distraction and focusing in the treatment of auditory hallucinations. *British Journal of Medical Psychology*, **71**(3), 339–349.

Hayes, S. C. (2004). Acceptance and commitment therapy, relational frame theory, and the third wave of behavioral and cognitive therapies. *Behavior Therapy*, **35**(4), 639–665.

Hayes, S. C., Strosahl, K. D., & Wilson, K. G. (1999). *Acceptance and Commitment Therapy: An Experiential Approach to Behavior Change*. New York: Guilford Press.

Hayes, S. C., Wilson, K. G., Gifford, E. V., Follette, V. M., & Strosahl, K. (1996). Experiential avoidance and behavioral disorders: a functional dimensional approach to diagnosis and treatment. *Journal of Consulting and Clinical Psychology*, **64**(6), 1152–1168.

Himadi, B., & Kaiser, J. (1991). Assessment of delusional beliefs during the modification of delusional verbalizations. *Behavioral Residential Treatment*, **6**(5), 355–366.

Holzel, B. K., et al. (2011). Mindfulness practice leads to increases in regional brain gray matter density. *Psychiatry Research*, **191**(1), 36–43.

Piet, J., & Hougaard, E. (2011). The effect of mindfulness-based cognitive therapy for prevention of relapse in recurrent major depressive disorder: a systematic review and meta-analysis. *Clinical Psychology Review*, **31**, 1032–1040.

Jacobson, N. S., et al. (1996). A component analysis of cognitive-behavioral treatment for depression. *Journal of Consulting and Clinical Psychology*, **64**(2), 295–304.

Kabat-Zinn, J. (1990). *Full Catastrophe Living: Using the Wisdom of Your Body and Mind to Face Stress, Pain, and Illness*. New York: Delacorte.

Keller, M. B., & Boland, R. J. (1998). Implications of failing to achieve successful long-term maintenance treatment of recurrent unipolar major depression. *Biological Psychiatry*, **44**(5), 348–360.

Kuyken, W., et al. (2015). Effectiveness and cost-effectiveness of mindfulness-based cognitive therapy compared with maintenance antidepressant treatment in the prevention of depressive relapse or recurrence (PREVENT): a randomised controlled trial. *The Lancet*, **386**(9988), 63–73.

Linehan, M. M., Kanter, J. W., & Comtois, K. A. (1999). Dialectical behavior therapy for borderline personality disorder: efficacy, specificity, and cost effectiveness. In: *Psychotherapy Indications and Outcomes*, ed. D. S. Janowsky. Washington, DC: American Psychiatric Press; pp. 93–118.

Linehan, M. (1993). *Cognitive-Behavioral Treatment of Borderline PersonalityDisorder*. New York: Guilford Press.

Safran, J. D., Greenberg, L. S., & Rice, L. N. (1988). Integrating psychotherapy research and practice: modeling the change process. *Psychotherapy: Theory, Research, Practice, Training*, **25**(1), 1–17.

Salkovskis, P. M., & Campbell, P. (1994). Thought suppression induces intrusion in naturally occurring negative intrusive thoughts. *Behaviour Research and Therapy*, **32**(1), 1–8.

Shea, M. T., et al. (1992). Course of depressive symptoms over follow-up: findings from the National Institute of Mental Health Treatment of Depression Collaborative Research Program. *Archives of General Psychiatry*, **49**(10), 782–787.

Wegner, D. M., Schneider, D. J., Carter, S. R., & White, T. L. (1987). Paradoxical effects of thought suppression. *Journal of Personality and Social Psychology*, **53**(1), 5.

Wierzbicki, M., & Pekarik, G. (1993). A meta-analysis of psychotherapy dropout. *Professional Psychology: Research and Practice*, **24**(2), 190–195.

Wisniewski, L., & Kelly, E. (2003). The application of dialectical behavior therapy to the treatment of eating disorders. *Cognitive and Behavioral Practice*, **10**(2), 131–138.

Chapter 14

Psychosocial rehabilitation

Mariam Ujeyl and Wulf Rössler

Introduction

It was in the early nineteenth century, during the age of Enlightenment, that the first mental health facilities appeared in Europe. Up to this time, mentally ill individuals had been kept together with criminals in prisons. These early asylums were generally located in remote rural areas, to facilitate recovery by removing the affected from their harmful social environments. This initially represented an improvement for the 'insane', who often encountered terrible living conditions, either in prisons or in their communities of origin. As no effective treatments were available, the new asylums were soon overcrowded, separated from and neglected by medicine. By the first half of the twentieth century, they had finally developed into the infamous 'snake pits' (Shorter, 2007). Wilhelm Griesinger (1817–1868), a professor of psychiatry and neurology at the Charité in Berlin, Germany, and also one of the most influential founders of brain research and modern university-based psychiatry, developed the concept of community-based care. As early as 1861, he advocated for the integration of the mentally ill into society and proposed short-term treatments in asylums close to the city that were linked with general hospitals (Griesinger, 1861; Rössler et al., 1994).

However, it took time until the end of the Second World War before the first wave of community-based care and the decline of the asylum, reflected in a closure of institutions accompanied by a dramatic reduction in hospital beds, began. Alongside changing societal views regarding civil rights and liberties, the concepts and structures of mental health care in all European and other high-income countries changed, resulting in a shift away from remote mental health institutions towards outpatient and community-based care (Shorter, 1997, 2007; Rössler & Drake, 2017). The underlying philosophy was to treat patients in their natural environment, instead of removing them from it. Whereas in the 1950s and 1960s mental health hospitals opened the 'back doors', the 1970s represented a more radical phase of deinstitutionalization, described by some as hospitals closing their 'front doors' (Turner-Crowson, 1993). However, community mental health followed different paths within and across countries (Feachem, 2000; Becker & Vazquez-Barquero, 2001), with some regions remaining 'overhospitalized' and others lacking comprehensive community-based alternatives despite rapid dehospitalization (Rutz, 2001), placing extra burden on families and risking homelessness or even reinstitutionalization for the most disabled (Lamb & Goertzel, 1971; Stelovich, 1979; Gralnick, 1985; Haug & Rössler, 1999; Munk-Joergensen, 1999; Leff, 2001).

The 1980s onwards represent the period of reform of mental health services with 'balanced care' approaches including both community- and hospital-based services that provide treatment close to home and specific to the diagnosis, needs, and priorities of each individual (Thornicroft & Tansella, 2004). It became clear that community-based treatment settings were not necessarily responsive to psychiatric patients or superior to hospital treatment, in terms of either symptom control or functioning (Anthony at al., 1986). Major developments then evolved from psychosocial rehabilitation (known synonymously as psychiatric rehabilitation; PR), a field and service within mental health systems that shifted the focus to the question of how (effectively), rather than of where, persons are being treated, and the primary outcome from symptom control to functional recovery (Bachrach, 1979; Farkas et al., 1987; Rössler, 2006; Farkas & Anthony, 2010).

PR's aim is to help individuals with severe and persistent mental illness to develop the skills needed to live in the community with the least amount of professional support (Anthony, 2002). To achieve this, PR builds on intervention strategies directed towards the individuals' competencies and towards introducing environmental changes to improve their quality of life (WHO, 1996; Rössler, 2006). Evidence-based models of PR to complement psychiatric treatment include supported housing, assertive community treatment (ACT), as well as individual placement and support (IPS) to help people obtain competitive employment. But challenges to effective PR remain, especially concerning stigma and segregation for people with severe mental illness (Rössler & Drake, 2017).

It was in the late 1940s when Joshua Bierer (1901–1984) opened up the first day clinic in Europe (London), thereby shifting treatment of the severely mentally ill from the hospital to the community. As Bierer shaped the idea that treatment has to include the entire environment and social relationships of a patient, his article on day hospitals (Bierer,1959) has been selected as a landmark paper, although he was only part of a movement that included other psychiatrists (Shorter, 1997).

Leonard Stein's and Mary Ann Test's approach to treatment in natural settings was particularly influential (Stein & Test, 1980). They developed and evaluated a community mental health treatment model for people with severe mental illness in the United States that became known as ACT. Their approach was a paradigm shift at that time (Bond & Drake, 2015).

It was Leona Bachrach in the USA who, in the late 1970s, had already stressed that deinstitutionalization could only realize its promises for long-term patients if programmes were in place that matched patients' individual needs and enhanced rehabilitation (Bachrach, 1978, 1979). Psychiatric rehabilitation shifted the treatment focus from symptom control to social inclusion by functional recovery in valued roles, such as work performance. In a review, she summarizes and discusses the basic concepts of PR, thereby preparing the ground for an interdisciplinary common definition, still absent at that time (Bachrach, 1992).

The process of psychiatric reforms proceeded very differently across countries, and not only in the USA has a lack of appropriate care in the community been linked to negative outcomes. Looking at six different European countries, Priebe et al. (2005) implies that reinstitutionalization has occurred since 1990, but suggests that this might have been driven mainly by factors outside mental health care provision, such as risk aversion (as indicated by the growing size of the prison population).

IPS provides an example of how the principles of psychiatric rehabilitation can successfully be implemented. People with severe mental illness are placed in competitive employment, thereby accessing services in non-psychiatric, non-stigmatized settings (Rössler & Drake, 2017). In a widely recognized, randomized trial in six European centres, Burns et al. (2007) were able to show that IPS doubled the rate of obtaining competitive employment compared with vocational services.

Psychiatric day hospitals

Main citation

Bierer, J. (1959). Theory and practice of psychiatric day hospitals. *The Lancet*, 274, 901–902.

Background

In the 1930s, the Mental Treatment Act in the United Kingdom prepared the ground for the transition to community-based psychiatry. It was during the Second World War when the psychiatrist Joshua Bierer, who trained in Austria in individual psychology with Alfred Adler, emigrated to the UK and began to establish group psychotherapy at a public mental hospital (Shorter, 1997; Cawley, 1992). He soon started the first therapeutic community, which was built on the principles of dynamic psychotherapy. These social clubs led to the founding in London, in 1946, of the Social Psychotherapy Centre, later renamed the Marlborough Day Hospital. This was the first day hospital in Europe. At the same time, Donald Ewen Cameron in Montreal had also established a day hospital, without knowledge of the existence of the London one (Bierer, 1980). In an important paper, Bierer outlined the conceptual basis and values of his vision of a day hospital (Bierer, 1959).

Methods

In Bierer's short article, that was published years after he had reported in detail on the progress of the day hospital in London (Bierer, 1951), he reviews the ideas underlying the original venture. He refers to the disadvantages of hospital treatment before laying out his theory of treating mental illness, then describes the practice of the day hospital, before discussing the implications of his experiences for future service planning.

Results

Bierer describes the Marlborough as a place where self-government and active cooperation of patients was encouraged, and where treatment was provided by a therapeutic team. The day hospital included a night hospital, where patients in need of physical therapy were treated. No patient was refused admission and diagnostic labels were avoided in favour of a 'full picture'. Importantly, faulty or inadequate relationships were seen as one of the causes of mental illness, and not their result. Treatment included 'occupational therapy, individual psychotherapy or group therapy ... group discussions, social club therapy, art, drama, or physical treatment (such as electro-convulsive therapy, lysergic acid, insulin, tranquilisers, abreaction' (Bierer, 1959, p. 902). Bierer suggested placing the day hospital in the centre of the area it served, separating the very ill from the not so ill, restricting the hospital from growing too big and thus losing its personal character, and avoiding discharging patients abruptly but, rather, transitioning them to therapeutic clubs.

Conclusions and critique

Bierer was the one who began psychiatric care in community settings in the UK and was also founder of the *International Journal of Social Psychiatry*. He shaped the idea that treatment has to include the entire environment and social relationships of a patient. With his commitment to community facilities and day hospitals, he promoted greater permeability between psychiatric institutions and society. Furthermore, he emphasized the capacity of all people with severe mental illness to participate actively in their treatment. As the first psychotherapist who was appointed to a post in a public hospital, he was both a pioneer of (group) psychotherapy and of social psychiatry at the same time. This alliance of the two subspecialties was commonplace at that time; it was only later that they developed along separate tracks (Holloway, 1992; Cawley, 1992; Clarke, 1997).

Despite his achievements, Bierer is hardly mentioned in the social psychiatric literature and had only a limited reputation compared with others in the field, such as Maxwell Jones, T. P. Rees, or Thomas Main. Critics argue that his approach remained speculative, that he failed to provide a conceptual underpinning for much of his work, and that a coherent strategy of care was missing at the Marlborough which, according to some, did not live up to its social and therapeutic claims, closing in 1978 (Clarke, 1997).

Assertive community treatment

Main citation

Stein, L. I. & Test, M. A. (1980). An alternative to mental health treatment. I: Conceptual model, treatment program, and clinical evaluation. *Archives of General Psychiatry*, 37, 392–397.

Background

Looking at the example of the USA in the mid-1970s, responsibility for mental health care was fragmented between mental health and the welfare sector, and likewise between many different agencies. In this situation, the concept of community support was developed, with significant influences coming from local services and 'model programmes' (Turner-Crowson, 1993). Stein and Test argued that hospital programmes were inferior to training and support initiatives in the community. Because of this inferiority, they conducted a randomized controlled study on treatment in natural settings, which became known as assertive community treatment (ACT). It was valued as paradigm-shifting, as it challenged many practices and beliefs (Test & Stein, 1976; Stein & Test, 1980).

Methodology

The study included 130 adults who sought admission for inpatient care. They were randomized either to 14 months of community treatment ('training in community living', TCL) or to hospital treatment for as long as necessary, before being integrated into existing community programmes. TCL included the availability of mental hospital ward staff 24 hours a day, individually tailored programmes based on coping skills and requirements for community living, assistance in daily-living activities and employment efforts, and assertive support (outreach) if a patient did not show up. Patients were followed over a 28-month period.

Results

In the hospital group, median length of stay was 17 days. Gains of the TCL group at 12-month follow-up (less symptomatology, less time in institutions, more time in sheltered employment, more satisfaction with life situation, higher medication compliance) mostly deteriorated after discontinuation of the programme. At the 28-month follow-up, time in the hospital doubled in the TCL group, but was stable in the comparator group. Advantages in symptomatology, life satisfaction, and compliance had disappeared.

Conclusions and critique

The authors concluded that it was possible to treat an unselected group of potential inpatients in the community, while at the same time enhancing their functioning and satisfaction with life. However, traditional community programmes for these patients seemed insufficient or inappropriate, as hospital use began to increase after weaning from TCL. It seemed that hospitals were forced to serve as the primary locus of care, rather than as specialized services.

Since then, ACT has been adapted to different settings with differing features. While numerous studies have shown that ACT can reduce time in the hospital, its impact on other outcomes, such as social functioning and symptoms, is less clear (Bond et al., 2001; Killaspy et al., 2006; Rössler, 2006). Recent studies in the UK, and in areas with good services in the USA, failed to show advantages over good-quality standard services that might have adopted many of the features originally pioneered by ACT (Bond & Drake, 2015; Burns, 2010). While some core components of ACT have been dropped over time (such as time-unlimited support; Finnerty et al., 2015), other elements have been identified as essential. These include small caseload size, regular visits at home, a high percentage of contacts at home, shared responsibility between health and social care and multidisciplinary teams including a psychiatrist (Rössler, 2006; Burns et al., 2006).

Psychosocial rehabilitation and psychiatry

Main citation

Bachrach, L. L. (1992). Psychosocial rehabilitation and psychiatry in the care of long-term patients. *American Journal of Psychiatry*, 149, 1455–1463.

Background

From very early on, physical rehabilitation recognized the importance of treating not only the physical illness but also its detrimental consequences on individuals' functional abilities and quality of life. In the mental health field, the concept of rehabilitation only gained importance after deinstitutionalization resulted in increasing numbers of persons with severe mental illness being discharged from hospitals (Anthony, 1992). The failure of the existing care system to rehabilitate those persons stimulated the growth of psychosocial rehabilitation (PR) (Anthony et al., 1986). By 1979 William Anthony had already formulated the mission of PR as being to ensure that a person with a psychiatric disability can perform his or her physical, emotional, and intellectual skills in order to live in the community with the least amount of intervention necessary from agents of the helping profession (Anthony, 1979). However, the term 'PR' quickly became extremely overused (Lamb, 1982), with negative and anti-professional practices identifying themselves as PR. In this situation, Bachrach (herself a proponent of PR since the 1950s) recognized the importance of providing a precise definition of PR. In 1992, she summarized and discussed its basic concepts.

Methods

In a review article, the author identified the mistrust between providers of PR and of psychiatric treatment as a threat to multidisciplinary care: on one side, the myth that PR is the only modality persons with long-term mental illness require; on the other side, the myth that rehabilitation philosophy is intrinsically anti-medical. To overcome this polarization, Bachrach analyses what constitutes the common ground of the two disciplines and describes the benefits that each may offer the other.

Results

Bachrach saw PR as a valuable support to psychiatry and identified eight fundamental concepts: (1) the goal to enable an individual to develop his or her fullest capacities; (2) a focus on environmental concerns; (3) an orientation towards the exploitation of individual strengths; (4) the aim to restore hope; (5) optimism about the vocational potential; (6) reaching beyond work activities; (7) an active involvement of the individual; and (8) the understanding of PR as an on-going process over time. At the same time, she identified practices that have arisen among non-psychiatric clinicians and violate these principles, and that compete with psychiatrists for limited resources. Such clinicians claim that PR is the only kind of treatment that persons with long-term mental illness require, resulting, for example, in the denial of illness expressed in anti-medical and anti-professional attitudes, in unrealistic expectations that pressured patients to perform, and in a practice of limiting programme admission to those who exactly fit in, while leaving others without alternatives.

Conclusions and critique

It is one of Bachrach's major contributions that she defined the philosophical foundation and conceptual basis of PR and, by doing this, tried to safeguard the field from being misunderstood. With her insight, she prepared the groundwork for an interdisciplinary common definition of PR and, thus, more cooperative treatment interventions by psychiatrists and PR personnel (Watts & Bennett, 1983; Bachrach, 1996, 2000). Bachrach was one among other important pioneers of PR—within and outside of clinical psychiatry—who promoted outcome measures beyond clinical conditions and direct effects of psychopathology; she established the view that environmental factors have to be modified to become more responsive to patients, and placed special emphasis on the vocational potential of the severely mentally ill (Watts & Bennett, 1983; Bachrach, 1996; Anthony et al., 1990; Rössler, 2006).

While there is no doubt that PR has since become accepted by the mental health field, the imprecise 'biopsychosocial' model that underlies the concepts of PR is judged by some to have hindered the application of more accurate and scientifically rooted diagnostic procedures that were introduced with the DSM-III in 1980 (Shorter, 1997). To date, the evidence base on interventions that constitute PR remains relatively limited. The emphasis is mostly on improving individuals' competencies rather than introducing environmental changes. In addition, implementation of services that have proven to be effective is low (Farkas & Anthony, 2010; Rössler & Drake, 2017; Liberman, 2006; Barbato, 2006).

Reinstitutionalization in mental health care

Main citation

Priebe, S., et al. (2005). Reinstitutionalisation in mental health care: comparison of data on service provision from six European countries. *British Medical Journal*, 330, 123–126.

Background

The reforms during the last decades of the twentieth century improved the care for persons with mental illness throughout industrial countries. However deinstitutionalization, with a reduction in the number of hospital beds and redistribution of patients, came with problems, as community care alone did not prove to be sufficient for all persons concerned. Unfortunately, psychiatric services' research was confronted with considerable methodological problems; an accompanying comprehensive assessment, that would show the extent to which the shift from hospital-based to community mental health care did meet the needs of patients, was omitted. Rather than comprehensive assessments, psychiatric bed rate and mean length of inpatient stay were used as indicators for progress in mental health reform (Salize et al., 2008). Already in 1999 Munk-Jorgenson argued that the process of deinstitutionalization might have gone too far, as it had resulted in adverse effects for patients and society. These adverse effects were indicated by increased suicide rates, criminal offending, and emergency admissions of persons with mental illness. In this respect, Stefan Priebe stated that reinstitutionalization already reflected a new international pattern (Priebe et al., 2003). To prove this, he and his colleagues compared data on changes in service provision in different European countries, covering not only general psychiatry but also forensic psychiatry and new forms of institutionalized mental health care.

Methods

Data from six European countries that had all undertaken major mental health reforms (England, Germany, Italy, the Netherlands, Spain, and Sweden) was collected. For the time period between 1990 and 2002, changes in the numbers of conventional psychiatric hospital beds were investigated. To see whether this was compensated for by reinstitutionalization, numbers of forensic hospital beds, involuntary hospital admissions, and places in residential care or supported housing were collected. Serving as a non-healthcare indicator of societal tendencies to risk containment, changes in the general prison population were also investigated.

Results

The number of general hospital beds did decrease in five countries (all but Italy). In all countries, an increase in the number of forensic beds and places in supported housing was observed. Changes in involuntary hospital admissions were inconsistent. Only in three countries (England, Spain, and Sweden) was the reduction in psychiatric hospital beds not compensated for by additional forensic beds or places in supported housing. In Italy and the Netherlands, the increase in forensic beds and supported housing has been much greater than the decrease in psychiatric bed numbers. In all countries, a substantial increase of the general prison population of between 16% and 104% was observed.

Conclusions and critique

With the evidence collected, the authors were able to quantify reinstitutionalization, and concluded that it was occurring in all countries investigated, despite wide differences across their health care systems. The results indicated that sectors were linked, and that changes in service provision in one sector (general psychiatric hospitals) affected other forms of institutionalized mental health care (forensic sector, supported housing) that to some degree compensated for the changes. Thereby, the results supported the view that the process of deinstitutionalization had already come to an end. However, the study results did not prove a causal relationship between changes in different sectors and also did not enable the authors to explain the historical and societal drivers of these changes (Chow & Priebe, 2016). However, as the prison population had substantially increased in parallel over the period investigated, it seemed that reinstitutionalization had been driven by risk aversion in European societies.

Following this article, further data-driven research into the phenomenon and causes of reinstitutionalization was published, and promoted the debate (Salize et al., 2008; Keown et al., 2011; Chow & Priebe, 2016). Because of the decreasing length of stay, fewer hospital beds do not necessarily result in fewer patients treated in hospitals (Pedersen & Kolstad, 2009). Thus, data on the number of places in institutions cannot provide sufficient evidence on whether patients might move from one sector to another. Rather, information on patient characteristics and long-term pathways is needed to ascertain if the provision of one institution influences utilization of another.

The effectiveness of supported employment for people with severe mental illness

Main citation

Burns, T., et al. (2007). The effectiveness of supported employment for people with severe mental illness: a randomised controlled trial. *The Lancet*, 370, 1146–1152.

Background

Employment is a major contributor to economic status, social position, and quality of life (Knapp et al., 2013). At the turn of the millennium, unemployment for persons with severe mental illness remained very high in Europe. The most widespread rehabilitation model focused on job skills' training to prepare patients for a return to employment ('train and place' model). However, an alternative model, in which patients were directly placed into occupation and then supported ('place and train'), had proven to be more effective in the United States (Gold et al., 2006; Drake et al., 1996; Latimer et al., 2006). As Europe differs in terms of welfare systems, labour market, and cultural attitudes, Tom Burns and colleauges, along with the EQOLISE Group, used a multicentre randomized controlled trial to investigate whether the most prominent 'place and train' model, known as individual placement and support (IPS), was superior to alternative services in achieving competitive employment in the European context.

Methods

Adults from six cities in the UK, Germany, Italy, Switzerland, the Netherlands, and Bulgaria were included if they had severe mental illness, major role dysfunction, and no competitive employment for at least one year. They were randomly assigned to IPS (n = 156) or traditional vocational services (n = 156) and followed over 18 months. IPS included helping participants develop realistic goals and seek appropriate employment within a given network. The primary outcome was the proportion of people entering competitive employment. The secondary outcomes included hours worked, number of days employed, job tenure, dropout from services, and hospital admissions.

Results

IPS was more effective than vocational service: 55% of people with IPS versus 28% of those with vocational services were at least one day in employment. IPS increased the number of hours worked (difference in hours 309) and number of days employed (difference in days 100). Service dropout rate was higher with vocational services than IPS (difference 32%), as was hospital admission rate (difference 11%). The effectiveness of IPS was significantly affected by local unemployment. Effectiveness, irrespective of service, was significantly affected by long-term unemployment, an increase in GDP, and the benefit trap (perceived or real financial disincentives to return to work).

Conclusions and critique

The study showed that IPS was superior to vocational training, and that its effectiveness can be transferred from the USA to the European context broadly undiminished. The rate of people that obtained competitive employment nearly doubled, and those assigned to IPS kept their jobs longer and worked more hours, without experiencing relapses resulting in psychiatric hospital admissions. The study contributed to the endorsement of IPS in Europe, thereby enabling people with severe mental illness to access services in non-psychiatric, non-stigmatized settings and offering them better chances to be independent and participate socially (Rössler & Drake, 2017; Killackey, 2008). In the German and Dutch centres, no significant differences between the interventions were found; the exact reason, beyond small sample sizes, remained unclear.

More than 50% of eligible patients refused to participate in the IPS trial, and greater disincentives to work impeded entry into the competitive workforce irrespective of service. This facilitated the debate on how to reach out to those who are currently unengaged, and raised the question of how values of social solidarity and incentives to work can best be reconciled to avoid the effects of a benefit trap (Latimer, 2008; Campbell et al., 2011; Burton, 2009). Limitations of studies on IPS include follow-up periods that are too short to address the durability of effects (Kinoshita et al., 2013).

Conclusion

The reforms during the last decades of the twentieth century improved the care for persons with mental illness throughout industrial countries. There is no doubt that the shift from mostly remote, hospital-based care to more balanced care (that includes outpatient and community mental health service provision) has been accomplished and has paved the way for better psychosocial rehabilitation. However, at the same time, a range of unanswered questions remain and point to the following obstacles that may impede further achievements towards functional recovery of the severely ill:

1.How does the more holistic approach of social psychiatry and the inevitably vague 'biopsychosocial' model of PR fit in modern diagnosis-specific treatment concepts? There is a risk that the emphasis on multidisciplinary teams, on functional recovery, and on the social environment competes against highly differentiated service provision, as well as against diagnosis-specific treatment approaches, if it is not integrated with these treatment methods but partly replaces them.

2.Is there still scope to achieve better responsiveness to the needs of the severely ill by further replacing inpatient time in general psychiatric hospitals with outpatient care? If so, it seems necessary to safeguard that further changes will not be to the detriment of the most severely ill. They might be 'shifted' (or reinstitutionalized) more readily to institutionalized mental health care settings that offer even less rehabilitation opportunities (as, for example, with decreasing length of inpatient stay, patients may be discharged in conditions that make them more likely to experience difficulties in performing their social roles). Any potential interplay between sectors needs to be investigated using comprehensive data.

3.What works for each particular population and setting? The examples of IPS and ACT have demonstrated that the (relative) effectiveness of model programmes may depend not only on the population addressed and components included, but also on variations between countries with respect to mental health service provision and social policy (e.g. social welfare system), thereby limiting regional and/or international generalizability of the available evidence.

4.How can PR be made more readily available for most of the mentally ill with functional disabilities? Better implementation of those approaches that have already proven to be effective seems needed. The attitude of the public towards psychiatry is mostly influenced by what PR accomplishes; thus it addresses the stigma associated with mental illness, which still impedes further progress in psychiatric reform.

References

Anthony, W. A. (1992). Issues and future policy perspectives: psychiatric rehabilitation. *Health Affairs*, **11**(3), 164–171.

Anthony, W. A. (1979). *The Principles of Psychiatric Rehabilitation*. Baltimore: University Park Press.

Anthony, W. A., Cohen, M., Farkas, M., & Gagne, C. (2002). *Psychiatric Rehabilitation*, 2nd edn. Boston: Boston University Center for Psychiatric Rehabilitation.

Anthony, W. A., Cohen, M., & Farkas, M. (1990). *Psychiatric Rehabilitation*. Boston: Boston University Center for Psychiatric Rehabilitation.

Anthony, W. A., Kennard, W. A., O'Brien, W. F, & Forbes, R. (1986). Psychiatric rehabilitation: past myths and current realities. *Community Mental Health Journal*, **22**(4), 249–264.

Bachrach, L. L. (2000). Psychosocial rehabilitation and psychiatry in the treatment of schizophrenia—what are the boundaries? *Acta Psychiatrica Scandinavia Supplement*, **407**, 6–10.

Bachrach, L. L. (1996). Psychosocial rehabilitation and psychiatry: what are the boundaries? *The Canadian Journal of Psychiatry*, **41**(1), 28–35.

Bachrach, L. L. (1992). Psychosocial rehabilitation and psychiatry in the care of long-term patients. *American Journal of Psychiatry*, **149**(11), 1455–1463.

Bachrach, L. L. (1979). Planning mental health services for chronic patients. *Hospital & Community Psychiatry*, **30**(69), 387–393.

Bachrach, L. L. (1978). A conceptual approach to deinstitutionalization. *Hospital & Community Psychiatry*, **29**(9), 573–578.

Barbato, A. (2006). Psychosocial rehabilitation and severe mental disorders: a public health approach. *World Psychiatry*, 5(3), 162–163.

Becker, I. & **Vázquez-Barquero, J. L.** (2001). The European perspective of psychiatric reform. *Acta Psychiatrica Scandinavia Supplement*, 410, 8–14.

Bierer, J. (1951). *The Day Hospital. An Experiment in Social Psychiatry and Syntho-Analytic Psychotherapy*. London: H. K. Lewis.

Bierer, J. (1959). Theory and practice of psychiatric day hospitals. *The Lancet*, **274** (7108), 901–902.

Bierer, J. (1980). From psychiatry to social and community psychiatry. *International Journal of Social Psychiatry*, **26**, 77–79.

Bond, G. R. & **Drake, R. E.** (2015). The critical ingredients of assertive community treatment. *World Psychiatry*, **14**(2), 240–242.

Bond, G. R., **Drake, R. E.**, **Mueser, K. T.**, & **Latimer, E.** (2001). Assertive community treatment for people with severe mental illness: critical ingredients and impact on patients. *Disease Management & Health Outcomes*, **9(3)**, 141–159.

Burns, T. (2010). The rise and fall of assertive community treatment? *International Review of Psychiatry*, 22, 130–137.

Burns, T., **Catty, J.**, & **Wright, C.** (2006). De-constructing home-based care for mental illness: can one identify the effective ingredients? *Acta Psychiatrica Scandinavia Supplement*, **429**, 33–35.

Burns, T., et al. (2007). The effectiveness of supported employment for people with severe mental illness: a randomised controlled trial. *The Lancet*, **370**(9593), 1146–1152.

Burton, J. D. (2009). Moving towards value-based supported employment programs. *Psychiatric Rehabilitation Journal*, **32**(4), 257–258.

Campbell, K., **Bond, G. R.**, & **Drake, R. E.** (2011). Who benefits from supported employment: a meta-analytic study. *Schizophrenia Bulletin*, **37**(2), 370–380.

Cawley, R. H. (1992). Bierer's precepts today and tomorrow. The Fifth Joshua Bierer Memorial Lecture delivered to the British Association for Social Psychiatry, 23 May 1991. *International Journal of Social Psychiatry*, **38**(2), 87–94.

Chow, W. S. & **Priebe, S.** (2016). How has the extent of institutional mental healthcare changed in Western Europe? Analysis of data since 1990. *BMJ Open*, **6(4)**, e010188. doi, 10.1136/bmjopen-2015-010188

Clarke, L. (1997). Joshua Bierer: striving for power. *History of Psychiatry*, **8**, 319–332.

Drake, R. E., **McHugo, G. J.**, **Becker, D. R.**, **Anthony, W. A.**, & **Clark, R. E.** (1996). The New Hampshire study of supported employment for people with severe mental illness. *Journal of Consulting and Clinical Psychology*, **64**(2), 391–399.

Farkas, M. & **Anthony, W. A.** (2010). Psychiatric rehabilitation interventions: a review. *International Review of Psychiatry*, **22**(2), 114–129.

Farkas, M. D., **Rogers, E. S.**, & **Thurer, S.** (1987). Rehabilitation outcome of long-term hospital patients left behind by deinstitutionalization. *Hospital & Community Psychiatry*, **38**(8), 864–870.

Feachem, R. G. (2000). Health systems: more evidence, more debate. *Bulletin of the World Health Organization*, **78**(6), 715.

Finnerty, M. T., et al. (2015). Clinicians perceptions of challenges and strategies of transition from assertive community treatment to less intensive services. *Community Mental Health Journal*, 51, 85–95.

Gold, P. B., **Meisler, N.**, **Santos, A. B.**, **Carnemolla, M. A.**, **Williams, O. H.**, & **Keleher, J.** (2006). Randomized trial of supported employment integrated with assertive community treatment for rural adults with severe mental illness. *Schizophrenia Bulletin*, **32**(2), 378–395.

Gralnick, A. (1985). Build a better state hospital: deinstitutionalization has failed. *Hospital & Community Psychiatry*, **36**(7), 738–741.

Griesinger, W. (1861). *Mental Pathology and Therapeutics*. New York: William Wood.

Haug, H. J. & Rössler, W. (1999). Deinstitutionalization of psychiatric patients in central Europe. *European Archives of Psychiatry and Clinical Neuroscience*, **249**, 115–122.

Holloway, F. (1992). Joshua Bierer and social psychiatry. *International Journal of Social Psychiatry*, **38**(2), 85–86.

Killaspy, H., et al. (2009). Randomised evaluation of assertive community treatment: 3-year outcomes. *British Journal of Psychiatry*, **195**(1), 81–82.

Killackey, E., Jackson, H. J., & McGorry, P. D. (2008). Vocational intervention in first-episode psychosis: individual placement and support v. treatment as usual. *British Journal of Psychiatry*, **193**(2), 114–120.

Kinoshita, Y., et al. (2013). Supported employment for adults with severe mental illness. *Cochrane Database of Systematic Reviews*, **13**(9), CD008297.

Knapp, M., et al. (2013). Supported employment: cost-effectiveness across six European sites. *World Psychiatry*, **12**(1), 60–68.

Keown, P., Weich, S., Bhui, K. S., & Scott, J. (2011). Association between provision of mental illness beds and rate of involuntary admissions in the NHS in England 1988–2008: ecological study. *British Medical Journal*, **343**, d3736.

Lamb, H. R. (1982). *Treating the Long-Term Mentally Ill: Beyond Deinstitutionalization*. San Francisco: Jossey-Bass.

Lamb, H. R. & Goertzel, V. (1971). Discharged mental patients—are they really in the community? *Archives of General Psychiatry*, **24**(1), 29–34.

Latimer, E. A. (2008). Individual placement and support programme increases rates of obtaining employment in people with severe mental illness. *Evidence-Based Mental Health*, **11**(2), 52.

Latimer, E. A., et al. (2006). Generalisability of the individual placement and support model of supported employment: results of a Canadian randomized controlled trial. *British Journal of Psychiatry*, **189**, 65–73.

Leff, J. (2001). Why is care in the community perceived as a failure? *British Journal of Psychiatry*, **179**(5), 381–383.

Liberman, R. P. (2006). Caveats for psychiatric rehabilitation. *World Psychiatry*, **5**(3), 158–159.

Munk-Jorgensen, P. (1999). Has deinstitutionalization gone too far? *European Archives of Psychiatry and Clinical Neuroscience*, **249**, 136–143.

Pedersen, P. B. & Kolstad, A. (2009). De-institutionalisation and trans-institutionalisation—changing trends of inpatient care in Norwegian mental health institutions 1950–2007. *International Journal of Mental Health Systems*, **3**(1). doi: 10.1186/1752-4458-3-28

Priebe, S. & Turner, T. (2003). Reinstitutionalisation in mental health care. This largely unnoticed process requires debate and evaluation. *British Medical Journal*, **326**, 175–176.

Priebe, S., et al. (2005). Reinstitutionalisation in mental health care: comparison of data on service provision from six European countries. *British Medical Journal*, **330**(7483), 123–126.

Rössler, W. (2006). Psychiatric rehabilitation today: an overview. *World Psychiatry*, **5**(3), 151–157.

Rössler, W. & Drake, R. E. (2017). Psychiatric rehabilitation in Europe. *Epidemiology and Psychiatric Sciences*, **19**, 1–7.

Rössler, W., Riecher-Rössler, A., & Meise, U. (1994). Wilhelm Griesinger and the concept of community care in 19th-century Germany. *Hospital & Community Psychiatry*, **45**(8), 818–822.

Rutz, W. (2001). Mental health in Europe: problems, advances and challenges. *Acta Psychiatrica Scandinavia Supplement*, **410**, 15–20.

Salize, H. J., Schanda, H., & Dressing, H. (2008). From the hospital into the community and back again—a trend towards re-institutionalisation in mental health care? *International Review of Psychiatry*, **20**(6), 527–534.

Shorter, E. (1997). *A History of Psychiatry. From the Era of the Asylum to the Age of Prozac.* New York: John Wiley.

Shorter, E. (2007). The historical development of mental health services in Europe. In:*Mental Health Policy and Practice across Europe*, ed. M. Knapp, D. McDaid, G. Thornicroft, & E. Mossialos. Maidenhead, UK: Open University Press/McGraw Hill.

Stein, L. I. & Test, M. A. (1980). An alternative to mental health treatment. I: Conceptual model, treatment program, and clinical evaluation. *Archives of General Psychiatry*, **37**, 392–397.

Stelovich, S. (1979). From the hospital to the prison: a step forward in deinstitutionalization? *Hospital & Community Psychiatry*, **30**, 618–620.

Test, M. A. & Stein, L. I. (1976). Practical guidelines for the community treatment of markedly impaired patients. *Community Mental Health Journal*, **12**(1), 72–82.

Thornicroft, G. & Tansella, M. (2004). Components of a modern mental health service: a pragmatic balance of community and hospital care: overview of systematic evidence. *British Journal of Psychiatry*, **185**, 283–290.

Turner-Crowson, J. (1993). *Reshaping Mental Health Services. Implications for Britain of US Experience (Research Report).* London: King's Fund.

Watts, F. N. & Bennett, D. H. (1983). Introduction: the concept of rehabilitation. In: *Theory and Practice of Psychiatric Rehabilitation*, ed. F. N Watts & D. H. Bennett. Chichester, England: John Wiley.

World Health Organization. (1996). *Psychosocial Rehabilitation: A Consensus Statement.* Geneva: World Health Organization.

Chapter 15

Social and community psychiatry

Neil Jordan

Introduction

Social and community psychiatry is a subspecialty within the field of psychiatry that focuses on the identification and treatment of mental health disorders in community-based (i.e. non-institutional) settings. This subspecialty evolved in the United States during the latter half of the twentieth century as a direct consequence of three major occurrences: (1) deinstitutionalization; (2) the biological psychiatry movement and the advent of psychotropic medications; and (3) the shift in financing of mental healthcare from states to public and private insurance programmes. Aided by the Community Mental Health Centers Act of 1963, the deinstitutionalization movement shifted the majority of psychiatric practice from state hospitals to community mental health centres, nursing homes, and other community settings. At the same time, the first generation of antipsychotic (e.g. chlorpromazine, haloperidol), antidepressant (e.g. imipramine, amitriptyline, nortriptyline), and stimulant (e.g. methylphenidate) medications increased the available options for treating mental health disorders. President Lyndon B. Johnson's Great Society Movement spurred federal legislation that created the Medicare and Medicaid public health insurance programmes in 1965, both of which provided coverage for certain psychiatric services and enabled many more Americans to afford mental health treatment. The Mental Health Parity and Addiction Equity Act of 2008 strengthened private health insurance coverage for psychiatric services. The combination of all three of these occurrences dramatically altered everyday practice for psychiatrists and other mental health providers in community practice.

The first significant challenge in reorienting psychiatric service delivery towards primarily community-based services was consideration of the prevalence and incidence of mental health disorders and describing the extent to which psychiatric services are received in different care settings. Regier et al.'s (1978) work made two important accomplishments: (1) it was the first paper to accurately estimate the prevalence of mental health disorders in the United States; and (2) it established that psychiatric services were more commonly delivered in the general medicine sector than in the specialty mental health sector.

As community psychiatry evolved, external factors such as managed care impacted the way that psychiatrists delivered mental health treatment. Olfson and colleagues (1999) were the first to use nationally representative data to demonstrate what many had reported anecdotally: psychotherapy use and visit duration had both decreased, while the use of psychotropic medications had increased.

Another consequence of health system reforms for psychiatric treatment was the evolution of primary care as an effective setting for mental healthcare, particularly for depression. Collaborative care models, where specialty mental health providers are integrated into the primary care clinic, were shown to significantly reduce depressive symptoms for patients with major depression (Katon et al., 1995, 1996). Building on those studies, Katon et al. (1999) demonstrated that a stepped care approach, in which patients with depressive disorders who were treated in primary care without improvement 'stepped up' to specialty mental healthcare, achieved better outcomes than continuation of usual primary care.

As the subspecialty of social and community psychiatry evolved, forcing the more precise measurement of disease prevalence and delineating further the context of treatment received, a subfield of social and community psychiatry also evolved. Known as cross-cultural psychiatry, this subfield focuses on understanding cultural and ethnic differences in mental health disorders, thus expanding our understanding of the prevalence and treatment of mental health disorders to include traditional ethnic or cultural contexts. Kleinman (1977) brought an anthropological lens to this subfield and makes the case that culture impacts the way that individuals talk about their mental health disorders and their willingness to engage in psychiatric treatment.

Prevalence of and treatment for mental health disorders by treatment sector

Main citation

Regier, D. A., Goldberg, I., & Taube, C. A. (1978). The de facto US mental health services system: a public health perspective. *Archives of General Psychiatry*, 35, 685–693.

Background

When Jimmy Carter's administration established the President's Commission on Mental Health, its first priority was to establish valid epidemiological data on the number of persons with a mental health disorder and the number of persons receiving mental health services (The White House, 1977). At that point in time, existing mental health services data allowed analysts to count the number of mental health service events (e.g. clinic visits, hospital admissions) but not the number of unique individuals receiving those mental health services (Public Health Service, 1977). In addition to being among the first to ever estimate the prevalence of mental health disorders and the number of persons receiving mental health services in specific sectors of the American mental health services system, Darrel Regier and colleagues also clearly defined these sectors for the first time.

Methods

The authors, all of whom worked for the National Institute of Mental Health's Division of Biometry and Epidemiology, gathered all existing data from a variety of sources. Sources of data included surveys of American mental health facilities, psychiatric halfway houses, and community residences; psychiatry and psychology visit data from the National Ambulatory Medical Care Survey and National Register of Health Service Providers in Psychology, respectively; and primary care data from the National Health Interview Survey. These data were organized into a one-year time frame. They then combined the data, eliminating redundancies in order to estimate the total number of persons with a mental health disorder treated in any facility during one year, receiving each type of service.

Results

Regier et al. identified four major sectors in which mental health services may be received: (1) specialty mental health, which primarily encompasses freestanding outpatient mental health clinics and community mental health agencies, private practice psychiatrists and psychologists, public mental hospitals, and general hospitals with a psychiatric unit; (2) general hospitals and nursing homes; (3) primary care and outpatient settings, known together as general medicine; and (4) what the authors refer to as the 'not in treatment/other human services' sector, although no survey or utilization data existed at the time to capture mental health service use received from 'other human services' providers. The authors estimated that at least 15% of the American population had a mental health disorder each year. They also estimated that only about one fifth of individuals with a mental health disorder received care in the specialty mental health sector. Identification and treatment for mental health disorders was much more common in the general medicine sector, where they estimated that three fifths of individuals with a mental health disorder received care. The remaining one fifth of individuals with a mental health disorder were not in treatment or received 'other human services'.

Conclusions and critique

Fortunately, we have a come long way since the 1970s in our ability to accurately assess the prevalence of mental health disorders in the American population and quantify the use of mental health services across all components of the mental health system of care. Regier et al.'s work set the stage for the National Comorbidity Survey (NCS), the first nationally representative survey of the prevalence of mental health disorders (Kessler et al., 1994), which is discussed in Chapter 2. Ron Kessler and colleagues went on to develop the National Comorbidity Survey Replication (NCS-R), which extended the NCS to assess treatment of mental health disorders (Wang et al., 2005). Unfortunately, neither the NCS nor the NCS-R has been administered since the early 2000s. Funded by the Substance Abuse and Mental Health Services Administration, the National Survey on Drug Use and Health (NSDUH) has been administered annually since 1971 (Department of Health and Human Services, 2019). The NSDUH assesses the prevalence of any mental health disorder, but as it is not designed to identify specific mental health disorder diagnoses, policymakers may wish to consider augmenting the NSDUH for this purpose.

Regier and colleagues were the first to point out the importance of epidemiological and mental health services research data for identifying mental health treatment needs. They were among the first to talk about mental health disorders as a public health problem, and they called for more support for mental health services research to ensure that policy-making related to mental health service delivery be data-driven.

Office-based psychiatric practice

Main citation

Olfson, M., Marcus, S. C., & Pincus, H. A. (1999). Trends in office-based psychiatric practice. *American Journal of Psychiatry*, 156, 451–457.

Background

Subjective data from the 1980s and 1990s indicates that the nature of office-based delivery of mental health services by psychiatrists changed notably during those decades. Administrative and fiscal mechanisms associated with managed care, such as lower physician fees, utilization management, and case management, were thought to have lessened the clinical roles of psychiatrists and eroded quality of mental healthcare. Some evidence suggested a reduction in psychotherapy and an increase in medication management, along with shorter visits (Bernstein, 1996; Schreter, 1997). However, since none of this evidence was drawn from nationally representative data, Mark Olfson and colleagues used a nationally representative sample of psychiatrists in office-based practice to analyse more objective changes in the nature of patients treated, treatments provided, and visit duration during 1985 and 1995. The authors hypothesized that from 1985 to 1995, psychotherapy use and visit duration had both decreased, while the use of psychotropic medications had increased.

Methods

Olfson et al. used the 1985 and 1995 National Ambulatory Medical Care Survey (NAMCS), an annual, nationally representative survey of physicians in office-based settings. The NAMCS captures information from patient visits including patient demographic information, diagnosis, receipt of medication or psychotherapy, length of visit, and payment source. The analysis was limited to visits to psychiatrists. The 1985 and 1995 NAMCS instruments were very similar.

Results

Relative to psychiatric visits in 1985, the 1995 sample included many more visits by older patients, patients who were not Caucasian, those with public health insurance, and patients whose care was paid for by a health maintenance organization (HMO). The 1995 sample also showed a higher proportion of patients receiving a psychotropic medication prescription (specifically those receiving an antidepressant, mood stabilizer, or stimulant) and a lower proportion of patients receiving psychotherapy, relative to the 1985 sample. The average duration of a visit to a psychiatrist fell by approximately 10%, from 43 minutes in 1985 to 38 minutes in 1995; by comparison, the average length of a visit to a primary care physician did not significantly decline across this ten-year period. Although patients who were not given a psychotropic medication prescription had shorter visits in 1995 than in 1985, patients receiving such a prescription did not experience a change over time in their average visit length. Two other groups of patients had notably shorter visits in 1995 than in 1985: patients who had previously received treatment from a psychiatrist and those who received psychotherapy during their visit.

Conclusions and critique

As hypothesized, Olfson and colleagues' analysis demonstrated what many were saying anecdotally: office-based psychiatrists provided shorter visits, more psychotropic medication prescriptions, and less psychotherapy in 1995 than they did in 1985. These changes suggest that office-based psychiatry may have been impacted by utilization constraints imposed by HMOs and other types of managed care insurance arrangements, which reduced the amount psychiatrists were reimbursed for providing office-based care. The increase in prescriptions for psychotropic medications may be partially explained by the expanded use of selective serotonin reuptake inhibitors, which began in the early 1990s and were better tolerated by patients than tricyclic antidepressants and monoamine oxidase inhibitors. The authors also noted that during the study period, psychiatric education developed in response to the evolution of psychopharmacological options: early-career psychiatrists were trained to appropriately prescribe and monitor psychotropic medications while using psychotherapy only in specific contexts (Beigel & Santiago, 1995). At the same time, evidence supporting the efficacy of brief psychotherapy visits for major depression was also mounting. Although the NAMCS does not allow us to determine whether an average person was less likely to receive a particular type of mental health service in 1995 than in 1985, this paper makes a compelling case that office-based psychiatric care was already pivoting toward the types of clinical psychiatric care that are most commonly offered today.

The findings from this study suggest several questions that should be addressed in future research. How has the relative use of psychotropic medications, psychotherapy, and medication management changed since Olfson et al. examined this question over 20 years ago? Has the duration of office visits continued to decline since 1995? Most importantly, how has the evolution of office-based, psychiatric treatments impacted clinical outcomes for patients with a mental health disorder?

Psychiatric treatment in primary care

Main citation

Katon, W., et al. (1999). Stepped collaborative care for primary care patients with persistent symptoms of depression: a randomized trial. *Archives of General Psychiatry*, 56, 1109–1115.

Background

During the 1990s, several studies demonstrated that depression among primary care patients was as high as 10% (Katon & Schulberg, 1992; Ormel et al., 1994). Given the decreased availability of specialty mental healthcare to primary care patients due to health system reforms (Wells, 1995), it became important to deploy community-based mental health specialty care as efficiently as possible. Wayne Katon, Michael Von Korff, and their colleagues from the University of Washington and Group Health Cooperative of Puget Sound (GHC), developed a collaborative care model for patients with major depressive disorder. Collaborative care models combine the integration of mental health professionals into the primary care clinic with patient psychoeducation to assist primary care physicians in providing evidence-based treatment of depressive disorders; such models have been shown to significantly reduce depressive symptoms for patients with major depressive disorder (Katon et al., 1995, 1996). Because some patients with major depressive disorder experience reduced symptoms via usual care, Katon and colleagues wondered whether an efficient approach would be to target collaborative care only to patients whose depressive symptoms did not resolve six to eight weeks after initiating routine treatment in primary care. Their hypothesis for this study was that patients who 'stepped up' from usual primary care treatment to collaborative care would receive more guideline-consistent antidepressant dose and duration, be more satisfied with their treatment, and achieve better outcomes over a six-month period than patients who continued with usual depression care.

Methods

This randomized controlled trial was carried out in four primary care clinics within GHC, a Seattle-based health management organization. The stepped collaborative care intervention arm included psychiatrist visits, telephone calls between visits, and antidepressant medication. The intervention arm also included a book and videotape developed by the research team to help patients understand the biological basis of depression, the mechanism of common treatments for depression, and how to partner with their doctor to treat their depression. Patients in the usual care arm had the option to cross over, by referral to GHC mental health services' arm, but otherwise continued receiving antidepressant prescriptions and more limited visits with their primary care physician.

Results

Study findings were consistent with the authors' hypotheses. Collaborative care patients were significantly more likely to have received guideline-consistent antidepressant dose and duration, to have rated the quality of their depression treatment as good to excellent, and to have recovered at three months and six months than patients who received usual care from their primary care physician.

Conclusions and critique

The study clearly demonstrated that collaborative care achieved outcomes for patients who were more difficult to treat beyond what they would have experienced with usual depression care. The authors attributed the success of the stepped collaborative care intervention to the use of targeted specialty visits, active monitoring of patients, and more robust follow-up care. Although collaborative care patients had fewer depressive symptoms at three and six months than their usual care counterparts, optimal outcome was achieved at three months, and the effect of collaborative care levelled off between three months and six months. This finding suggests that a different approach may be required to treat patients whose depressive symptoms persist beyond six months. Although the study findings are limited by a lack of racial and socioeconomic heterogeneity in the study setting and its implementation in a health system where it is relatively easy to integrate primary care with specialty care, subsequent studies have demonstrated that collaborative care for major depressive disorder is a highly effective treatment approach in other treatment settings (Bauer et al., 2011; Fortney et al., 2013). Future research should test the effectiveness of collaborative care for other mood disorders such as anxiety and post-traumatic stress disorder.

Cross-cultural psychiatry

Main citation

Kleinman, A. M. (1977). Depression, somatization, and the 'new cross-cultural psychiatry'. *Social Science & Medicine*, 11, 3–10.

Background

Cross-cultural psychiatry (sometimes referred to as transcultural psychiatry or cultural psychiatry) is a subfield of psychiatry focused on understanding cultural and ethnic differences in mental health disorders, their prevalence across cultures, and different modalities of treatment among different cultural contexts. Much of the early work in this subfield assumed that Western mental health diagnostic categories were universal and did not carefully consider whether culture impacts depressive disorders and other mental health disorders. Arthur Kleinman, a psychiatrist with a master's degree in social anthropology, asserted that a particular anthropological insight must be applied here: culture not only shapes illness as an experience, but it also shapes the way that people conceive of illness. For example, several studies have reported that Chinese patients with mental health disorders tend to present with somatic symptoms instead of psychological symptoms (Rin et al., 1973), and Kleinman and others have reported a similar phenomenon among Chinese patients with depression in the United States. Conversely, somatization in the presence of depressive symptoms occurs, but is much less common, in the United States.

Kleinman proposes a 'new' cross-cultural psychiatry that uses anthropological data and ethnographical methods to assess the relationship between culture and illness, and in this landmark paper he provides evidence to demonstrate the impact of Chinese culture on how Chinese persons with depressive disorders talk about their depressive symptoms.

Methods

Kleinman used a case-study approach to describe somatization among Chinese patients with depressive disorders. He described the cases of two persons living in Taiwan and one Chinese male living in Boston; Kleinman indicated that these three cases were typical of many Chinese patients with depressive disorders whom he had treated and studied.

Results

There were several consistent themes across the three cases. Despite clearly presenting with common depressive symptoms (e.g. fatigue, loss of energy, insomnia, weight loss), all three patients would not talk about their psychological symptoms with the psychiatrist. The three patients had different ways of talking about their depression. For example, one patient (and his family) described his problem as due to 'wind' and 'not enough blood'. Details about each patient's course of psychiatric treatment are also provided.

Conclusions and critique

Kleinman makes an interesting case for the ways in which Chinese cultural norms impact the way that Chinese persons with depression talk about their illness and their treatment. A case-study approach limits generalizability, but Kleinman's findings are consistent with prior literature. He also points out that other literature stresses the importance of distinguishing two closely related aspects of sickness: disease and illness. Disease reflects maladaptation or malfunctioning of biological or psychological processes; illness is a cultural construct that represents a personal or cultural reaction to disease. Kleinman goes on to say that treatment of disease can be called cure, while treatment of an illness can be referred to as healing. The healing language is a precursor to the notion of recovery from a mental health disorder, which refers to the idea that individuals with a mental health disorder can get well, stay well, and fulfil their life goals by developing a recovery plan (see MentalHealth.gov website). In summary, Kleinman's work supports the notion that cross-cultural psychiatry should use both epidemiological and anthropological methods to examine questions about the relationship between culture, mental health disorders, and illness in general. Future research should test and evaluate combinations of specific epidemiological and anthropological methods to determine which combinations best help us understand cross-cultural differences in mental health disorders.

Conclusion

As described throughout this chapter, the evolution of social and community psychiatry during the past 50 or more years has dramatically altered the way that psychiatric care is provided to persons with mental health disorders. Regier and colleagues' work set the stage for better measurement of where psychiatric services are delivered. Olfson and colleagues documented what has been a gradual change in the delivery of psychiatric services: shorter office visits, less psychotherapy use, and more psychotropic medication use. Katon and colleagues' research showed that collaborative depression care in primary care settings is an effective way to deploy scarce specialty mental health resources. Kleinman's work in cross-cultural psychiatry demonstrates that culture affects both the ways that people talk about their mental health disorders and their willingness to engage in psychiatric treatment. It is clear that the field of social and community psychiatry is here to stay.

There are many more recent phenomena that may impact the delivery of community-based psychiatric care:

1. As mobile technology becomes increasingly widespread in the general population globally and among persons with serious mental illness (Glick et al., 2016), to what extent can mobile technology (mHealth) be used to successfully and cost effectively deliver community-based psychiatric services? mHealth has the potential to reach subpopulations with mental health disorders who have typically been hardest to engage in psychiatric treatment.
2. Community mental health agencies (CMHAs) are increasingly implementing electronic health records (EHRs), which facilitate coordination of mental health and primary care services (Larrison et al., 2018). Has the increased use of EHRs improved the quality and outcomes of care for persons who receive psychiatric care from CMHAs?
3. Collaborative care has been effective at improving outcomes for persons with major depressive disorder. Can collaborative care also be successfully used for persons with other psychiatric illnesses, including bipolar disorder (Kilbourne et al., 2017), post-traumatic stress disorder (Fortney et al., 2015), and schizophrenia (Kilbourne et al., 2017)? Another notable advantage of coordinating primary care and mental health specialty care for persons with psychiatric illness is the increased opportunity to provide treatment for common comorbid medical conditions such as cardiovascular disease and respiratory disease. Treating comorbid medical conditions is essential given that persons with schizophrenia are seven to ten times more likely to die from chronic obstructive pulmonary disease, influenza, and pneumonia than persons in the general population (Olfson et al., 2015).
4. Although Kleinman's work led to cultural competency initiatives that have been used to help psychiatry residents understand the beliefs and behaviours of ethnic minority and immigrant patients (Qureshi et al., 2008), cultural competency alone may be insufficient for helping these patients who also experience structural barriers to mental health (e.g. living in a neighbourhood with gun violence, which may lead to anxiety or a trauma-related disorder). Several psychiatry residency training programmes are developing structural-competency rotations to help residents understand the structural determinants of mental health and provide skills that can be used in community-based practice settings. For example, Yale University residents participate in a community programme in which they are required to survive on two dollars per day or find fresh produce in a

low-income neighbourhood, factors that increase the risk of mental illness. The goal of this programme is to help residents develop the habit of being aware of patients' living conditions and other structural barriers to mental health (Hansen et al., 2018).

References

Bauer, A. M., et al. (2011). Implementation of collaborative depression management at community-based primary care clinics: an evaluation. *Psychiatric Services*, **62**, 1047–1053.

Beigel, A., & **Santiago, J. M.** (1995). Redefining the general psychiatrist values, reforms, and issues for psychiatric residency education. *Psychiatric Services*, **46**, 769–774.

Bernstein, D. B. (1996). Does managed care permit appropriate use of psychotherapy? *Psychiatric Services*, **47**, 971–974.

Department of Health and Human Services, Substance Abuse and Mental Health Services Administration, Center for Behavioral Health Statistics and Quality. (2019). *National Survey on Drug Use and Health 2017* (NSDUH-2017-DS0001). Retrieved from Substance Abuse and Mental Health Data Archive, at https://datafiles.samhsa.gov/

Fortney, J. C., et al. (2013). Practice-based versus telemedicine-based collaborative care for depression in rural federally qualified health centers: a pragmatic randomized comparative effectiveness trial. *American Journal of Psychiatry*, **170**, 414–425.

Fortney, J. C., et al. (2015). Telemedicine-based collaborative care for posttraumatic stress disorder: a randomized clinical trial. *Journal of the American Medical Association: Psychiatry*, **72**(1), 58–67.

Glick, G., **Druss, B.**, **Pina, J.**, **Lally, C.**, & **Conde, M.** (2016). Use of mobile technology in a community mental health setting. *Journal of Telemedicine and Telecare*, **22**, 430–435.

Hansen, H., **Braslow, J.**, & **Rohrbaugh, R. M.** (2018). From cultural to structural competency—training psychiatry residents to act on social determinants of health and institutional racism. *Journal of the American Medical Association: Psychiatry*, **75**(2), 117–118.

Katon, W., & **Schulberg, H.** (1992). Epidemiology of depression in primary care. *General Hospital Psychiatry*, **14**, 237–247.

Katon, W., et al. (1995). Collaborative management to achieve treatment guidelines: impact on depression in primary care. *Journal of the American Medical Association*, **273**, 1026–1031.

Katon, W., et al. (1996). A multifaceted intervention to improve treatment of depression in primary care. *Archives of General Psychiatry*, **53**, 924–932.

Katon, W., et al. (1999). Stepped collaborative care for primary care patients with persistent symptoms of depression: a randomized trial. *Archives of General Psychiatry*, **56**, 1109–1115.

Kessler, R. C., et al. (1994). Lifetime and 12-month prevalence of DSM-III-R psychiatric disorders in the United States: results from the National Comorbidity Survey. *Archives of General Psychiatry*, **51**, 8–19.

Kilbourne, A. M., et al. (2017). Improving physical health in patients with chronic mental disorders: twelve-month results from a randomized controlled collaborative care trial. *Journal of Clinical Psychiatry*, **78**(1), 129–137.

Kleinman, A. M. (1977). Depression, somatization, and the 'new cross-cultural psychiatry'. *Social Science & Medicine*, **11**, 3–10.

Larrison, C. R., **Xiang, X.**, **Gustafson, M.**, **Lardiere, M. R.**, & **Jordan, N.** (2018). Implementation of electronic health records among community mental health agencies. *Journal of Behavioral Health Services & Research*, **45**(1), 133–142. doi:10.1007/s11414-017-9556-9

MentalHealth.gov [website]. Available at: https://www.mentalhealth.gov/basics/recovery-possible, (accessed 4 August 2018).

Olfson, M., Gerhard, T., Huang, C., Crystal, S., & Stroup, T. S. (2015). Premature mortality among adults with schizophrenia in the United States. *Journal of the American Medical Association: Psychiatry*, **72**(12), 1172–1181.

Olfson, M., Marcus, S. C., & Pincus, H. A. (1999). Trends in office-based psychiatric practice. *American Journal of Psychiatry*, **156**(3), 451–457.

Ormel, J., Von Korff, M., Usun, T. B., Pini, S., Korten, A., & Oldehinkel, T. (1994). Common mental disorders and disabilities across culture: results from the WHO Collaborative Study on Psychological Problems in General Health Care. *Journal of the American Medical Association*, **272**, 1741–1748.

Public Health Service. (1977). *Health Statistics Plan, Fiscal Years 1978–1982.* Washington: US Department of Health, Education, and Welfare.

Qureshi, A., Collazos, F., Ramos, M., & Casas, M. (2008). Cultural competency training in psychiatry. *European Psychiatry*, **23**(Suppl 1), 49–58.

Regier, D. A., Goldberg, I., & Taube, C. A. (1978). The de facto US mental health services system: a public health perspective. *Archives of General Psychiatry*, **35**(6), 685–693.

Rin, H., Schooler, C., & Caudill, W. A. (1973). Symptomatology and hospitalization: culture, social structure and psychopathology in Taiwan and Japan. *Journal of Nervous and Mental Disease*, **157**(4), 296–312.

Schreter, R. K. (1997). Coping with the crisis in psychiatric training. *Psychiatry*, **60**, 51–59.

Wang, P. S., Lane, M., Kessler, R. C., Olfson, M., Pincus, H. A., & Wells, K. B. (2005). Twelve-month use of mental health services in the US: results from the National Comorbidity Survey Replication (NCS-R). *Archives of General Psychiatry*, **62**(6), 629–640.

Wells, K. B. (1995). Cost-containment and mental health experiences from US studies. *British Journal of Psychiatry*, 27(Suppl), 43–51.

White House. (1977). Executive Order No. 11973—President's Commission on Mental Health. Office of the White House Press Secretary.

Chapter 16

Child and adolescent psychiatry and psychology

Mark R. Dadds, Yixin Jiang, Valsamma Eapen, and Stephen Scott

Introduction

References to mental illness in children were rare in the scientific and medical literature before 1900. By the end of the nineteenth century, however, many psychiatry textbooks included sections on children. In 1887, the German psychiatrist Hermann Emminghaus published one of the first treatises on child psychiatry (*Psychic Disturbances in Childhood*). In 1899, the term 'child psychiatry' was used (in French) as a subtitle in Marcel Manheimer's monograph *Les Troubles Mentaux de l'Enfance*. In the USA, Lightner Witmer established the world's first psychological clinic at the University of Pennsylvania in 1896 (see Parry-Jones, 1989 and Rey et al., 2015 for elaborated histories of child psychotherapy).

However, it was not until the early twentieth century that child psychotherapy began with the work of Sigmund Freud. In creating psychoanalysis, he redefined sexuality to include its infantile forms, including the Oedipus complex, as a central tenet of psychoanalysis and his 'Analysis of a phobia in a five-year-old boy' (Little Hans) (Freud, 1909). During the 1920s, Melanie Klein and Anna Freud began to explore how Freud's work with adults could be extended to help troubled children. They argued that through play, the internal world of the child could be understood and difficulties addressed. In the 1920s, behaviourism was taking hold in the USA and pioneers such as John Watson and Mary Cover Jones developed theories and experimental methods to understand how psychopathological behaviour could be learned and unlearned. At the same time, the Child Guidance Movement emerged in Chicago, with a focus on treating and preventing juvenile delinquency.

Through the twentieth century, the field of child psychotherapy rapidly expanded and adopted an increasingly scientific approach. This chapter presents some landmark papers that have shaped this transition. The review emphasizes papers with empirical evidence and adopts a broad definition of psychotherapy that includes both symptom reduction and enhancement of developmental trajectories, regardless of whether the work is undertaken directly with the child, or through the parent, family, and social milieu.

Space constraints led to the omission of many landmark papers that were clearly worthy of being included, a notable one being Michael Rutter's grand review of the state of child psychological treatments (Rutter, 1982). While that paper appeared during the age of dominance of psychodynamic therapy, it marked the shift within family, behavioural, and cognitive therapies toward embracing the new idea of the child as a social agent embedded in an ecological system. Further, this paper was the first to ask: 'What does NOT work in child psychotherapy?' Another omission is one of the first review papers attempting to quantify the evidence base for child psychotherapies: a meta-analysis of 150 outcome studies published between 1983 and 1993, which was conducted by Weisz et al. (1995).

Other papers have been landmarks at the public-health level. These include Marmot (2008) on the social determinants of health, Knapp (1997) on economic evaluation of psychotherapies, and Garcia et al.'s (2016) work on the health benefits of early child-care settings. While they would have been controversial choices, they represent an important development in child psychotherapy—that mental health is in part determined by the broad ecology of child development (Bronfenbrenner & Ceci, 1994). Finally, the Multimodal Treatment Study of Children with ADHD (Jensen et al., 1999) was not at the forefront of any new ideas or techniques but represented an important step in child psychotherapy—the recognition that large, multi-site, randomized controlled trials are needed to produce clear and generalizable data on treatment effectiveness, as discussed in Chapter 10.

Notwithstanding these exceptions, it is proposed that the final chosen list represents a group of work that marks the best of our history and should be acknowledged as the cornerstones on which our rapidly developing field is built. Cover Jones' paper is a culmination of the innovative but fraught case studies by Freud (Little Hans) and Watson (Little Albert), in which she first uses observational methods to overcome fear in young children using theoretically driven methods. Lovaas' work with autism has received more than its fair share of negative portrayals since its dissemination; however, few treatments have surpassed its success in improving social competence. As a result, applied behaviour analysis has become a mainstay evidence-based intervention for young children with autism. Children with aggressive and antisocial behaviour were historically excluded from psychiatric practice and study. However, the Oregon Social Learning Center Group, led by Patterson and Reid, was part of an innovative movement that saw antisocial behaviour as firmly embedded in the moment-to-moment interactions of the family, developed observational methods for verifying their models, and translated them into readily transportable parenting interventions that have now become one of the great achievements of child psychotherapy. Similarly, the early family therapists saw eating disorders as embedded in problematic family interactions, and the first attempt to operationalize family therapy into a testable model by Russell et al. (1987) is featured.

Another important area within child psychotherapy is attachment theory, and so the first meta-analysis that summarized and quantified treatment effects is included. It is notable for addressing the causal relationship between sensitive parenting and child attachment, an issue noted as being still unresolved in terms of specificity to attachment processes. Finally, the work of Olds et al. on the Family Nurse Partnership is featured. It is especially innovative for focusing on methods for prevention and early intervention for at-risk parents and child abuse and neglect. It represents one of the first and most influential attempts to get out of the clinic and into the home environment of vulnerable children.

Overcoming fear: Freud, Watson, and the first evidence-based approach

Main citations

Jones, M. C. (1924a). The elimination of children's fears. *Journal of Experimental Psychology*, 7, 382–390.
Jones, M. C. (1924b). A laboratory study of fear: the case of Peter. *Journal of Genetic Psychology*, 31, 308–315.

Background

Sigmund Freud had first written about the causes and treatment of childhood phobias and their putative association with the Oedipus complex in his case of Little Hans. This was followed by John Watson's now infamous Little Albert experiment that used classical conditioning to teach an infant to fear a previously innocuous white rodent and other objects. Mary Cover Jones was a researcher in Watson's lab and advanced this work by asking if the learning model could be used for therapeutic purposes. Thus, she was the first to test whether young children could be taught to overcome fear using a series of experiments based on Watson's conditioning models.

Methods

Cover Jones' (1924a) paper includes a case series of 70 children (aged three months to seven years) who showed normal development and health, but a marked degree of fear to stimuli/situations such as being left alone, being in a dark room, animals like rabbits and frogs, and loud sounds. Various methods, often in combination, were tested for their ability to eliminate the fears, including: ignoring the fear; verbal, positive reappraisal of the fear-object; repeated presentation of the fearful stimuli; repressing overt fear expressions; distraction with a substitute activity; social imitation/modelling; and associating the fear-object with a positive stimulus (i.e. direct conditioning). Most famously, the case of Peter illustrated this last approach (see Jones, 1924b). The infant Peter, whilst hungry, was placed in a high chair and given his favourite food, candy, to eat. His fear-object, a rabbit, was then brought in, which evoked a negative response from Peter. The rabbit was then moved away gradually until it was at a sufficient distance so as not to interfere with the child's eating. The fear-object was then slowly brought closer to build tolerance as Peter engaged in the positive activity of eating candy.

Results

Among the different reported case studies, direct conditioning and social imitation/modelling were shown to be successful approaches. The other methods were sometimes effective but not reliably so, unless used in combination with other approaches.

Conclusions and critique

This study was seminal for demonstrating that fear responses in infants can be unlearned. Interestingly, the paper remarked that none of the aforementioned approaches were used in a pure form, but the aim was usually to cure fear 'by the group of devices most appropriate at any given stage of treatment' (Jones, 1924a, p. 390). This sort of technical pragmatism is quite consistent with the way that the field has developed since. After Cover Jones, several theorists tried to specify relatively pure techniques for how deconditioning fear should occur (e.g. Wolpe, 1961, with 'systematic desensitization'); however, decades of research have demonstrated that deconditioning is a complex process that can entail a range of behavioural, cognitive, verbal, and social processes (Milad & Quirk, 2011). Further, the work is seminal for its attempted use of controlled experimental, observational methods rather than the reliance on assumed theory that characterized the psychoanalytic movement. Cover Jones rightly became known as 'the mother of behaviour therapy'; deconditioning techniques such as exposure and desensitization are now a mainstay of psychotherapy.

The first evidence base for behavioural treatment for children with autism

Main citation

Lovaas, O. I. (1987). Behavioral treatment and normal educational and intellectual functioning in young autistic children. *Journal of Consulting and Clinical Psychology*, 55, 3–9.

Background

In 1911, Eugen Bleuler was the first person to use the term autism, referring to a group of symptoms related to schizophrenia. In 1943, Leo Kanner published his landmark paper that identified children with highly withdrawn and repetitive behaviour. At about the same time, Hans Asperger identified a similar condition. By the 1950s, psychiatrists had developed elaborate psychodynamic explanations for the condition, regarding it as an analogue to the emotional withdrawal seen in abused/institutionalized children (Baker, 2010). Bruno Bettelheim, a psychoanalyst in Chicago, brought these ideas to a wide audience in his 1967 book *The Empty Fortress* (Bettleheim, 1967). These models of autism were shown to be deeply flawed, and effective interventions for autism remained elusive.

With the rise of Skinnerian behaviourism in the USA, operant learning theory was being enthusiastically applied to a range of behavioural disorders. Ferster (1961) first proposed

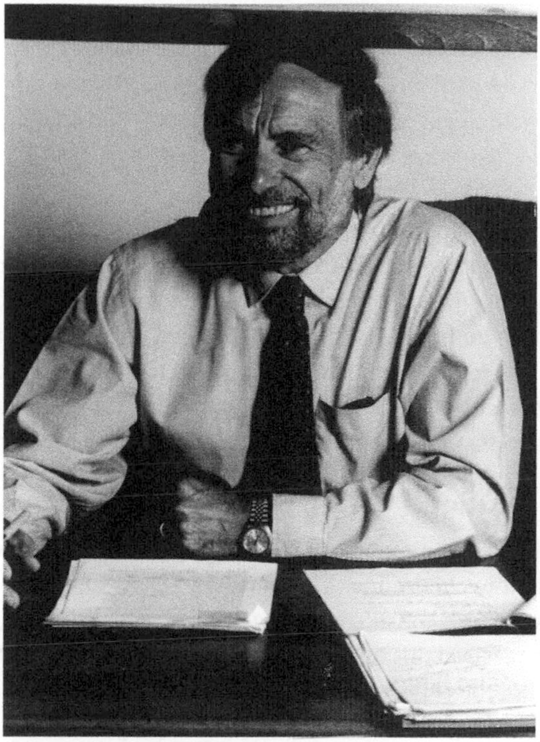

Figure 16.1 O. Ivan Lovaas in the 1980s.
Reproduced with permission from the Lovaas Institute.

a behavioural learning framework to help understand childhood autism. This prompted much work on operant methods for reducing aberrant behaviours and promoting pro-social behaviour, generally using single case studies. Ivan Lovaas (see Figure 16.1) was the first to conduct a randomized controlled trial of an intensive, behavioural modification treatment. His 1974 paper described the key features of an intervention focusing on behaviour instead of underlying disease or aetiology. Treatment involves isolating and understanding one behaviour at a time, identifying the conditions that control it, and modifying the behaviour using reinforcement learning. These techniques are used for reducing self-destructive behaviours, teaching and reinforcing appropriate behaviours, shaping language skills, and generalizing learning across contexts.

Methods

In his 1987 study, 59 very young children (under four years old) with autism were allocated to three groups: a treatment group who received intensive, long-term behaviour modification (more than 40 hours of one-to-one treatment per week involving all significant persons in all significant environments); and two control groups (one followed in Lovaas' clinic and one in an external clinic) who received ten hours or less of one-to-one treatment per week. All groups received treatment for two or more years, up to six years of age. Pre-treatment assessments included mental age; observations of self-stimulatory behaviours, appropriate play, and word use during free play; parent interview to determine overall child pathology; and age at first diagnosis and treatment. Post-treatment assessments included first-grade class placement and IQ.

Results

At follow-up, 47% of children in the treatment group achieved normal intellectual and educational functioning, normal-range IQ, and successful first-grade performance (compared to 2% of children in the control groups); 40% had mild intellectual impairment and required special classes for language delay (compared to 45% in the control groups); and 10% had severe intellectual impairment and required special classes for children with autism (compared to 53% in the control groups).

Conclusions and critique

Lovaas' (1987) study was the first controlled trial of an intensive, behavioural modification treatment applied to children with autism. The results famously (and perhaps, controversially, as autism is still considered a largely intractable condition) show that nearly half of children who received this intensive early intervention went on to live independent lives. For nearly half of the children in his treatment group, the treatment resulted in improvements to a broad range of observed behaviours and good schooling outcomes—the treatment allowed some children to catch up with normal peers by first grade. The poor outcomes of the children in the control group negate spontaneous improvement as an explanation for the outcomes of the treatment group.

It should be noted that the groups were not strictly randomized, with the paper noting that this could not be fully achieved due to staff shortages, parent protests, and other ethical considerations. Lovaas was also quite realistic in noting that treatment gains were only achieved slowly, as a result of long-term, intensive intervention. He also noted that for some children, the gains were reversible, and that other residual deficits (not identified in the classroom setting) often remained.

The work has not been without its critics and negative portrayals, with claims that data for effectiveness are exaggerated (see Morris, 2009) and that the operant strategies of reward and negative consequence are odious and unethical (e.g. Moser & Grant, 1965). Despite this, it is interesting to note that core interventions and outcomes for children with autism have not greatly improved since this work; its techniques and principles remain core pillars of contemporary treatments. In the last few years, new forms of parent-mediated treatments that focus on the child's development of social communicative skills are also showing potential for improving the core deficits for autism (e.g. Pickles et al., 2016). These, along with applied behavioural analysis, form the core of early interventions that stem from Lovaas' early model of interpersonal therapies and have the potential to minimize the lifelong impairments associated with autism.

The first family-based approach to childhood aggression and conduct problems

Main citation

Patterson, G. R. & Reid, J. B. (1973). Intervention for families of aggressive boys: a replication study. *Behaviour Research and Therapy*, 11, 383–394.

Background

Although the Child Guidance Movement in the early twentieth century developed to prevent and treat juvenile delinquency, disorders of conduct (delinquency, aggression, antisocial behaviour) typically did not respond to traditional psychotherapeutic models and thus were historically excluded from mental health clinics, especially those using psychanalytical approaches. During the 1960s, a number of innovative thinkers were beginning to apply social learning theory to family processes, the context in which children learned prosocial versus conduct problem behaviours (e.g. Hawkins et al., 1966; Wahler et al., 1965; Patterson & Brodsky, 1966). Social learning theory grew out of Skinnerian operant theory and retained its core focus on environmental context and reinforcement history, but included human cognition and interpersonal process as extra explanatory factors (e.g. Bandura, 1977). Researchers Gerry Patterson and John Reid (1973), as shown in Figure 16.2, were the first to present a comprehensive model of how social learning processes could be applied to family interactions, especially those implicated in the

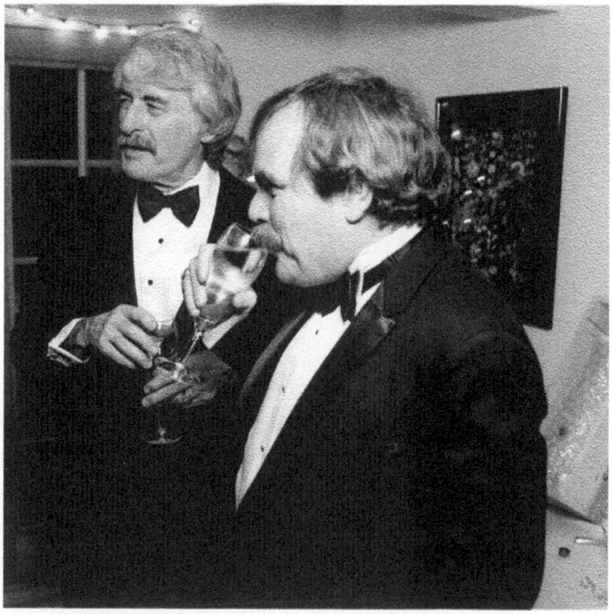

Figure 16.2 Jerry Patterson (left) and John Reid (right) in a formal moment.

development and maintenance of child aggressive and antisocial behaviour (Coercive Family Process or Coercion Theory; Patterson, 1982). The model explained the development of problems and offered methods for observing the behaviours in their natural settings and strategies for correcting the child's problems through parent training. In this paper, the authors present systematic observational data using multiple outcome criteria for the treatment of multiple cases. The study replicates and expands upon earlier unpublished data by Patterson and colleagues (1973) that trained parents to alter aggressive behaviour in their children.

Methods

The sample consisted of 11 consecutive referrals by community agencies of boys (5–12 years old) who displayed high rates of aggressive, non-compliant behaviour. Their parents completed a training programme that involved studying didactic material and attending 8 to 12 weekly group meetings with therapists to observe and alter their child's behaviour based on learning theory. Treatment effects were assessed via observers conducting home visits at baseline and throughout the intervention to collect data on child and family social interactions, via parent reports of problematic behaviours during observation days, and via mothers' global ratings of improvement in their child's behaviour 5 to 12 months after treatment. Finally, the researchers recorded the amount of professional time required for treatment for each family, which included all contact with the family (consultations, staff conferences, telephone contact, or home visit travel).

Results

At the end of the treatment, there were significant reductions (average of 61% from baseline) in observed deviant child behaviour and moderate reductions in parent-reported problem behaviours (see Figure 16.3). Furthermore, at 5 to 12 months post-treatment, mothers reported marked global improvements beyond what was expected: increased happiness in their children, better family functioning, and more positive feelings toward their children. In a nod to the future emphasis on health economics, the authors reported that the average amount of professional time spent with families was 31.4 hours.

Conclusions and critique

This influential study was the first to demonstrate the effectiveness of a family-based treatment for aggressive behaviour by using systematic multi-informant data across multiple outcomes. A number of case studies had appeared describing operant methods for treating conduct problems in children (e.g. Hawkins et al., 1966; Wahler et al., 1965), including some by Patterson (Patterson & Brodsky, 1966); however, this was the first study to conduct a systematic group analysis using more robust methods. The intervention was also the first to show durability of change at the end of treatment and at 5–12 months' follow-up. The study is the first to report cost–benefit analyses. Although the study did not have a control group, subsequent work has confirmed the effectiveness of these

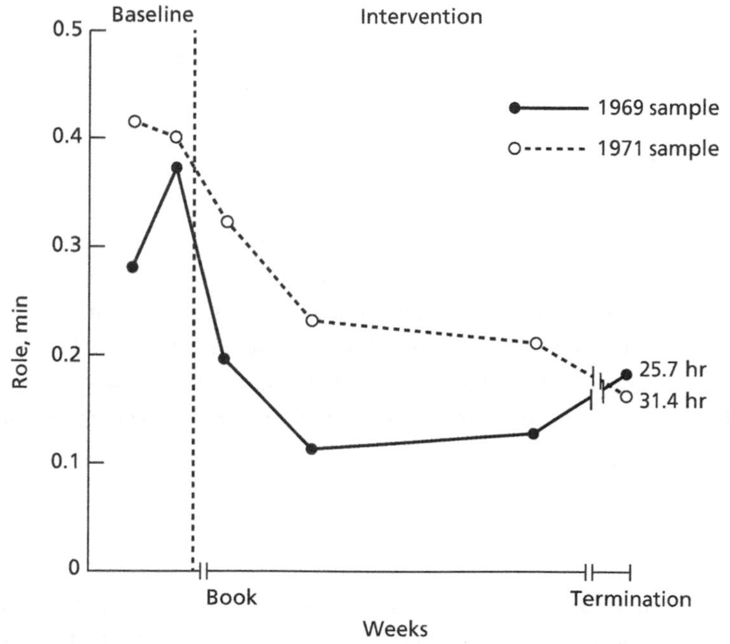

Figure 16.3 Direct observations showing the rate per minute of targeted child behaviours during treatment for two samples.

Reprinted from *Behaviour Research and Therapy*, 11, 4, Patterson GR and Reid JB, Intervention for families of aggressive boys: A replication study, pp. 383–394. Copyright (1973) with permission from Elsevier. DOI: http://dx.doi.org/10.1016/0005-7967(73)90096-X

techniques using rigorous designs (Furlong et al., 2012). By the time of an influential 1998 review (Brestan & Eyber, 1998) there had been 29 years of research and 82 studies involving 5,272 children attesting to the effectiveness of this approach. Thanks to this pioneering study and related research, behavioural parent training has become one of the great achievements of child mental health sciences.

Family therapy for anorexia nervosa and bulimia nervosa

Main citation

Russell, G. F., Szmukler, G. I., Dare, C., & Eisler, I. (1987). An evaluation of family therapy in anorexia nervosa and bulimia nervosa. *Archives of General Psychiatry*, 44, 1047–1056.

Secondary citations

Minuchin, S., Baker, L., Rosman, B. L., Liebman, R., Milman, L., & Todd, T. C. (1975). A conceptual model of psychosomatic illness in children: family organization and family therapy. *Archives of General Psychiatry*, 32, 1031–1038.

Selvini Palazzoli, M. (1978). *Self-Starvation: From Individual to Family Therapy in the Treatment of Anorexia Nervosa*, trans. A. Pomerans. New York: Jason Aronson.

Background

The search for effective treatments for anorexia nervosa has been an important priority for clinical psychiatry and psychology, especially given increasing prevalence throughout the twentieth century in most Western countries. By the 1980s there had been a growing emphasis on family-based treatments in clinical practice. This had been stimulated by the family therapy literature, including the influential writings of Salvatore Minuchin at the Philadelphia Child Guidance Clinic and Mara Selvini Palazzoli in Milan. Both groups developed models to explain family processes in the aetiology of anorexia nervosa, and both reported successful outcomes from their family therapies. Neither, however, substantiated their claims with controlled trials or follow-up assessments. Russell et al. formulated family therapy into a systemized and replicable method, facilitating the first controlled trial comparing family therapy with individual therapy for anorexia nervosa and bulimia nervosa.

Methods

The study recruited 57 patients with anorexia nervosa and 23 with bulimia nervosa from Maudsley Hospital in London, where they had been admitted for weight restoration. The patients were randomized to family therapy or control treatment. Treatments were provided as outpatient hourly sessions over the course of one year, occurring fortnightly for the first three months, then every three weeks, with some flexibility according to the patients' needs and compliance. Family therapy involved meeting with all family members of the patient and focused on helping the parents manage their child's symptoms and weight. Individual therapy involved non-specific supportive, educational, and problem-centred therapy. Outcomes, assessed one year after treatment, included body weight, menstrual function, clinical assessment, need for readmission to hospital, and psychological adjustment.

Results

Randomization and all statistical analyses were conducted according to subgroups:

1. age of onset of anorexia <19 years and duration of illness <3 years (21 patients);
2. age of onset of anorexia <19 years and duration of illness >3 years (15 patients);
3. age of onset of anorexia >19 years (21 patients);
4. patients with bulimia nervosa (23 patients).

Results differed by subgroup such that, after one year, family therapy was found to be more effective (better clinical outcome, maintenance of normal weight, and more weight gain) than individual therapy, when illness was not chronic and had begun before the age of 19 years. Individual supportive therapy was found to hold greater value for older patients (>19 years) and resulted in more weight gain than family therapy, but the improvement still fell short of clinical recovery in most patients. Notably, relatively few patients had fully recovered from either anorexia or bulimia nervosa, as judged by good clinical outcomes on the Morgan and Russell categories (Morgan & Russell, 1975) at one-year follow-up. There was also no significant difference between therapies on the likelihood of readmission.

Conclusions and critique

Family-based interventions are now a routine part of care for anorexia, thanks to the pioneering efforts of Minuchin, Selvini Palazzoli, and the Institute of Psychiatry team who led this study. The study provided the first controlled evidence for the efficacy of family therapy for eating disorders. In contrast to the overly positive case-study results presented by the early family therapists (e.g. Minuchin et al., 1975), these results did not universally favour the family-based approach. That is, in an auspicious nod to the now common findings for psychotherapy (that results rarely apply equally across patients), outcomes differed according to the individual characteristics of the patients and their history with the disorder. The authors were also overtly realistic about the findings, carefully reporting dropout data, problems with group matching, noting that few patients had fully recovered from their illnesses, and that the one-year follow-up was too short to assess the eventual prognosis of both anorexia and bulimia nervosa, which are often chronic conditions. Despite this, the study provided a critical step forward in establishing the family-based approach as a core treatment for eating disorders in young people. It also stands as a forerunner to more contemporary evidence-based treatments of eating disorders (led by, for example, Christopher Fairburn, William Stewart Agras, G. Terrence Wilson, Daniel Le Grange).

Translating attachment theory into treatments: a work in progress?

Main citation

Bakermans-Kranenburg, M. J., van IJzendoorn, M. H., & Juffer, F. (2003). Less is more: meta-analyses of sensitivity and attachment interventions in early childhood. *Psychological Bulletin*, 129, 195–215.

Background

Since its inception in the 1960s by John Bowlby, attachment theory has been an influential framework for understanding child development. Its central premise is that the developing child requires a secure, predictable psychological base from which to develop into a healthy, independent adult. This psychological base was defined as stemming from the predictable and ongoing availability of a responsive, sensitive caregiver. The development of objective measures of child attachment, based on the parent–child patterns of separation and rapprochement, proved a massive impetus for research in this area (Ainsworth & Bell, 1970). The development of evidence-based attachment interventions lagged behind the growing theoretical scope and empirical research in attachment theory. Exceptions were the innovative work by clinical researchers such as Mary Dozier and Charlie Zeanah, who led the formulation of attachment-based psychotherapies. In 2003, Bakermans-Kranenburg et al. presented the first meta-analysis of studies on interventions for enhancing parental sensitivity and attachment security. Their paper also addressed questions of causal relationships between parental sensitivity and child attachment security.

Methods

The meta-analyses involved studies that aimed at enhancing parental sensitivity or children's attachment security, included observational measures of changes in parental behaviour, and started before children's mean age of 54 months. Studies were coded for numerous aspects including study design, sample characteristics, the nature of the intervention, and the nature of the outcome (sensitivity and attachment) measures.

Results

The review identified 88 intervention effects on parental sensitivity and/or attachment security across 70 studies (n = 9957 families). Of these, 51 studies attempted to enhance maternal sensitivity and included a randomized control group. The mean intervention effect was found to be significant and moderate (d = 0.33). For attachment security, there were 23 studies involving a randomized control group, and the mean intervention effect was significant but small (d = 0.20). For both maternal sensitivity and attachment security, more effective interventions generally had a clear-cut behavioural focus (that is, they promoted specific caregiver behaviours), used parental sensitivity as the goal, had fewer sessions, and were started beyond six months of age for the child. Sample characteristics (such as socioeconomic status or family risk factors) did not moderate the effectiveness of the interventions. Of the 24 studies that assessed both maternal sensitivity and attachment security, the studies with the largest effect sizes for sensitivity were also most effective in enhancing attachment security.

Conclusions and critique

Attachment theory has provided a rich vein of knowledge for understanding child development and psychopathology. Compared to other forms of family and behaviour therapy, however, it has not been widely influential in terms of extensively disseminated evidence-based psychotherapies, although there have been innovative exceptions (e.g. Dozier, 2003; Zeanah et al., 2011). This meta-analysis was the first to synthesize findings from experimental intervention studies and establish the effectiveness of interventions for enhancing parental sensitivity and, to a lesser extent, infant attachment security. The most effective interventions were those that were more behaviourally focused on enhancing parental sensitivity. Moreover, contrary to common assumptions, the more effective interventions did not necessarily include a large number of sessions nor start early in life or pre-birth.

Importantly, the results provide evidence to substantiate a causal link between parental sensitivity and infant attachment security. However, they raise questions about the specificity of attachment-based constructs. Recent studies have shown that parenting interventions stemming from the work of Patterson and colleagues (reviewed earlier) produce similar changes in parental sensitivity and child attachment through the use of social learning theory, without specifically employing attachment constructs (Blizzard et al., 2017; O'Connor et al., 2013). This raises critical questions for the ongoing design of new treatments based on attachment theory. It is hoped that more research on this area will see the full potential of attachment theory being translated into new and powerful psychotherapeutic interventions.

'We'll come to you': a first evaluation of nurse home visitations

Main citation

Olds, D. L., Henderson, C. R., Chamberlin, R., & Tatelbaum, R. (1986). Preventing child abuse and neglect: a randomized trial of nurse home visitation. *Pediatrics*, 78, 65–78.

Secondary citations

Olds, D. L., et al. (1997). Long-term effects of home visitation on maternal life course and child abuse and neglect: fifteen-year follow-up of a randomized trial. *Journal of the American Medical Association*, 278, 637–643.
Olds, D., et al. (1998). Long-term effects of nurse home visitation on children's criminal and antisocial behavior: 15-year follow-up of a randomized controlled trial. *Journal of the American Medical Association*, 280, 1238–1244.

Background

The middle of the twentieth century witnessed increasing attention to the importance of preventing child abuse and neglect, which has a deleterious impact on nearly all facets of child development and health. Evidence was lacking, however, in terms of the best preventative approaches. Four previous controlled trials (O'Connor et al., 1980; Siegel et al., 1980; Lealman et al., 1983; Gray et al., 1979 [cited by Olds et al., 1986]) involving early and extended post-partum mother–child contact, drop-in centres, home visitations, or intensive paediatric consultation had produced mixed results. The nurse-visitation series of studies, led by David Olds (Figure 16.4), evaluated a comprehensive programme of supportive prenatal and infancy home visitation by nurses as a method of preventing a wide range of health and developmental problems in children born to at-risk families.

Methods

This randomized controlled trial targeted first-time mothers who were either teenagers, unmarried, or of low socioeconomic status (SES) in a semi-rural community in New York State. Four hundred mothers were randomized into four different treatment groups: (1) a control group (where the child was screened for developmental problems at ages one and

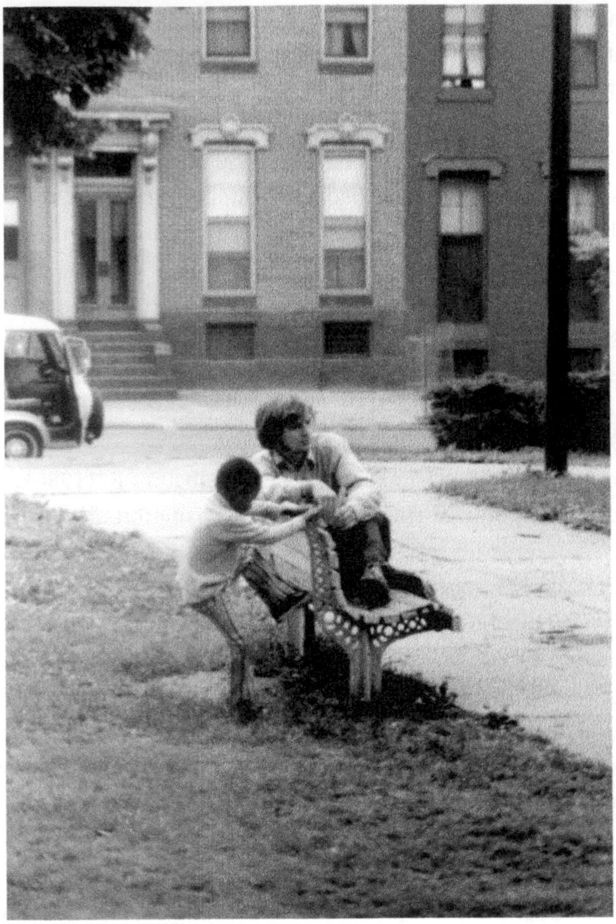

Figure 16.4 David Olds in the 1970s.
Reproduced with permission from David Olds © 2017.

two); (2) child development screening plus free transportation to regular prenatal and child healthcare at local clinics; (3) the aforementioned services plus nurse home visitation during pregnancy; and (4) the aforementioned services plus nurse home visitation during pregnancy (average of nine visits) and child's first two years of life (average of 23 visits). The nurse home visitations focused on parent education about fetal/infant development and parenting (e.g. responsive caregiving); involvement of family members and friends in childcare and supporting the mother; and linking family members to other services. Interviews, infant assessments (including developmental tests and home observations), and review of medical records and child abuse and neglect registries were conducted at registration (prior to thirtieth week of pregnancy) and at 6, 10, 12, 22, and 24 months of the infant's life. Follow-up studies (Olds et al., 1997, 1998) were conducted when the children were 15 years old. In these studies, assessments included maternal outcomes and child outcomes. Data were analysed with a number of approaches including general linear modelling using intent-to-treat samples.

Results

For women with the highest risk of caregiving dysfunction (i.e. unmarried or low SES), those visited by a nurse had significantly fewer instances of verified child abuse and neglect during the child's first two years of life. These women were observed to restrict and punish their child less frequently at home and provide more appropriate play; they had fewer emergency room visits for their infants; and they reported less crying and fussiness and improved cognitive development in their babies. Babies of all nurse-visited women, regardless of family risk status, were less frequently seen at emergency room and by physicians (e.g. for accidents and poisoning). Mothers who were only visited during pregnancy exhibited levels of functioning in between the control group and mothers who were visited during pregnancy and postnatally, indicating a dose–response relationship for level of home visitation.

At 15-year follow-up (Olds et al., 1997), women in the home-visit group, regardless of SES status, were less likely to be identified as perpetrators of child abuse and neglect. Among women who were unmarried or of low SES at initial enrolment, home visits were associated with fewer subsequent children, more time between first and second pregnancies, fewer months of receiving family welfare, fewer behavioural impairments due to alcohol and drug use, and fewer arrests. Outcomes for children at 15-year follow-up were positive as well (Olds et al., 1998). Relative to the comparison groups, adolescents of high-risk women who received nurse visits pre- and postnatally reported fewer instances of running away, arrests, convictions and violations, lifetime sex partners, and cigarettes smoked per day, as well as lower consumption of alcohol. This aligned with parent reports of fewer child behavioural problems related to use of alcohol and drugs.

Conclusions and critique

For pregnant women identified as vulnerable and at risk for abuse and neglect, nurse home visitations during pregnancy and during the infant's first two years of life were shown to be effective in reducing later child abuse and neglect. The programme also yielded numerous immediate and long-term benefits for both mother and child (for mental health, physical health, family functioning, and societal role functioning).

While the home visitation programme was expensive, preliminary cost–benefit analysis revealed that these initial costs are offset by minimizing foster care placements, hospitalizations, emergency room visits, and child protective service involvement; by reducing family size, use of welfare services, and maternal and child criminality; and, not in the least, by reducing human suffering. A recent analysis showed that the family–nurse partnership model is one of the most cost-effective interventions yet developed for child health outcomes (London School of Economics, 2007). While not all home visitation programmes have been universally effective (e.g. Robling et al., 2016), the nurse visitation studies represent one of the most convincing longitudinal datasets supporting the efficacy and cost-effectiveness of early intervention. The study was seminal in driving research, dissemination, and policy development of similar programmes, and the provision of visitation services to at-risk mothers remains one of the core elements of interventions to maximize child outcomes and prevent abuse and neglect.

Conclusion

This chapter has canvassed several landmark papers in the history of child psychotherapy. Notable is the variability in design from case studies to small innovative observation studies, to large and complex randomized controlled trials with long follow-up periods. Not all of these research designs are surviving; the case study is almost extinct, in favour of the randomized controlled trial. To sacrifice innovation in search of size and instant data on outcomes would be, in our opinion, a backward step. Science is a logic that takes many forms rather than a prescribed set of designs. Hopefully, the chapter's take on this rather diverse history helps keep such diversity of methods and innovation alive.

In terms of substance, the relatively brief history of child psychotherapy has witnessed the emergence of effective treatments for childhood anxiety, conduct, and eating disorders, as well programmes for improving general parenting skills and environments. While laudable, these psychotherapies are far from optimal. Even the most effective treatments, such as behavioural parent training for conduct problems, still only produce clinically significant change in approximately 50% of cases (Brestan & Eyberg, 1998); for autism, outcomes are far less optimistic. Their 'reach' remains a problem; only a small percentage of children, even in the most developed nations on earth, accesses effective evidence-based interventions (Sawyer et al., 2001).

While one would be forgiven for wishing more had been achieved in child mental health, it is instructive to reflect on the likely experiences of a family seeking help with early-onset behavioural and emotional problems, one hundred years ago and now. Over the past century, studies have shown the benefits accrued from the individual tailoring of treatments, the involvement of the family and the child's broader ecology, the delivery of brief targeted intervention delivered early, and the use of varied designs to develop and evaluate effectiveness. These axiomatic guidelines can continue to guide the aims of the next century.

References

Ainsworth, M. D. & **Bell, S. M.** (1970). Attachment, exploration, and separation: Illustrated by the behavior of one-year-olds in a strange situation. *Child Development*, **41**, 49–61.

Baker, J. P. (2010). Autism in 1959: Joey the mechanical boy. *Pediatrics*, **125**, 1101–1103

Bakermans-Kranenburg, M. J., **Van IJzendoorn, M. H.**, & **Juffer, F.** (2003). Less is more: meta-analyses of sensitivity and attachment interventions in early childhood. *Psychological Bulletin*, **129**, 195–215.

Bandura, A. (1977). *Social Learning Theory*. Oxford, England: Prentice-Hall.

Bettelheim, B. (1967). *The Empty Fortress: Infantile Autism and the Birth of the Self.* New York: Free Press.

Blizzard, A. M., Barroso, N. E., Ramos, F. G., Graziano, P. A., & Bagner, D. M. (2017). Behavioral parent training in infancy: what about the parent–infant relationship? *Journal of Clinical Child & Adolescent Psychology*, **17**, 1–13.

Brestan, E. V. & Eyberg, S. M. (1998). Effective psychosocial treatments of conduct-disordered children and adolescents: 29 years, 82 studies, and 5,272 kids. *Journal of Clinical Child Psychology*, **27**, 180–189.

Bronfenbrenner, U. & Ceci, S. J. (1994). Nature–nurture reconceptualized in developmental perspective: a bioecological model. *Psychological Review*, **101**, 568–586.

Dozier, M. (2003). Attachment-based treatment for vulnerable children. *Attachment and Human Development*, **5**, 253–257.

Ferster, C. B. (1961). Positive reinforcement and behavioural deficits of autistic children. *Child Development*, **32**, 437–456.

Freud, S. (1909). Analysis of a phobia of a five-year old boy. In: *The Pelican Library, Volume 8, Case Histories*, pp. 169–306

Furlong, M., McGilloway, S., Bywater, T., Hutchings, J., Smith, S. M., & Donnelly, M. (2012). Behavioural and cognitive-behavioural group-based parenting programmes for early-onset conduct problems in children aged 3 to 12 years. *Cochrane Database of Systematic Reviews*, CD008225. doi:10.1002/14651858.CD008225.pub2

García, J. L., Heckman, J. J., Leaf, D. E., & Prados, M. J. (2016). *The life-cycle benefits of an influential early childhood program*. National Bureau of Economic Research Working Paper No. 22993. Available at: http://www.nber.org/papers/w22993

Gray, J., Cutler, C., Dean, J., & Kempe, C. H. (1979). Prediction and prevention of child abuse and neglect. *Journal of Social Issues*, **35**, 127–139.

Hawkins, R. P., Peterson, R. F., Schweid, E., & Bijou, S. W. (1966). Behavior therapy in the home: amelioration of problem parent–child relations with the parent in a therapeutic role. *Journal of Experimental Psychology*, **4**, 99–107.

Jensen, P. S. (1999). A 14-month randomized clinical trial of treatment strategies for attention-deficit/hyperactivity disorder. *Archives of General Psychiatry*, **56**, 1073–1086.

Jones, M. C. (1924a). The elimination of children's fears. *Journal of Experimental Psychology*, 7, 382–390.

Jones, M. C. (1924b). A laboratory study of fear: the case of Peter. *Journal of Genetic Psychology*, **31**, 308–315.

Knapp, M. (1997). Economic evaluations and interventions for children and adolescents with mental health problems. *Journal of Child Psychology and Psychiatry*, **38**(1), 3–25.

Lealman, G, et al. (1983). Prediction and prevention of child abuse. An empty hope? *Lancet*, **1**, 1423–1424

London School of Economics. (2007). *Cost benefit analysis of interventions with parents*. Research Report DCSF-RW008. London, UK: Department for Children, Schools and Families.

Lovaas, O. I. (1987). Behavioral treatment and normal educational and intellectual functioning in young autistic children. *Journal of Consulting and Clinical Psychology*, **55**, 3–9.

Marmot, M., Friel, S., Bell, R., Houweling, T. A., Taylor, S., & Commission on Social Determinants of Health. (2008). Closing the gap in a generation: health equity through action on the social determinants of health. *Lancet*, **372**(9650), 1661–1669.

Milad, M. R. & Quirk, G. J. (2011). Fear extinction as a model for translational neuroscience: ten years of progress. *Annual Review of Psychology*, **63**, 129–151.

Minuchin, S., Baker, L., Rosman, B. L., Liebman, R., Milman, L., & Todd, T. C. (1975). A conceptual model of psychosomatic illness in children: family organization and family therapy. *Archives of General Psychiatry*, **32**, 1031–1038.

Morgan, H. G. & Russell, G. F. M. (1975). Value of family background and clinical features as predictors of long-term outcome in anorexia nervosa: four-year follow-up study of 41 patients. *Psychological Medicine*, 5, 355–371.

Morris, E. K. (2009). A case study in the misrepresentation of applied behavior analysis in autism: the Gernsbacher Lectures. *Behavior Analysis*, **32**, 205–240.

Moser, D. & Grant, A. (1965). Screams, slaps and love. *Life*, **58** (18), 90–101.

O'Connor, S, Vietze, P. M., Sherrod, K. B., Sandler, H. M, & Altemeier III, W. A. (1980). Reduced incidence of parenting inadequacy following rooming-in. *Pediatrics*, **66**, 176–182.

O'Connor, T. G., Matias, C., Futh, A., Tantam, G., & Scott, S. (2013). Social learning theory parenting intervention promotes attachment-based caregiving in young children: randomized clinical trial. *Journal of Clinical Child & Adolescent Psychology*, **42**, 358–370.

Olds, D. L., Henderson, C. R., Chamberlin, R., & Tatelbaum, R. (1986). Preventing child abuse and neglect: a randomized trial of nurse home visitation. *Pediatrics*, **78**, 65–78.

Olds, D. L., et al. (1997). Long-term effects of home visitation on maternal life course and child abuse and neglect: fifteen-year follow-up of a randomized trial. *Journal of the American Medical Association*, **278**, 637–643.

Olds, D. L., et al. (1998). Long-term effects of nurse home visitation on children's criminal and antisocial behavior: 15-year follow-up of a randomized controlled trial. *Journal of the American Medical Association*, **280**, 1238–1244.

Parry-Jones, W. L. (1989). The history of child and adolescent psychiatry: its present day relevance. *Journal of Child Psychology and Psychiatry*, **30**, 3–11.

Patterson, G. R. (1982). *Coercive Family Process*. Eugene, OR: Castalia.

Patterson, G.R. & Brodsky, G. (1966). A behaviour modification program for a child with multiple problem behaviours. *Journal of Child Psychology and Psychiatry*, 7, 277–295.

Patterson, G. R., Cobb, J. A., & Ray, R.S. (1973). A social engineering technology for retraining the families of aggressive boys. In: *Issues and Trends in Behaviour Therapy*, ed. H. E. Adams & I. P. Unikel. Springfield, Illinois: Charles C. Thomas.

Patterson, G. R. & Reid, J. B. (1973). Intervention for families of aggressive boys: a replication study. *Behaviour Research and Therapy*, **11**, 383–394.

Pickles, A., et al. (2016). Parent-mediated social communication therapy for young children with autism (PACT): long-term follow-up of a randomised controlled trial. *The Lancet*, **388**, 2501–2509.

Rey, J. M., et al. (2015). History of child and adolescent psychiatry. In: *IACAPAP e-Textbook of Child and Adolescent Mental Health*, ed. J. M. Rey. Geneva: International Association for Child and Adolescent Psychiatry and Allied Professions.

Robling, M., et al. (2016). Effectiveness of a nurse-led intensive home-visitation programme for first-time teenage mothers (Building Blocks): a pragmatic randomised controlled trial. *The Lancet*, **387**, 146–155.

Russell, G. F., Szmukler, G. I., Dare, C., & Eisler, I. (1987). An evaluation of family therapy in anorexia nervosa and bulimia nervosa. *Archives of General Psychiatry*, **44**, 1047–1056.

Rutter, M. (1982). Psychological therapies in child psychiatry: issues and prospects. *Psychological Medicine*, **12**, 723–740.

Sawyer, M. G., et al. (2001). The mental health of young people in Australia: key findings from the Child and Adolescent Component of the National Survey of Mental Health and Well-being. *Australian and New Zealand Journal of Psychiatry*, **35**, 806–814.

Selvini Palazzoli, M. (1978). *Self-Starvation: From Individual to Family Therapy in the Treatment of Anorexia Nervosa*, trans. A. Pomerans. New York: Jason Aronson.

Siegel, E., Bauman, K. E., Schaefer, E. S., Saunders, M. M., & Ingram, D. D. (1980). Hospital and home support during infancy: impact on maternal attachment, child abuse and neglect, and health care utilization. *Pediatrics* **66**, 183–190.

Wahler, R. G., Winkle, G. H., Peterson, R. F., & Morrison, D. C. (1965). Mothers as behavior therapists for their own children. *Behavior Research & Therapy*, **3**, 113–124.

Weisz, J. R., Weiss, B., Han, S. S., Granger, D. A., & Morton, T. (1995). Effects of psychotherapy with children and adolescents revisited: a meta-analysis of treatment outcome studies. *Psychological Bulletin*, **117**(3), 450.

Wolpe, J. (1961). The systematic desensitization treatment of neuroses. *Journal of Nervous and Mental Disease*, **132**, 189–203.

Zeanah, C. H., Berlin, L. J., & Boris, N. W. (2011). Practitioner review: clinical applications of attachment theory and research for infants and young children. *Journal of Child Psychology and Psychiatry and Allied Disciplines*, **52**, 819–833.

Section V

Somatic treatments

Chapter 17

Electroconvulsive therapy

Keith G. Rasmussen

Introduction

The early to mid-twentieth century was a time of much experimentation with new psychiatric treatments. Examples include insulin coma therapy, malarial fever therapy, and frontal lobotomy. Insulin coma therapy had no rational basis—it was used in psychiatry merely because insulin had been discovered (Shorter & Healy, 2007). Though dangerous, it probably did have a beneficial effect in some patients. Malarial fever therapy was used for neurosyphilis by Julius Wagner von Jauregg (Shorter & Healy, 2007) and probably actually worked, but the development of antibiotics assuaged its use. Frontal lobotomies became quite popular, and António Egas Moniz even won a Nobel Prize for his work in this area. However, this treatment too fell out of popularity because of lack of reliable success, extreme risk of complications, and unacceptable side-effects.

A lasting treatment from this era did not emerge until Ladislas J. Meduna, a Hungarian neuroscientist and clinician born in 1896, began inducing seizures in psychiatric patients in 1934. Working in psychiatric and brain research in Budapest in the late 1920s through to the late 1930s, Meduna reasoned, based on his histological studies of glial cells in the brains of patients with schizophrenia and epilepsy, that some type of biological antagonism exists between the two syndromes. He concluded that inducing seizures in patients with schizophrenia could be curative. It was fortuitous that catatonic patients were considered schizophrenic in those days, because the first patients he chose to treat this way had catatonia, which as it turns out is one of the most dramatic conditions to respond to convulsive therapy. Meduna utilized chemicals to induce his seizures—first camphor, then pentylenetetrazol. The technique was dramatically effective and spread around the world (Shorter & Healy, 2007). Thus, convulsive therapy was born.

However, chemically induced seizures were unreliably produced, with patients often waiting an excruciating length of time for the seizure to occur, and occasionally, much-delayed seizures would occur at inconvenient times. Another method of seizure induction was needed, and that is the story to which this chapter is devoted.

The electric shock

Main citation

Cerletti, U. & Bini, L. (1938). Un nuevo metodo di shockterapie 'L'ettroshock'. *Bollettino Accademia Medica Roma*, 64, 136–138.

Background

Ugo Cerletti, born in Conegliano, Italy, in 1877, was a neuropsychiatrist at the Sapienza University of Rome during the 1930s. He had studied during his training with some of the great neuropsychiatric researchers of his time, including Alois Alzheimer, Pierre Marie, Franz Nissl, and Emil Kraepelin. In Rome, he became aware of Meduna's pharmacological seizure induction method. Inspired by his own epilepsy research inducing seizures in dogs with electrical stimuli, he set about developing an electrical method of seizure induction that would be safe for humans, as a replacement for pharmacologically induced seizures. Lucio Bini, a psychiatrist colleague of his at Sapienza, provided much-needed technical assistance in developing a machine that would send an electrical current safely through electrodes applied to the patient's head to induce a seizure without killing the patient.

Methods

The authors describe the problems associated with Meduna's pharmacologically induced seizures and the history of the notion that electrical stimuli could be used to cause seizures safely and reliably. Details of the device are not provided, but it can be deduced that the current was a sinewave form based on the municipal electrical supply. The number of patients and their clinical information are not specified.

Results

Cerletti and Bini focus on safety and reliability of seizure induction and description of the types of seizures induced. If a powerful enough electrical stimulus is passed through two electrodes placed on each side of the head in the temporal region, a seizure rapidly ensues that is tonic-clonic and lasts a minute or so. The seizure is followed by a brief period of unconsciousness and then awakening with no memory of the procedure. The patients did not complain of discomfort. It was better tolerated and more reliable than the pharmacological method. No psychopathological outcome data were presented.

Conclusions and critique

What followed the publication of the electrical technique for seizure induction in 1938 is nothing less than astonishing. This new method, ultimately termed electroconvulsive therapy (ECT), spread throughout the world at breakneck pace. Sanitoria could easily and safely treat some of their most severely ill patients, something beforehand considered impossible.

The psychiatric literature from the 1940s abounds with publications about this new technique. Research focused on identifying likely treatment responders and optimal treatment delivery. Patients with schizophrenic psychoses, mania, catatonia, and severe depression responded best, whereas neurotically depressed and anxiety-disordered patients did not respond as well. Efficacy was established through clinical experience as reported in large case series—the concept of placebo-controlled trials was not well elaborated at that time. It was also discovered that multiple treatments were needed for maximal effect, not just one. Thrice weekly became the standard treatment frequency, with courses of treatments usually spanning two to six weeks. ECT unmodified by anaesthesia and muscular paralysis (that is, ECT with a full convulsive fit) ran a high risk of bone fractures. Abram Elting Bennett (1940) demonstrated that convulsive movements could be dramatically reduced with the addition of curare and anaesthesia.

There was a lot of enthusiasm for ECT during its first decades. In addition to its reliable induction of seizures, easy administration, and apparent medical safety, the treatment was quite simply the most dramatically effective psychiatric treatment ever invented. There was a big drawback, however, and it is to that issue that we now turn.

Amnesia

Main citation

Janis, I. L. (1950). Psychologic effects of electric convulsive treatments. I: Post-treatment amnesias. *Journal of Nervous and Mental Disease*, 111, 359–382.

Background

Patients undergoing ECT were often noted to forget autobiographical information, including names, dates, life events, addresses, and the like. Patients sometimes complained bitterly about this effect. The literature almost ignored this side-effect until the publication of this seminal paper in 1950. Irving L. Janis was a doctoral student in psychology at Columbia University who became interested in psychological mechanisms of ECT effects. He devised a method of investigating autobiographical memory that is still used today.

Methods

If autobiographical memory is to be tested, how does one construct a standardized test? How does one test the ability to recall events of the past when people have different life memories? Janis devised a non-quantitative questionnaire in which multiple domains of personal experience were explored. Some of the content areas included questions about schools attended, jobs undertaken, psychiatric history, relationships, and childhood experiences. Patients' answers, including details of life events, were carefully recorded before a course of ECT was commenced. A non-ECT control group was included. Approximately a month after the end of the ECT courses, and after approximately an equivalent time period in the non-ECT controls, the interviews were repeated. Thus, Janis could compare test-retest recall in the two groups and presumably control for normal forgetting as well as the effects of ECT.

Results

There were 19 ECT patients and 11 non-ECT control patients with schizophrenia or depression. At baseline, there were no between-group differences in patterns of answering the autobiographical questions either in terms of number of events recalled or number of details per event. In the non-ECT controls, there were no differences in answers 10–12 weeks later. However, in every one of the ECT patients, there were substantial gaps in recall: even with reminders, or even after showing patients in writing what their previous answers were, patients could not recall some life events. Repeat testing about a month later showed continued gaps, but not as many, thus demonstrating that with the passage of time, some recovery of recall does occur. This indicates that the forgotten memories were not necessarily 'wiped out' from the brain, but rather, accessing those memories became more difficult. Better recall after ECT with the passage of time has been replicated (Lisanby et al., 2000).

There were other notable findings. Janis found that recent life events were more likely to be forgotten than remote ones. Also, even though noticeable gaps in memories of life events occurred in all ECT patients, the patients all recalled far more of such events than they forgot. In other words, there was no evidence of 'memory wipe out' occurring across the board. Most life memories remained intact. Emotional significance of a memory did not seem correlated with whether it was forgotten or recalled after ECT.

Conclusions and critique

A modern course of ECT usually consists of 6–12 treatments. The patients in Janis' series received an average of about 18 treatments. Even so, patients recalled more of their lives than they forgot.

In the decades since Janis' report, there have been many studies of the amnesic effects of ECT. The methodology of studying autobiographical memories in modern times is strikingly similar to that of Janis. Standardized autobiographical memory interviews have been designed, with questions about one's past (Kopelman et al., 1990; McElhiney et al., 1995). Scores can be quantified and thus subjected to statistical analysis. This has allowed much research to investigate various methods of reducing memory impairment with ECT, and Janis' groundbreaking efforts were pivotal to that effort.

Thus, circa the early 1950s, two things were clear about ECT: it worked, but it caused memory impairment. This begged the question of whether something could be done about it, and this is the subject of our next landmark paper.

Unilateral electrode placement

Main citation

Lancaster, N. P., Steinert, R. R., & Frost, I. (1958). Unilateral electro-convulsive therapy. *Journal of Mental Science*, 104, 221–227.

Background

ECT involves the placement of two electrodes, each connected to the ECT machine, on the patient's head. In the early years of ECT practice, the electrodes were placed in the temporal regions on each side of the head, termed bilateral placement.

Neville Peel Lancaster was a consultant psychiatrist at Barrow Hospital in Bristol, England. Reuben Ralph Steinert was a psychiatric trainee, and Isaac Frost, a consultant at Deva Hospital in Chester, England. They reasoned that since, in most people, the left hemisphere was dominant for language, perhaps application of the ECT electrodes to the non-dominant right side would cause less memory impairment. The question at hand was relatively simply stated: would use of one-sided, which they termed unilateral, placement result in the same clinical results as the then standard bilateral placement, while causing less memory impairment? Their seminal study changed the course of ECT history.

Methods

The authors treated depressed patients, 15 with the usual bilateral format and 28 with the new unilateral format, in which one electrode was placed on the right temporal fossa while the other one was placed roughly over the right parietal region. While the assignment to the groups does not appear to have been random, the investigators did utilize three innovations that have since become standard in clinical psychiatric research in ECT: use of a quantifiable depression severity rating scale, use of a memory test, and blind outcome assessment (i.e. the investigator testing depression severity or memory did not know which treatment the patient had had). For depression severity, a rating of zero (nil or not present) to three (extreme) was given for each of nine depressive symptoms (such as insomnia, guilt, retardation). The 'depressive quotient' consisted of the sum of scores for the nine items. The testing for depression outcome was done at baseline and after four ECT treatments were finished. For memory, ability to recall a sentence with four items, presented just prior to treatment, was tested along with global orientation. This was completed after each treatment.

Results

The unilaterally treated group seemed to experience the same outcome on the depression scale, though the clinical impression of the treating psychiatrists was that the bilaterally treated patients experienced more improvement. The unilaterally treated patients performed much better on the sentence recall and orientation tests than did the bilaterally treated patients. The authors concluded that unilateral placement was advised for people in whom memory issues would be particularly problematic, and that bilateral placement was preferable for those with particularly severe clinical states of depression or psychosis.

Conclusions and critique

This paper received a lot of attention, and over the next several decades there have been innumerable replication attempts to determine if in fact unilateral electrode placement confers the same antidepressant properties, but with less memory dysfunction, than bilateral placement (Janicak et al., 1985). There has been a raging debate splitting the ECT community into two camps: those who insist right unilateral placement is equivalent to bilateral, and those who insist that bilateral is better. It turns out the story is more complicated than electrode placement alone (see the section 'Not all seizures are created equal'). For now, however, we turn to the increasing emphasis in psychiatry on proving the efficacy of psychiatric treatments with placebo-controlled clinical trials. But how does one conduct a 'placebo'-controlled trial with ECT? Let us now find out.

Sham electroconvulsive therapy

Main citation

Johnstone, E. C., et al. (1980). The Northwick Park electroconvulsive therapy trial. *The Lancet*, 2, 1317–1320.

Background

For several decades, the prevailing belief in the efficacy of ECT was based on case series and clinical lore. However, the standard in clinical medicine is the placebo-controlled trial. This type of study is relatively easy with medications, where identical-looking placebo pills can be used. But how should one perform a 'placebo'-controlled trial with ECT?

Eve C. Johnstone and colleagues at Northwick Park Hospital in Middlesex, England, utilized a procedure termed 'sham ECT', whereby anaesthesia was administered without seizure induction. The idea with sham ECT was to induce anaesthesia as well as muscular paralysis and then ventilate the patient until resumption of spontaneous respirations occurred. Patients who consented to the study were randomly assigned to real versus sham ECT, without being told which one they were receiving. Outcomes for depressive severity could then be compared. The value of such trials inherently relies on patients not knowing whether they are receiving sham or real ECT.

Methods

The investigators randomly assigned 70 inpatients with depression to twice-weekly sham or real treatments for four weeks (thus, eight sessions total). Electrode placement was bilateral, and the electrical stimulus was sinewave, which was still commonly used at that time. Depression severity was quantified with the Hamilton Depression Rating Scale (Hamilton, 1960). The ratings were conducted at baseline and weekly for four weeks, and then repeated at one and six months post-treatment. The primary outcome was improvement on this rating scale.

Results

At baseline, the real and sham ECT groups had equal scores. At the end of four weeks, the real ECT group had lower scores, meaning lesser depression severity. However, the size of this difference was rather small, and the sham group had enjoyed impressive reductions in depression severity in their own right. Thus, the trial did indeed provide evidence of efficacy for ECT beyond placebo, but the magnitude of the difference raised questions about whether this supra-placebo efficacy was clinically worth the cognitive effects of the treatment. At the end of four weeks of treatment, the real ECT group mean score was about 20, which on the Hamilton scale is consistent with moderately severe depression. Thus, even though those scores were a lot lower than at baseline (where scores were about 50), most patients still were not in remission from their depressive episode.

Conclusions and critique

The Northwick Park trial was meticulously well designed. All depressed patients were diagnosed with standardized diagnostic instruments, and the psychopathological features were consonant with those thought to presage a particularly good response to ECT (Carney et al., 1965). The psychiatric field was baffled not at the level of response of the ECT group, which was impressive, but at that of the sham group, which was also impressive. What could account for these results? It is not necessarily a placebo response. Ironically, what is commonly called a 'placebo'-controlled study does not in fact test for the placebo response itself. There are multiple mechanisms whereby a patient improves in regard to a disease process: effects of the treatment, effects of other interventions such as psychotherapy, the natural history of the disease, the placebo response, and error in measurement. In the Northwick Park trial, the patients' expectations or beliefs in whether they were receiving real or sham ECT were not assessed, so the reader cannot assume it was placebo effects accounting for the improvement in depression in the sham group. All patients in the trial were inpatients and thus received whatever milieu therapy interventions were offered, such as group therapy or family sessions. It is likely the latter factor played a role in the patients' improvement. Thus, a clinical recommendation might be that ECT should be reserved for depressed patients who do not respond to such interventions.

Also, even though the patients enjoyed substantial reductions in depression severity, most did not achieve the remission which is expected of ECT. In the real ECT group, this probably was due to only having received eight treatments (many depressed patients need several more than that to achieve maximal response), and the twice-weekly versus the more standard thrice-weekly schedule probably also caused lesser improvement in the real ECT group. Thus, the patients in the Northwick Park trial were undertreated with real ECT. Additionally, in another publication (Clinical Research Centre, 1984), the research group analysed data for psychotic versus non-psychotic patients and found that the difference between real and sham treatments was bigger in the psychotically depressed group. Psychotic depression is considered an especially ECT-responsive type of depression (Petrides et al., 2001).

In sum, the Northwick Park trial, though with somewhat equivocal results, introduced the use of modern scientific methods to assess the efficacy of ECT and thus stands as a landmark in the history of this treatment. The time period of this study was the early

1980s, and the ECT field was ripe for capitalizing on technological developments in electrical stimulus delivery. It is to this topic that we now turn our attention.

Not all seizures are created equal

Main citation

Sackeim, H. A., Decina, P., Kanzler, M., Kerr, B., & Malitz, S. (1987). Effects of electrode placement on the efficacy of titrated, low-dose ECT. *American Journal of Psychiatry*, 144, 1449–1455.

Background

The electrical stimulus in early decades of ECT practice was a sinewave formation, which is what emanates from municipal power supplies. It was in the 1940s when Wladimir Liberson, a Russian immigrant to the United States who had been involved in research using electrical stimuli to excite nervous tissue, became aware of the usage of the sinewave formation for ECT devices. He was rather aghast, as he knew perfectly well that this stimulus was much greater than was minimally needed to excite neurons. He devised an ECT machine that delivered what he termed 'brief-stimulus therapy', meaning that the machine took the sinewave stimulus from the electrical supply and converted it into a series of brief pulses of electricity (Liberson, 1948). He was able to induce seizures in humans with much less total electrical charge than using the sinewave stimulus. Unfortunately, brief-stimulus technique, later termed 'brief-pulse square-wave', was not incorporated into popular use until about the 1970s. The brief-pulse square-wave stimulus allowed quantification of the electrical charge, or electrical dose, administered to the patient. It also introduced four modifiable parameters: duration of each pulse in milliseconds, duration of the interval between pulses, duration of the total pulse train, and current of each pulse in amperes (millicoulombs per millisecond).

In this landmark paper, the psychologist Harold Sackeim and colleagues at Columbia University describe a technique that fundamentally changed ECT delivery throughout the world. Utilizing a machine with the brief-pulse square-wave stimulus, they devised a method of introducing the smallest amount of electrical charge necessary to induce a seizure in each patient. At the first session, the smallest amount of charge the machine could deliver was used. If the patient had a seizure, no further stimulations were administered. If the patient did not have a seizure, then the amount (or dose) of electricity was increased (by increasing the frequency of pulses) and a re-stimulation given. If no seizure ensued, then a further increase in dose was administered, and so on, until each patient had a seizure. The minimal amount of electrical charge needed to induce a seizure, termed 'the seizure threshold', was calculated for each patient based on the four stimulus parameters and was found to vary substantially among patients. This technique of seizure-threshold determination allowed each patient to receive only the minimal amount of electricity needed to elicit a seizure. Nobody had done this before. The idea was that by using the lowest amount of electrical charge to induce seizures, the memory side-effects could be minimized. The main purpose of the paper was to compare unilateral versus bilateral electrode placement for efficacy, utilizing this seizure-threshold method.

Methods

The investigators compared unilateral versus bilateral electrode placement in a randomized fashion in patients with severe depression scheduled for ECT. Patients with substance abuse or an organic brain syndrome were excluded. The minimal amount of electricity needed to induce a seizure was used (a method the authors called 'low-dose' ECT). Patients were followed with serial depression rating scale scores and were treated until they experienced an at least 50% reduction in the scores or until there was no response after ten treatments. Statistical analysis focused on comparison of the depression rating scale scores post-treatment and proportion of patients in each group who achieved response status.

Results

Utilizing low-dose ECT and comparing unilateral with bilateral electrode placement, the response rates were more than twice as high in the bilateral group, even though seizure duration was equal between the two groups. The bilateral group enjoyed a 70% response rate compared to 28% for unilateral placement.

Conclusions and critique

This study established the standard for technique in ECT studies in the modern era. First, there must be random assignment to groups, blind evaluation of outcome, and precise criteria established for response. Second, there must be brief-pulse square-wave electrical stimulation, not sinewave, and sufficient information about stimulus parameters must be provided to allow for calculation of electrical charge used. Third, there must be seizure-threshold determination at the first session with an explanation for how electrical dose was determined at future sessions. These are the obligatory elements of a modern ECT clinical study. The fact that unilateral placement was so markedly inferior to bilateral could be explained by the fact that the lowest possible electrical dose was used to induce seizures. In the large unilateral versus bilateral literature that predated this study, electrical dosing had not been specified. It was theorized that higher electrical doses may have been used in unilateral groups in previous studies where it was equal to bilateral for efficacy, and that these higher doses resulted in greater efficacy. However, this was just a theory, and it needed scientific testing.

The same group, in a follow-up study (Sackeim et al., 1993), replicated the first but added two additional groups: half of each electrode placement group were treated after the first session with a dose of electricity two and a half times greater than the seizure-threshold dose. Thus, there were four groups in total: unilateral versus bilateral, and low-dose versus high-dose. The same depression rating scale was used to assess therapeutic outcome. The purpose of the study was to see if higher electrical doses resulted in greater therapeutic efficacy. The response rates for the low-dose groups were quite similar to the first study (17% for low-dose unilateral and 65% for low-dose bilateral). However, high-dose unilateral placement resulted in 43% response rates while those for high-dose bilateral were 63%. Thus, for unilateral placement, there was a clinically significant increase in efficacy with higher electrical doses, although the efficacy still did not match that of bilateral placement. For bilateral placement, higher electrical doses did not result in increased response rates.

Two other developments in ECT technique presented by this group further elaborated these issues. A third study (Sackeim et al., 2000) utilized three levels of electrical dosing for unilateral ECT: low-dose, two and a half times threshold, and six times threshold. These were compared to a bilateral group, and the highest level of electrical dosing in the unilateral group, six times threshold, did indeed match bilateral for efficacy and caused lesser degrees of amnesia. This has become the standard dosing for unilateral ECT. Additionally, a later study (Sackeim et al., 2008) modified the electrical stimulus further by utilizing what was called an ultra-brief pulse width. The reader will recall that duration of each electrical pulse is one stimulus parameter that can be controlled with modern ECT devices. The ultra-brief pulse-width technique turned out to cause even less memory impairment than the previous standard, longer pulse widths, and this technique has now become quite commonly used in ECT practice.

There were multiple important and influential findings in these studies. First, seizure duration did not correlate with efficacy, reflecting the dictum that 'not all seizures are created equal' (Sackeim et al., 1984). Second, it was possible to quantify the electrical stimulus and use the lowest amount of electricity to individualize the electrical dose on a case-by-case basis, thus lowering cognitive side-effects. This method of quantifying the electrical dose and determining seizure threshold has become the standard of care for both clinical practice and research in the ECT field. Sinewave stimulation or brief-pulse square-wave stimulation without calculating electrical doses is no longer acceptable. This development has undoubtedly reduced the burden of memory impairment with ECT. Additionally, the demonstration that different forms of ECT resulted in different efficacy rates probably constitutes the best evidence yet, even greater than the sham ECT studies, of the inherent efficacy of ECT beyond placebo effects. This is because if one assumes that the lowest efficacy type of ECT, namely low-dose unilateral, would not have been outperformed by a sham group (had there been one), which is a very realistic assumption, then one can consider that group to essentially be a 'placebo' group. Finally, the finding that high-dose unilateral ECT heightens the remission rates, while still preserving a better cognitive side-effect profile, has led to greater acceptance of unilateral electrode placement in the ECT field.

Preventing relapse with continuation electroconvulsive therapy

Main citation

Kellner, C. H., et al. (2006). Continuation electroconvulsive therapy versus pharmacotherapy for relapse prevention in major depression: a multisite study from the Consortium for Research in Electroconvulsive Therapy (CORE). *Archives of General Psychiatry*, 63, 1337–1344.

Background

Up to now in this chapter, the focus has been on the acute treatment of depression with ECT. A typical course of ECT consists of thrice-weekly treatments administered over a few weeks. Remission rates are high, but over the ensuing months and years, relapse rates are also high. A recent review of this topic found overall six-month relapse rates for depression to be around 50% after initially successful acute ECT (Jelovac et al., 2013). Relapse prevention has been a consistent challenge in ECT practice. One method that received some early attention was continuation ECT, in which the course of treatments is not abruptly stopped after the thrice-weekly phase leads to remission but, rather, is continued at spaced intervals for weeks to months or longer. The intertreatment interval during continuation ECT has varied but usually starts with weekly treatments for a few weeks, eventually progressing to every other week, and ultimately to once a month. This technique did not have a good evidence basis until the groundbreaking study of Charles Kellner and colleagues in the Consortium for Research on ECT (CORE) herein presented.

Methods

In this study, 201 patients with major depression treated with thrice-weekly ECT treatments until remission occurred were randomized to receive six months of either an antidepressant medication regimen or continuation ECT. The former was a combination of lithium and nortriptyline titrated to blood levels of 0.7 mEq/L and 125 ng/mL, respectively. The latter was administered once a week for four treatments, then once every other week for four treatments, then monthly for two months, to achieve a six-month period of treatment. Standardized depression rating scales were used to assess relapse rates, since all patients started the randomized phase of the study with very low scores. The purpose of the study was to see if continuation ECT treatments compared favourably to pharmacotherapy in relapse prevention capability.

Results

There were essentially three ways of looking at the outcomes during the six months of the trial: sustained remission rates (i.e. patients who remained well for the six-month observation period), relapse rates, and dropout rates. In the pharmacotherapy group, percentages for these three outcomes were, respectively, 46.3%, 31.6%, and 22.1%. For the continuation ECT group, the percentages were 46.1%, 37.1%, and 16.8%. None of the intergroup differences were statistically significant. Thus, patients' clinical outcomes were equal for treatment with continuation ECT as with an aggressive medication regimen.

Conclusions and critique

Clinicians have known for a long time that relapses are common after an initially successful ECT course. A post-ECT pharmacotherapy study (Sackeim et al., 2001) demonstrated that the addition of lithium carbonate to an antidepressant substantially reduced relapse rates, but the role of continuation ECT was relatively unstudied. For several decades, continuation ECT had been utilized by clinicians as an attempt to prevent relapse. However, controlled trial evidence was lacking. The Kellner study provided that evidence and, indeed, continuation ECT was highly effective in preventing relapses, thus justifying its use. In the years since this trial, further data have elaborated the role of continuation ECT combined with pharmacotherapy to result in even lesser degrees of relapse (Kellner et al., 2016). Continuation ECT has now become an accepted option to prevent relapses after successful acute-phase ECT.

Conclusion

This chapter described the development of this highly effective treatment modality in psychiatry. While most of the papers highlighted here focus on its effects for depression, it is important to remember that ECT is effective for other psychiatric conditions as well, such as catatonia, mania, and psychosis. Though the field has come far in fine-tuning this technique, several key questions remain unanswered:

1. *What is the mechanism of action of ECT?* Ever since the dramatic efficacy of induced seizures for psychiatric disorders was discovered in the 1930s, investigators have speculated on putative mechanisms of action. In the 1940s and 1950s, consistent with the predominance of psychoanalysis in American psychiatry, theories focused on psychodynamic processes such as 'satisfaction of unconscious masochism'. With the advent of 'biological psychiatry' in the 1960s, the theories have become more biologically sophisticated, incorporating neurotransmitters, neurohormones, neuroplasticity, and neurocircuitry (the last of which is of intense modern interest). Yet, any kind of convincing theory has been elusive. A method of studying the intact functioning brain, especially at the microscopic level, is needed, as cellular changes (indicative of neuroplasticity) are undoubtedly of importance. Unfortunately, thousands of studies on the biological effects of induced seizures in animals have yielded limited insight and the field desperately awaits a safe, sophisticated method of study in humans.

2. *Can the efficacy of ECT be matched with another neurostimulatory procedure?* The search continues for an intervention that can mimic the neurobiological effect of ECT, whatever that may be, without necessitating anaesthesia, inducing a seizure, or causing cognitive impairment. Methods like transcranial magnetic stimulation (TMS), transcranial direct

current stimulation (tDCS), vagus nerve stimulation (VNS), and deep brain stimulation (DBS) are in various stages of development (and discussed in Chapters 18 and 19), but none thus far matches the efficacy of ECT. TMS, in particular, seems an attractive alternative given its negligible side-effects, lack of cognitive impairment, wide availability, and convenience. Regrettably, it is therapeutically weak. tDCS devices are actually available over the internet, but studies of this ultra-low current stimulation suggest barely supra-placebo efficacy. VNS and DBS, disconcertingly invasive, with surgical implantation of electrical devices, have failed thus far to offer true benefit. It will probably take elaboration of the neurobiological mechanism of ECT first before a good alternative can be developed.

3. *Should the unilateral ultra-brief technique be used for all depressed patients?* As discussed in this chapter, the unilateral ultra-brief technique of ECT has enjoyed widespread popularity by demonstrating fairly good efficacy while sparing cognitive side-effects. Not all patients respond to it, however, and it is not yet known how to utilize this technique optimally. For example, what electrical dose should be used—six times threshold or even higher, such as eight to ten times threshold? Also, when should non-responding patients be switched to another method—after four, six, or eight treatments? And what should the next technical step be for these non-responders: even higher electrical doses or changing to bilateral electrode placement? Surprisingly, these questions that are relatively simple to test have not been submitted to controlled clinical research.

4. *What is the best method of preventing relapse after a successful course of acute-phase ECT?* Post-ECT relapse is now one of the most problematic aspects of ECT practice, given that modern techniques have dramatically reduced acute memory concerns. It is clinically easier for most patients to be treated over the next few months (the highest-risk time period for relapse) with medications alone. However, recent data suggest that combining medications with continuation ECT may enhance sustained remission rates. However, continuation ECT is unavailable for patients who do not live near an ECT service, it is inconvenient for those who need to take days off from work in order to receive it, and it may not be reimbursed by the patient's health plan. Thus, the ECT field needs to specify the clinical predictors of which patients are the best candidates for continuation ECT; these may include demographic factors, qualitative features of the depressive episode, or variables related to the longitudinal course of illness (such as number of prior episodes, duration of current episode, or age at onset of the first episode).

References

Bennett, A. E. (1940). Preventing traumatic complications in convulsive shock therapy by curare. *Journal of the American Medical Association*, **114**(4), 322–324.

Carney, M. W.P., Roth, M., & **Garside, R. F.** (1965). The diagnosis of depressive syndromes and the prediction of ECT response. *British Journal of Psychiatry*, **111**, 659–674.

Clinical Research Centre, Division of Psychiatry. (1984). The Northwick Park ECT trial. Predictors of response to real and simulated ECT. *British Journal of Psychiatry*, **144**, 227–237.

Hamilton, M. (1960). A rating scale for depression. *Journal of Neurology, Neurosurgery and Psychiatry*, **23**, 56–62.

Janicak, P. G., et al. (1985). Efficacy of ECT: a meta-analysis. *American Journal of Psychiatry*, **142**(3), 297–302.

Jelovac, A., Kolshus, E., & McLoughlin, D. M. (2013). Relapse following successful electroconvulsive therapy for major depression: a meta-analysis. *Neuropsychopharmacology*, **38**, 2467–2474.

Kellner, C. H., et al. (2016). A novel strategy for continuation ECT in geriatric depression: phase 2 of the PRIDE study. *American Journal of Psychiatry*, **173**(11), 1110–1118.

Kopelman, M., Wilson, B., & Baddeley, A. (1990). *The Autobiographical Memory Interview*. London: Thames Valley Test Company, Harcourt Assessment.

Liberson, W. T. (1948). Brief stimulus therapy. Physiological and clinical observations. *American Journal of Psychiatry*, **105**, 28–29.

Lisanby, S. H., et al. (2000). The effects of electroconvulsive therapy on memory of autobiographical and public events *Archives of General Psychiatry*, **57**, 581–590.

McElhiney, M. C., et al. (1995). Autobiographical memory and mood: effects of electroconvulsive therapy. *Neuropsychology*, **9**(4), 501–517.

Petrides, G., et al. (2001). ECT remission rates in psychotic versus nonpsychotic depressed patients: a report from CORE. *Journal of ECT*, (4), 244–253.

Sackeim, H. A. (1984). Not all seizures are created equal. *Behavioral and Brain Science*, 7(1), 32–33.

Sackeim, H. A., et al. (1993). Effects of stimulus intensity and electrode placement on the efficacy and cognitive effects of electroconvulsive therapy. *New England Journal of Medicine*, **328**(12), 839–846.

Sackeim, H. A., et al. (2000). A prospective, randomized, double-blind comparison of bilateral and right unilateral electroconvulsive therapy at different stimulus intensities. *Archives of General Psychiatry*, **57**(5), 425–434.

Sackeim, H. A., et al. (2001). Continuation pharmacotherapy in the prevention of relapse following electroconvulsive therapy: a randomized controlled trial. *Journal of the American Medical Association*, **285**(10), 1299–1307.

Sackeim, H. A., et al. (2008). Effects of pulse width and electrode placement on the efficacy and cognitive effects of electroconvulsive therapy. *Brain Stimulation*, **1**(2), 71–83.

Shorter, E. & Healy, D. (2007). *Shock Therapy. A History of Electroconvulsive Treatment in Mental Illness*. New Brunswick, New Jersey: Rutgers University Press.

Chapter 18

Non-convulsive brain stimulation

Kevin A. Caulfield and Mark S. George

Introduction

While a full history of non-invasive brain stimulation is beyond the scope of this chapter, we present, in the context of other psychotherapies, a brief history of the emergence of the brain-stimulation approach. Non-invasive brain stimulation first arose on a foundation of psychopharmacological advancements in the 1920s and 1930s. In 1927, Manfred Sakel in Berlin, Germany, observed that giving psychotic patients an overdose of insulin caused seizures that could effectively treat schizophrenia (Sakel, 1937). In parallel, Ladislaus von Meduna, a physician working in Budapest, Hungary, in 1934, used pentylenetetrazol (metrazol) to induce convulsions to remediate psychosis (Meduna, 1999; Gazdag et al., 2009). Meduna's findings intrigued Ugo Cerletti, an Italian epileptologist, who believed that seizures were an effective therapy for schizophrenia but that the effects of metrazol were too difficult to control. In response, Cerletti rigorously developed electroconvulsive therapy (ECT) to produce seizures by passing high-voltage electricity between two electrodes placed on the scalp (Endler, 1988). He first tested ECT on dogs in 1936, and eventually, on a patient with schizophrenia in 1938. Psychiatrists quickly realized the utility of ECT as a treatment for depression, and modern clinical trials have very high remission rates of around 70% in acute psychotically depressed patients (Petrides et al., 2001).

Subsequently developed medications and technologies have used ECT as a touchstone, with the benefits of each treatment weighed against its side-effects in comparison to ECT. With the rise of antidepressants in the 1960s, particularly tricyclic antidepressants (TCAs) and monoamine oxidase inhibitors (MAOIs), and growing public reaction to the side-effects of ECT (most notably, retrograde amnesia), ECT became less widely used. However, psychiatrists quickly became concerned about the side-effects of some antidepressants (including Parkinsonism and cardiovascular side-effects from antipsychotics and TCAs, respectively), leading to a renewed interest in ECT and to developing new forms of non-invasive brain-stimulation technology to treat psychiatric conditions.

In 1980, at Queen Square in London, Patrick Merton, Bert Morton, and other colleagues began using transcranial electrical stimulation (TES), a form of non-invasive brain stimulation that sends a weaker current (approximately 60–100 milliamps of current compared with 700–900 milliamps in ECT) across two electrodes in humans, attempting to elicit muscle movements and phosphenes (flashes of light) from stimulating through the skull into the cortex (Merton et al., 1982; Merton & Morton, 1980). While TES effectively caused hand twitches and phosphenes, this method of stimulation was uncomfortable and even painful, limiting its further investigation as a therapeutic device and resulting in an ongoing need for a more tolerable method of transcranially stimulating the brain.

Five years after Merton and Morton published their seminal TES paper (1980), Anthony (Tony) Barker and his team at Sheffield, in the United Kingdom, created a breakthrough brain-stimulation device (Barket et al., 1985), developing a way to use electromagnetic (as opposed to electrical) stimulation to excite the cortex. This technique, called transcranial magnetic stimulation (TMS), used the principles of Faraday's Law by inducing electrical current in the brain from brief electromagnetic pulses of current produced in a coil of wire held over the scalp. In contrast to ECT and TES, TMS not only reached the cortex but was also relatively pain-free. However, the therapeutic potential of TMS was initially limited by the lack of a way to identify brain-stimulation targets for clinical application.

The neuroimaging revolution of the 1980s and 1990s was the key that unlocked the therapeutic potential of TMS, especially in psychiatry. New neuroimaging methods, such as positron emission tomography (PET) and magnetic resonance imaging (MRI), allowed scientists to observe, for the first time, the structural and functional status of the brain, in health and pathology, and in real time (i.e. before death). Armed with this information, neuroscientists now had a 'map' of where, potentially, to apply transcranial brain stimulation in different psychiatric conditions.

In 1994, psychiatrists began to use TMS in medication-resistant depression (as defined by inadequate clinical response to two or more pharmacological therapies). Multiple large-scale, double-blind clinical trials, including the Optimization of TMS for the Treatment of Depression (OPT-TMS) trial published in 2010 (George et al., 2010), firmly established its efficacy in the acute treatment of depression. In 2008, the Food and Drug Administration (FDA) in the United States was first to clear a TMS device, and now five TMS devices are FDA approved for the acute treatment of depression. Concurrent with the wider use of TMS in the United States, the United Kingdom's National Institute for Health and Care Excellence (NICE) approved the use of TMS in 2015.

Neuroscientists have now developed additional non-invasive brain-stimulation techniques to build on the widespread use of TMS for depression. Over time, there has been a trend toward newer technologies that have lower stimulation intensities. (See Figure 18.1 for a summary of the strength of stimulation current for each technology in the first year of therapeutic use, at the level of the scalp.) These stimulation methods include vagus nerve stimulation (VNS), which became FDA-cleared for treating depression in 2005, and, most recently, transcranial direct current stimulation (tDCS) and transcranial alternating current stimulation (tACS).

In this chapter, we present five landmark papers that outline the theoretical reasoning, clinical implementation, and future directions of non-invasive, transcranial brain stimulation. First, we present Barker's seminal TMS paper from 1985. Next, we highlight a representative neuroimaging paper from 1994 that contributed to the foundation for TMS

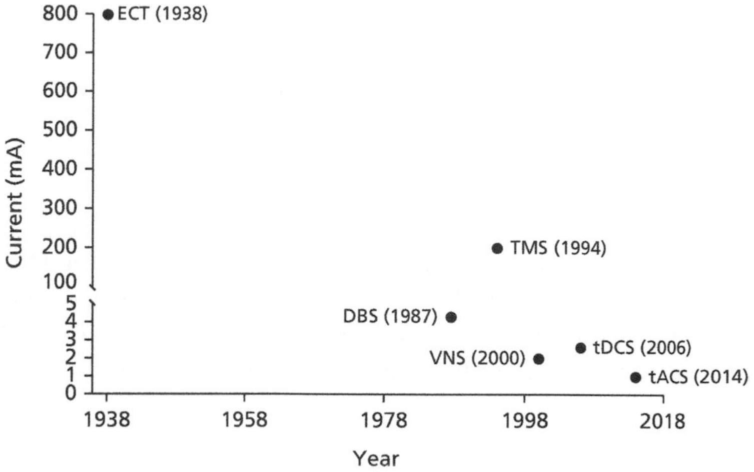

Figure 18.1 Graph depicting how newer forms of non-invasive brain stimulation have trended toward using increasingly less electrical current to effect changes in the brain.

in depression. Our third selection, the OPT-TMS trial published in 2010, was a pivotal multisite, double-blind, sham (placebo)-controlled trial that used neuroimaging observations to inform cortical targets for TMS, on the path to widescale clinical applications of TMS for depression. Fourth, we sought to convey the excitement about coordinating transcranial stimulation with the brain's intrinsic rhythms in an emerging technology (tACS), published in 2010. Lastly, we discuss the multisite, double-blind, sham-controlled trial from 2005 that heavily contributed to VNS being cleared for the treatment of depression. In each of these areas, we performed literature searches with citation scores to identify candidate papers, and chose the papers in this chapter.

A new transcranial technique

Main citation

Barker, A. T., Jalinous, R., & Freeston, I. L. (1985). Non-invasive magnetic stimulation of the human motor cortex. *Lancet*, 325, 1106–1107.

Background

In the early 1980s, neuroscientists were beginning to probe the brain using non-invasive, transcranial techniques. Transcranial electrical stimulation (TES), pioneered by Merton and colleagues at Queen Square in London, was first applied directly over peripheral muscle nerve fibres, followed by stimulation over the motor cortex (Merton et al., 1982; Merton & Morton, 1980). Merton et al. found that electrical stimulation over the motor cortex could reliably produce muscle action potentials in the hand and leg (adductor pollicis and tibialis anterior). However, they also discovered that electrical stimulation over the cortex, particularly over occipital regions, could be intolerable due to pain.

Therefore, there was a compelling reason to find another, hopefully less painful, method to transcranially stimulate the brain.

In contrast to electrical stimulation, electromagnetic stimulation is a relatively painless way of non-invasively stimulating the brain. Transcranial magnetic stimulation (TMS) draws on the principles of Faraday's law of induction, in which quick changes in electrical current through a coiled wire can produce a transient magnetic field. Neuroscientists first used this technique in *in vitro* frog muscle (Kolin et al., 1959) and over *in vivo* peripheral nerves in humans (Polson et al., 1982), but it remained unclear whether TMS over the human cortex could cause neuronal firing. The paper presented here, cited over 3,800 times, was the first application of magnetic stimulation over the human cortex. From this novel stimulation technique, a new basic and clinical neuroscience field was born.

Methods

In the early 1980s, Anthony (Tony) Barker and his colleagues were working in Sheffield, England, with a clinical group trying to stimulate the spine (dorsal roots). Barker was tasked with creating a TMS device with sufficient power to reach the spine. Over several years and many failed machines (and some big explosions), Barker was able to create capacitors that could store a charge and then discharge it rapidly enough to cause neuronal depolarization. They found this could stimulate the spinal cord as they wished, and also realized it could likely reach the surface of the brain, if applied over the scalp. Barker then collaborated with Merton and Morton to actually do this. The researchers stimulated the motor cortex over the region associated with the contralateral thumb and recorded muscle action potentials using surface electrodes on the thumb. For comparison, Barker et al. also stimulated the ulnar nerve at the elbow and recorded from the same electrodes.

Results

Stimulation over the motor cortex and ulnar nerve at the elbow elicited similar muscular action potentials.

Conclusions and critique

This landmark paper demonstrated for the first time that it is possible to effectively and rather painlessly stimulate cortical structures using TMS. It thus clearly launched a revolution. Barker and colleagues produced twitching in a specific area of the hand in awake, alert human volunteers by applying TMS to the motor cortex. Today, TMS has become a vital tool in neuroscience, since depending on stimulation parameters, specific brain areas can either be excited or inhibited. Thus, Barker's original demonstration of a non-invasive and pain-free method of stimulating specific brain areas has evolved into a critical tool in basic neuroscience investigation, in the study of brain abnormalities in disease states, and in the treatment of neurological and psychiatric conditions. Since 1985, there have been several thousand publications involving TMS. This discovery has sent ripples forward, creating an entire field of researchers using TMS to understand how the brain works and how to change the brain in order to treat diseases like depression.

Transient mood states induce regional changes in brain activity

Main citation

George, M. S., Ketter, T.A., Parekh, P.I., Horwitz, B., Herscovitch, P, & Post, R.M. (1995). Brain activity during transient sadness and happiness in healthy women. *American Journal of Psychiatry*, 152, 341–351.

Background

Early brain research was reliant on neurological damage (O'Reardon et al., 2007) to ascribe function to different brain regions. Early studies in the nineteenth century were informative, showing that there are loci of cortical areas corresponding to various neurological functions (Harlow, 1868). However, the interpretations and applications of these studies were limited by the scarcity of these incidents, the varying regions and volume of brain damage from trauma or stroke, and the inability to visualize the brain-damaged regions before death. This need to focus on single cases, brain injury, and autopsy posed an impasse to a nascent field of psychiatry, as any associations drawn between affective state and brain damage were unavoidably retrospective.

This changed in the 1980s. Armed with emerging imaging techniques allowing *in vivo* studies of the brain, neuroscientists began to identify how the brain is organized in cortical–subcortical–thalamic loops (Alexander et al., 1986). Within this organizational framework that was clear for motor, sensory, and visual systems, scientists postulated that there may be prefrontal or orbitofrontal subcortical limbic circuits that were involved in emotion regulation. Several researchers at the time began to test whether the prefrontal cortex was a crucial neural locus of affect whose perturbation was linked with affective pathology, again using clinical strokes (Robinson et al., 1984) or lesions (Kellner et al., 1991) (knockout) as the method of study. The crucial tool of neuroimaging allowed researchers to not only look at structural abnormalities but also examine the functionally active brain regions during different tasks.

This landmark paper used positron emission tomography (PET), a neuroimaging technique utilizing a radioactive tracer to track and measure blood flow to different brain regions, to determine the functionally active brain regions during an affective task (George et al., 1995). This study evaluated brain activity during transient sadness in healthy adults. Later work built on this and compared these changes in health to those seen in patients with clinical depression (George et al., 1996, 1997, 1999). This study is but one among several that examined real-time, task-dependent changes in brain activity in varying emotional states (Pardo et al., 1993; Mayberg et al., 1995, 1997, 1999).

Methods

Eleven non-depressed women each listed neutral, happy, and sad memories prior to PET scanning. (Interestingly, almost all the sad events involved the loss of a loved one or pet.) In the scanner, participants recalled their listed memories while being primed with neutral, happy, or sad faces, with each scan acquired over 60 seconds. (Everyone cried during the sadness induction.) A radioactive tracer ($H_2{}^{15}O$ PET) was injected immediately prior to each memory recall, and sufficient time between tasks ensured adequate radioactive decay of the previous tracers to avoid carry-over. Varying areas of regional cerebral blood flow in each task were calculated using reductive comparisons between each emotion state (i.e. sad minus neutral, happy minus neutral, and sad versus happy).

Results

Brain activity during sadness (compared to neutral) was greater in limbic and paralimbic structures, including the medial prefrontal cortex; left lateral prefrontal cortex; bilateral anterior cingulate, fornix, insula, thalamus; and bilateral putamen and caudate. In contrast, the happy task minus the neutral task had no increased activity, with decreases in the bilateral midtemporal cortex, right prefrontal cortex, and right superior temporal gyrus. For the direct comparison between sad and happy tasks, there was greater activity in sadness in the right anterior cingulate and bilateral prefrontal cortex, thalamus, and basal ganglia.

Conclusions and critique

This manuscript, cited over 850 times, clearly demonstrated that specific brain regions change their activity during temporary sadness. Emotions arise from activity in discrete brain circuits involving both cortical and subcortical/limbic regions. This study could not distinguish whether the brain regions were causing the sadness or were activated in response to the sadness. However, it was a landmark paper in terms of clearly establishing the link between regional brain activity and mood regulation. Later PET studies examining brain activity in patients with depression showed similar prefrontal hypoactivity as in this study of transient sadness; these areas reverted to typical levels of activity in patients who came out of depression, suggesting mutable and revertible physiology between affective health and pathology (George, 1994; Nobler et al., 1994, 2000). Now, there were clear potential targets for therapeutic interventions, and researchers began to use targeted brain stimulation.

Optimization of TMS (Transcranial Magnetic Stimulation) for the Treatment of Depression Study (OPT-TMS)

Main citation

George, M. S., et al. (2010). Daily left prefrontal transcranial magnetic stimulation therapy for major depressive disorder: a sham-controlled randomized trial. *Archives of General Psychiatry*, 67, 507–516.

Background

Piecing together converging lines of evidence from functional neuroimaging experiments (like the one discussed previously), stroke studies, and the stimulation location producing optimal response to ECT, Mark George and other neuropsychiatrists identified the left prefrontal cortex as a potential treatment target for depression. In 1995, these researchers demonstrated that over the course of daily TMS sessions, high-frequency (20 Hz) stimulation for 800 total pulses per session, applied over the presumed location of the left prefrontal cortex (approximately 5 cm anterior to the motor cortex) at an intensity of 80% of the resting motor threshold (rMT), significantly improved depressive symptoms in two out of six medication-resistant patients (George et al., 1995). While these results were revelatory, larger clinical evaluations of TMS using sham-controlled designs were still necessary to pin down the ideal stimulation parameters, including the standardization of how to determine the stimulation target in the prefrontal cortex, the number of pulses applied within each TMS session, the intensity of stimulation, and how to individually dose the intensity of the treatment.

The paper presented in this chapter established a set of TMS treatment guidelines that were rigorously evaluated on a large scale in a multisite, sham-controlled experimental design.

Methods

This multisite, sham-controlled trial enrolled 190 patients with medication-resistant depression (as defined by inadequate response to two or more pharmacological therapies) in an adaptive treatment design of three weeks' duration. Participants who had a 30% or greater improvement in depression during the fixed treatment period, whether from active or sham stimulation, continued their treatment condition for up to three weeks longer, while those with a lower than 30% improvement exited to receive active TMS treatment without breaking the blind concerning their initial treatment. The researchers acquired a rMT (the amount of stimulation to cause a muscle twitch 50% of the time) for each participant on a weekly basis, and the treatment was administered at 120% of the rMT to ensure that stimulation was delivered suprathreshold. In each session, stimulation was applied at 10 Hz (10 pulses per second) for 4 seconds, with 26 seconds between each stimulation train (grouping of TMS pulses), for a total of 3,000 pulses per session. The stimulation target was 5 cm or 6 cm anterior to the scalp location of the rMT. The primary and secondary outcomes were the number of remitters and responders to the treatment (defined by a Hamilton Scale for Depression score of three or fewer, or a 50% or greater reduction in score, respectively).

This NIH-funded, industry-independent clinical trial of daily prefrontal TMS was also the first truly double-blind TMS trial. Prior to this study, even the best sham systems did not control for the differential pain of stimulation, the noise induced by the coils, or the 'twitch' of scalp muscles underneath the coil. Any competent treater could quickly figure out which patients were getting real or sham treatment. Thus, unblinded treaters were in the same room as the patients for as long as 30 hours. The OPT-TMS study perfected a new form of sham that mimicked the pain and produced the same twitch (Borckardt et al., 2006, 2008a, 2008b). Both patients and treaters wore noise-cancelling earbuds.

Results

The rates of remission and response were significantly higher in the active-treatment condition (14.1% versus 5.1% for remission; 15% versus 5% for response). Further analyses showed that active stimulation participants were 4.2 times more likely to reach remission, and 4.6 times more likely to reach response criteria.

The active open-label trial following the acute double-blind phase also yielded positive results, with 29.9% of patients reaching remission (Mantovani et al., 2012; McDonald et al., 2011). Notably, this cohort was comprised of active and sham participants, with the remitters being almost equivalently from each group (30.2% from the active TMS condition and 29.6% from the sham TMS condition), suggesting that prolonged treatment can lead to improved outcome even for those not initially having a robust response to TMS. The sham TMS system sufficiently blinded the patients, clinical providers, and raters, who rarely reported they were 'extremely confident' in their treatment condition guess (only 14% of patients, and no treaters or raters).

Conclusions and critique

This landmark paper demonstrated (in a true double-blind, industry-independent design) that a circuit-based, non-invasive, and non-convulsive stimulation method could treat depression. It helped establish safe and effective stimulation parameters (such as the frequency, location, and duration of treatment) for TMS treatment in depression. The finding that active TMS to the left prefrontal cortex had greater remission and response rates than sham stimulation firmly contributed to the body of literature that has now led to FDA clearance of TMS for depression, for first one device (Neuronetics) (O'Reardon et al., 2007) and, more recently, five more (Brainsway (Levkovitz et al., 2015), Magstim, MagVenture, Nexstim, and Neurosoft). There are likely more than 20 TMS manufacturers around the world.

There is ongoing discussion about the ways to optimize TMS treatment for depression. Drawing on findings of chronic hyperactivation in the right prefrontal cortex due to depression, some researchers have suggested that an alternative to high-frequency, excitatory TMS over the left prefrontal cortex would be to stimulate using low-frequency (1 Hz), inhibitory TMS over right prefrontal areas. A growing body of evidence supports this treatment strategy (Klein et al., 1999), although it has not yet been included in the FDA-cleared treatment parameters. Other TMS treatment protocols using high-frequency stimulation have safely altered the parameters without affecting treatment efficacy, using higher-frequency (18 Hz) stimulation with shorter trains (2 seconds) and intertrain intervals (20 seconds), and fewer total pulses per session (1,980 pulses) (Levkovitz et al., 2015). Further investigations into other pulsed-pattern stimulation methods, such as theta-burst stimulation (TMS delivered in bursts of three 50 Hz pulses at the theta frequency of 5Hz), and their effect on cortical activation are in progress (Huang et al., 2005), with promising early results (Williams et al., 2018).

Weak electric fields enhance and entrain slow oscillations *in vitro*

Main citation

Frohlich, F. & McCormick, D. A. (2010). Endogenous electric fields may guide neocortical network activity. *Neuron*, 67, 129–143.

Background

Since the early 2000s, neuroscientists have had a renewed interest in transcranial electrical stimulation (TES). Unlike Merton and Morton's form of TES (Merton et al., 1982), modern TES methods, including transcranial direct current stimulation (tDCS) and transcranial alternating current stimulation (tACS), deliver a much weaker, less painful current through the scalp (1–2 mA versus 60–100 mA in Merton and Morton's study). tDCS and tACS do not cause neuronal firing but, rather, raise the neuronal resting state to be closer to activation (tDCS) or entrain natural sinewave oscillations to an external waveform (tACS). Sinewave oscillations are a particularly enticing stimulation method as it is hypothesized that to draw upon a global feedback sinewave oscillation signal causes network-wide synchronization. By tapping into this circuit via tACS, there is widespread therapeutic potential, with early evidence from network-based stimulation parameters in TMS (i.e. stimulation frequency matched to each patient's alpha rhythm of 8–12 Hz) showing clinical promise for treating schizophrenia (Jin et al., 2006) and depression (Leuchter et al., 2013, 2015; Jin & Phillips, 2014). tDCS and tACS are additionally appealing as they carry low health risks (in contrast to TMS, which carries a minimal risk of acute seizure; no labs or clinics have ever reported a seizure from TES (Bikson et al., 2016)) and are much cheaper and thus easier to implement on a widespread scale (a TMS system for clinical treatments can cost upwards of $60,000 whereas some tDCS devices cost only $30).

The landmark paper we present here, published by Flavio Frohlich and David McCormick in 2010 and cited over 400 times, rigorously tested different parameters of TES protocols (tDCS and tACS) using *in vivo* and *in vitro* animal models. While modern TES had been used prior to its publication, this paper defined the mechanisms for what causes endogenous brain oscillations, as well as how tDCS and tACS can alter cortical excitability and entrain oscillatory activity (i.e. use tACS to synchronize endogenous brain oscillations to an exogenous brain-stimulation source).

Methods

In vivo experiments

Frohlich and McCormick used anaesthetized male ferrets for *in vivo* experiments, largely because ferrets have extensive gyri while rodents do not. The authors recorded extracellular voltage fluctuations from 16 electrodes positioned between the cranium and retracted muscle.

In vitro experiments

The researchers took seven *in vitro* visual cortex slices from two male ferrets, recording electrical activity with 14 electrodes. Exogenous electric fields (EFs) were applied through two wires placed perpendicular to the cortex.

Results

In vivo experiments

Frohlich and McCormick found that an endogenous EF directly synchronizes slow-wave oscillations. This endogenous EF accompanies the multi-unit neuronal firing (up state) and quiescence (down state) that characterizes endogenous slow oscillations.

In vitro experiments

In vitro visual cortex exhibited spontaneous physiological activity (up and down states) that resembled endogenous slow-wave oscillations. A series of experiments demonstrated that weak exogenous EFs, applied with *in vivo* amplitudes, can cause membrane depolarizations. Subsequent experiments showed that constant electric fields that mimicked tDCS caused faster firing rates that scaled with intensity (compared to 0 mV/mm stimulation, 2.0 and 4.0 mV/mm stimulation caused significantly shorter up states and longer down states).

Next, the authors tested the effects of exogenous sinewave EFs (tACS-like activity) at 0 (control), 0.5, 1.0, 2.0, and 4.0 mV/mm on the timing and regularity of *in vitro* network oscillations. Sinewave EFs were matched to endogenous oscillation frequency. Central peaks of the oscillatory structure, reflecting heightened overall activity levels, significantly increased for each amplitude.

A second tACS experiment tested how 4.0 mV/mm stimulation at different periods (at 67%, 100%, or 133% of the endogenous network-period duration) affects the oscillation period. The applied 4.0 mV/mm field changed the oscillation frequency of the network, regardless of how different the intrinsic and applied frequencies were. However, these data were not replicated with lower amplitudes (i.e. 2.0 mV/mm and below), suggesting that weaker exogenous EFs can only entrain slow oscillations close to their intrinsic frequencies (a concept referred to as 'Arnold's tongue' (Frohlich, 2015)).

Subsequent experiments probed the mechanism of entrainment by analysing how exogenous EFs can affect preferred phase (alignment of individual up states with the exogenous EF sinewaves, in degrees). Zero degrees denoted complete alignment between an up state and the sinewave. Frohlich and McCormick found that external EFs entrain preferred phase, as evidenced by conversion to phases that were closer to 0 degrees. Amazingly, the phase reverted to its original amount of degrees offset from the entrained preferred phase when the EF was turned off.

Frohlich and McCormick also wanted to establish the existence of a feedback loop between neuronal activity and endogenous EF by using positive or negative feedback. Positive feedback enhanced the rhythmic structure of slow oscillations such that up and down state duration variability was minimized. Negative feedback, which opposed the natural EF, had the opposite effect; the variability of the up and down states both increased.

Tying these *in vitro* findings back to *in vivo* cortical activity, the authors tested what effect naturalistic EFs have on *in vitro* cortex. These temporally naturalistic EFs strongly modulated *in vitro* cortical activity, even at very low EFs such as 0.5 mV/mm and exponentially increasing between 0 and 4.0 mV/mm. That is, *one can directly change brain-firing activity with external stimulation that is orders of magnitude too weak to depolarize a neuron.* For ECT, the stimulus must be massive, and enough to induce a seizure. TMS was considered radical in that the stimulus was not strong enough to routinely cause a seizure, and yet it had therapeutic effects. The Frohlich manuscript extended this spectrum by showing that even very weak but precisely timed and oscillating stimuli could directly change brain activity.

Conclusions and critique

Frohlich and McCormick had several key findings that heightened interest in tDCS and tACS, and informed future studies and stimulation parameters. First, the authors explained how endogenous slow oscillations are formed and the mechanism through which exogenous EFs can modulate cortical activity. Specifically, they provided the mechanism for tACS, demonstrating that alternating sinewave activity can regulate and amplify network-wide weak intrinsic EFs to elicit changes in cortical activity.

Furthermore, the authors delineated several notable variables that can impact the efficacy of TES. For instance, it appears important, for weak stimuli, that the exogenous EF stimulation period matches the natural frequency of each person's endogenous EF. Stimulation that deviated too far from naturalistic conditions (e.g. stimulating at a sinewave period of 5 seconds when the naturalistic oscillatory pattern was a period of 3.1 seconds) did not result in significant entrainment. Frohlich and McCormick also found that stimulating at higher intensities in tDCS-like stimulation resulted in greater changes in cortical activity. While the authors did not test stimulation intensities above 4 mV/mm, it appears that higher intensities result in greater cortical activation.

With the mechanism underlying several forms of TES in hand, researchers have continued to characterize the variables that can alter its effects in humans. For instance, building upon Frohlich and McCormick's stimulation directly over the cortex, neuroscientists have modelled how much TES non-invasively reaches the human cortex from two electrodes placed on the scalp, using structural MRI to calculate that 2 mA of tDCS results in 0.1 A/m^2 of intracranial current density (Miranda et al., 2006, 2013). In addition, researchers have recently demonstrated that using multiple small, EEG-sized electrodes can improve the focality of TES (Faria et al., 2009; Dmochowski et al., 2011), especially in a 4 x 1 'ring' configuration (one central anodal electrode encircled with four surrounding cathodal electrodes) (Datta et al., 2009).

For neuropsychiatric conditions, TES has had small yet promising effects. Anodal tDCS over the left dorsolateral prefrontal cortex (DLPFC) has been tested in depression and schizophrenia, with mixed results to date. For example, a recent meta-analysis for tDCS in depression, including only randomized, sham-controlled, double-blind studies lasting between 5 and 15 sessions, found significantly higher response (34% to 19%) and remission (23.1% to 12.7%) rates in active versus sham tDCS (Brunoni et al., 2016). Unfortunately, a recent well-conducted international trial failed to find a difference (Loo et al., 2018). Similarly, a review detailing the effects of tDCS for schizophrenia demonstrated small to medium effects of anodal tDCS on attention, memory, processing speed, social cognition, and cognitive ability (Mervis et al., 2017).

Vagus nerve stimulation for depression

Main citation

George, M. S., et al. (2005). A one-year comparison of vagus nerve stimulation with treatment as usual for treatment-resistant depression. *Biological Psychiatry*, 58, 364–373.

Background

The vagus nerve, named for its wandering and far-reaching synapses between the brain, heart, lungs, and digestive tract, has a long history of neuroscientific study. Animal studies in the 1930s laid the groundwork for interventional therapies in humans by characterizing vagus nerve fibres as predominantly afferent, with 80% of vagus nerve signals terminating in the brain (Foley & Dubois, 1937). Further experiments substantiated these data, with *in vivo* electrical stimulation of the feline vagus nerve resulting in changes in electroencephalogram (EEG) activity recorded directly from the surface of the cerebral cortex (Bailey & Bremer, 1938).

The basis for therapeutic vagus nerve stimulation (VNS) in humans was born out of a robust understanding of structurally connected areas of the rodent brain. Many studies, taken in conjunction, have characterized the path of afferent vagal fibres ascending from the peripheral nervous system and terminating in the nucleus tractus solitarius (NTS) in the medulla, which feeds into the noradrenergic nucleus locus coeruleus (LC) (van Bockstaele et al., 1989, 1999a, 1999b). LC neurons extend throughout the cortex, with strong noradrenergic innervation in the orbitofrontal cortex and insula, including areas that neuroscientists have somatotopically affiliated with limbic information (Aston-Jones, 2004). Thus, there is a feasible mechanism for the vagus nerve, via NTS synapses, regulating emotion through norephinephrine release (George & Ashton-Jones, 2010).

Building on pioneering animal work in the mid-1980s demonstrating the anticonvulsive utility of VNS in animals (Zabara, 1985a, 1985b, 1992), multiple research groups demonstrated the therapeutic antiepileptic utility of VNS in humans (Penry & Dean, 1990; Ben-Menachem et al., 1994; Handforth et al., 1998). As neurologists began using VNS for epilepsy on a wider scale, anecdotal mood improvements secondary to anticonvulsive activity and PET imaging studies (Henry et al., 1998) hinted at its potential therapeutic value for depression. Pilot research into the use of VNS for depression began to reveal such therapeutic potential. These early VNS studies showed antidepressant response rates as high as 30–40%, a remarkable finding given the prior degree of treatment resistance in these patients (Rush et al., 2000; Sackeim et al., 2001). Further research suggested a therapeutic VNS benefit that increased over the course of one (Dmochowski et al., 2011) to two years (Datta et al., 2009), which belied conventional wisdom. However, not all VNS studies had clear-cut results. One randomized, sham-controlled study reported relatively similar efficacy between VNS and sham, with response rates of 15.2% and 10% respectively (Rush et al., 2005), creating a compelling need to definitively evaluate the therapeutic potential of VNS for depression.

The landmark study we present here, cited over 300 times, aimed to conclusively evaluate the efficacy of VNS and tested the durability of VNS effects over a one-year period, using an appropriately matched control group. Published in 2005, this study directly contributed to the FDA clearance of VNS for depression in the same year.

Methods

Researchers recruited 205 treatment-resistant depression patients (as defined by no response to two or more pharmacological therapies) for a one-year, VNS plus treatment as usual (TAU) study. These patients were particularly treatment-resistant, with an average duration of depression prior to enrolment of 25 years and with a high proportion having been hospitalized or having undergone ECT treatment. TAU allowed changes in medication, psychotherapy, and non-pharmacological treatments such as TMS or ECT. The control cohort that only received TAU had 124 participants. Primary and secondary analyses examined score changes in commonly used depression inventories (the 30-item Inventory of Depressive Symptomatology–Self-Report, IDS-SR_{30} (primary outcome); the 24-item Hamilton Rating Scale for Depression, $HRSD_{24}$; the Clinical Global Impression–Improvement, CGI-I). Differences between the VNS plus TAU and TAU groups were evaluated at baseline and every three months until the end of the study.

Results

The primary analysis showed that VNS plus TAU patients had a significant decrease in IDS-SR_{30} scores at one year. Consistent with other studies, improvements in depressive symptoms from VNS plus TAU and TAU diverged, starting at three months post-onset of VNS and further widening over time. At the end of one year, compared to TAU controls, the VNS plus TAU population had significantly higher rates of response (21.7% versus 11.6%) and remission (15% versus 3.6%). So, having a VNS device on top of other medication treatments increased the chances of remission fivefold. Secondary outcomes corroborated the change in IDS-SR_{30} scores.

Conclusions and critique

This landmark paper came at a time when VNS was being evaluated as a treatment for depression. VNS efficacy on a smaller scale had been promising (Marangell et al., 2002; Nahas et al., 2005), but was limited by small sample sizes and no appropriate control group in longitudinal VNS studies. This paper was the first to evaluate VNS on a larger scale (one year) against an appropriately matched TAU group, with strong evidence that VNS has therapeutic potential with strong durability over the course of one year. Neuroscientists have since replicated the clinical value of VNS for depression, with durable antidepressant effects over the course of five years (Aaronson et al., 2017).

Other VNS studies have investigated the optimal treatment dosage. Multiple VNS settings affecting dosage, including current, pulse width, frequency, and duty cycle (amount of time 'on' and 'off'), may impact the efficacy of VNS treatment (Aaronson et al., 2013). Thus, investigating the optimal stimulation parameters seems to be a fruitful contribution to the therapeutic VNS literature.

Lastly, there is a developing non-invasive approach to targeting the vagus nerve called 'transcutaneous VNS' or 'tVNS' (taVNS for auricular, and tcVNS for cervical). Reasoning that the auricular branch of the vagus nerve runs close to the middle-third and lower-third surface of the ear, researchers have successfully stimulated the vagus nerve using ear clips (Fallgatter et al., 2003), showing that taVNS can cause increased blood flow to vagal afferent pathways in functional imaging experiments (Dietrich et al., 2008; Kraus et al., 2007), and that taVNS can change resting-state functional connectivity in depressed patients (Fang et al., 2016; Liu et al., 2016). Preliminary clinical evidence for taVNS in depression has also been promising, with higher rates of response and remission in taVNS conditions over sham stimulation conditions (Hein et al., 2013; Rong et al., 2016).

Conclusion

In sum, non-invasive, transcranial brain-stimulation methods are a new and enticing investigative and therapeutic tool in psychiatry. There are many future directions for this field of neuroscience, with the following key unanswered questions:

1. *Are there useful biomarkers of change produced by brain-stimulation methods that can be used to dose or titrate stimulation?* It is currently difficult to predict whether a patient will respond well to TMS treatment. It would be useful to have biomarkers of change that can accurately predict how a patient will respond to TMS treatment prior to starting the treatment or inform how to best adjust the treatment parameters once treatment has started.

2. *What are the best patterns of stimulation that can produce long-term and lasting therapeutic changes?* Ideally, more refined non-invasive brain stimulation would be so effective as to permanently remediate brain activity in depression without the need for additional stimulation. In lieu of a longer-lasting or permanent therapeutic response, perhaps a parallel strategy would be to investigate strategies to make it easier for patients to receive ongoing treatment to retain the clinical response from non-invasive brain stimulation. For instance, while the cost, safety, and complexity of TMS machines currently require patients to travel to a clinic for treatment, other cheaper, safer, and simpler to use non-invasive approaches (such as taVNS or tACS) could potentially allow patients to safely administer maintenance treatments to themselves at home, under the guidance of their psychiatrists.

3. *What is the best method for non-invasively stimulating precise or diffuse regions anywhere in the brain (the holy grail)?* There is an ongoing debate about how to best target deep brain areas. One strategy in TMS is to stimulate with greater intensity, such as by using an H-coil that broadly stimulates the brain with high electromagnetic fields at overlapping areas of the coil (Roth et al., 2002). Another technique in TMS is to stimulate superficial brain areas that are structurally (measured by diffusion tensor imaging; DTI) or functionally (measured by resting state functional MRI; rsfMRI) connected to deeper, downstream areas of interest. Researchers have already demonstrated the theoretical potential of these techniques in treating diseases with subcortical pathology, such as being able to predict that patients with stronger functional connectivity between the DLPFC and limbic system may be likelier to respond to extant TMS treatments for depression (Drysdale et al., 2017). Lastly, there are emerging technologies with immense clinical potential for stimulating precise subcortical brain regions, such as low-intensity focused ultrasound pulsation (LIFUP) (Legon et al., 2014) and temporally interfering electric fields (Grossman et al., 2017) that can non-invasively and deeply stimulate without affecting the cortex between the stimulation device and the deep-brain target.

References

Aaronson, S. T., et al. (2013). Vagus nerve stimulation therapy randomized to different amounts of electrical charge for treatment-resistant depression: acute and chronic effects. *Brain Stimulation*, **6**(4), 631–640.

Aaronson, S. T., et al. (2017). A 5-year observational study of patients with treatment-resistant depression treated with vagus nerve stimulation or treatment as usual: comparison of response, remission, and suicidality. *American Journal of Psychiatry*, **174**(7), 640–648.

Alexander, G. E., DeLong, M. R., & Strick, P. L. (1986). Parallel organization of functionally segregated circuits linking basal ganglia and cortex. *Annual Reviews in Neuroscience*, **9**, 357–381.

Aston-Jones, G. (2004). Locus coeruleus, A5 and A7 noradrenergic cell groups. In: *The Rat Nervous System*, 3rd edn, ed. G. Paxinos. London: Academic Press; pp. 259–294.

Bailey, P. & Bremer, F. (1938). A sensory cortical representation of the vagus nerve: with a note on the effects of low blood pressure on the cortical electrogram. *Journal of Neurophysiology*, **1**(5), 405–412.

Barker, A. T., Jalinous, R., & Freeston, I. L. (1985). Non-invasive magnetic stimulation of the human motor cortex. *Lancet* **325**, 1106–1107.

Ben-Menachem, E., et al. (1994). Vagus nerve stimulation for treatment of partial seizures: 1. A controlled study of effect on seizures. *Epilepsia*, **35**(3), 616–626.

Bikson, M., et al. (2016). Safety of transcranial direct current stimulation: evidence based update 2016. *Brain Stimulation*, **9**(5), 641–661.

Borckardt, J. J., et al. (2006). Reducing pain and unpleasantness during repetitive transcranial magnetic stimulation. *Journal of ECT*, **22**(4), 259–264.

Borckardt, J. J., et al. (2008a). Focal electrically administered therapy: device parameter effects on stimulus perception in humans. *Journal of ECT*, **25**(2), 91–98.

Borckardt, J., et al. (2008b). Development and evaluation of a portable sham TMS system. *Brain Stimulation*, **1**(1), 52–59.

Brunoni, A. R., et al. (2016). Transcranial direct current stimulation for acute major depressive episodes: meta-analysis of individual patient data. *British Journal of Psychiatry*, **208**(6), 522–531.

Datta, A., Bansal, V., Diaz, J., Patel, J., Reato, D., & Bikson, M. (2009). Gyri-precise head model of transcranial DC stimulation: improved spatial focality using a ring electrode versus conventional rectangular pad. *Brain Stimulation*, **2** (4), 201–207.

Dietrich, S., et al. (2008). A novel transcutaneous vagus nerve stimulation leads to brainstem and cerebral activations measured by functional MRI [Funktionelle magnetresonanztomographie zeigt aktivierungen des hirnstamms und weiterer zerebraler strukturen unter transkutaner vagusnervstimulation]. *Biomedical Engineering [Biomedizinische Technik]*, **53**(3), 104–111.

Dmochowski, J. P., Datta, A., Bikson, M., Su, Y., & Parra, L. C. (2011). Optimized multi-electrode stimulation increases focality and intensity at target. *Journal of Neural Engineering*, **8**(4), 046011.

Drysdale, A. T., et al. (2017). Resting-state connectivity biomarkers define neurophysiological subtypes of depression. *Nature Medicine*, **23**(1), 28–38.

Endler, N. S. (1988). The origins of electroconvulsive therapy (ECT). *Convulsive Therapy*, **4**(1), 5–23.

Fallgatter, A., et al. (2003). Far field potentials from the brain stem after transcutaneous vagus nerve stimulation. *Journal of Neural Transmission*, **110**(12), 1437–1443.

Fang, J., et al. (2016). Transcutaneous vagus nerve stimulation modulates default mode network in major depressive disorder. *Biological Psychiatry*, **79**(4), 266–273.

Faria, P., Leal, A., & Miranda, P. C. (2009). *Comparing different electrode configurations using the 10-10 international system in tDCS: a finite element model analysis.* Paper presented at the Annual International Conference of the IEEE Engineering in Medicine and Biology Society. September 2009, 1596–1599. doi: 10.1109/IEMBS.2009.5334121

Fink, M. (1999). Ladislas J. Meduna M.D., 1896–1964. *American Journal of Psychiatry*, **156**(11), 1807.

Foley, J. O. & DuBois, F. S. (1937). Quantitative studies of the vagus nerve in the cat. I. The ratio of sensory to motor fibers. *Journal of Comparative Neurology*, **67**(1), 49–67.

Frohlich, F. (2015). Tuning out the blues—thalamo-cortical rhythms as a successful target for treating depression. *Brain Stimulation*, **8**(6), 1007–1009.

Gazdag, G., Bitter, I., Ungvari, G. S., Baran, B., & Fink, M. (2009). Laszlo Meduna's pilot studies with camphor inductions of seizures: the first 11 patients. *Journal of ECT*, **25**(1), 3–11.

George, M. S. & Aston-Jones, G. (2010). Noninvasive techniques for probing neurocircuitry and treating illness: vagus nerve stimulation (VNS), transcranial magnetic stimulation (TMS) and transcranial direct current stimulation (tDCS). *Neuropsychopharmacology*, **35**(1), 301–316.

George, M. S. (1994). An introduction to the emerging neuroanatomy of depression. *Psychiatric Annals*, **24**, 635–636.

George, M. S., et al. (1995). Daily repetitive transcranial magnetic stimulation (rTMS) improves mood in depression. *NeuroReport*, **6**, 1853–1856.

George, M. S., et al. (1997). Blunted left cingulate activation in mood disorder subjects during a response interference task (the stroop). *Journal of Neuropsychiatry and Clinical Neurosciences*, **9**, 55–63.

George, M. S., et al. (2010). Daily left prefrontal transcranial magnetic stimulation therapy for major depressive disorder: a sham-controlled randomized trial. *Archives of General Psychiatry*, **67**(5), 507–516.

George, M. S., Ketter, T. A., Parekh, P. I., Herscovitch, P., & Post, R. M. (1996). Gender differences in regional cerebral blood flow during transient self-induced sadness or happiness. *Biological Psychiatry*, **40**(9), 859–871.

George, M. S., Ketter, T. A., Parekh, P. I., Horwitz, B., Herscovitch, P., & Post, R. M. (1995). Brain activity during transient sadness and happiness in healthy women. *American Journal of Psychiatry*, **152**, 341–351.

George, M. S., Nahas, Z., Lomarov, M., Bohning, D. E., & Kellner, C. (1999). How knowledge of regional brain dysfunction in depression will enable new somatic treatments in the next millennium. *CNS Spectrums*, **4**(7), 53–61.

Grossman, N., et al. (2017). Noninvasive deep brain stimulation via temporally interfering electric fields. *Cell*, **169**(6), 1029–1041.

Handforth, A., et al. (1998). Vagus nerve stimulation therapy for partial-onset seizures A randomized active-control trial. *Neurology*, **51**(1), 48–55.

Harlow. J. M. (1868). Recovery after severe injury to the head. *Publications of the Massachusetts Medical Society*, **2**, 327–346.

Hein, E., et al. (2013). Auricular transcutaneous electrical nerve stimulation in depressed patients: a randomized controlled pilot study. *Journal of Neural Transmission*, **120**(5), 821–827.

Henry, T. R., et al. (1998). Brain blood flow alterations induced by therapeutic vagus nerve stimulation in partial epilepsy: I. Acute effects at high and low levels of stimulation. *Epilepsia*, **39**(9), 983–990.

Huang, Y-Z., Edwards, M. J., Rounis, E., Bhatia, K. P., & Rothwell. J. C. (2005). Theta burst stimulation of the human motor cortex. *Neuron*, **45**(2), 201–206.

Jin, Y. & Phillips, B. (2014). A pilot study of the use of EEG-based synchronized transcranial magnetic stimulation (sTMS) for treatment of major depression. *BMC Psychiatry*, **14**(1), 13.

Jin, Y., et al. (2006). Therapeutic effects of individualized alpha frequency transcranial magnetic stimulation (alphaTMS) on the negative symptoms of schizophrenia. *Schizophrenia Bulletin*, **32**(3), 556–561.

Kellner, C. H., Goust, J. M., George, M. S., & Bernstein, H. (1991). An MRI investigation into mood disorders in multiple sclerosis patients. *Biological Psychiatry*, **29**, 564s.

Klein, E., et al. (1999). Therapeutic efficacy of right prefrontal slow repetitive transcranial magnetic stimulation in major depression: a double-blind controlled study. *Archives of General Psychiatry*, **56**, 315–320.

Kolin, A., Brill, N. Q., & Broberg. P. J. (1959). Stimulation of irritable tissues by means of an alternating magnetic field. *Proceedings of the Society for Experimental Biology and Medicine*, **102**(1), 251–253.

Kraus, T., Hösl, K., Kiess, O., Schanze, A., Kornhuber, J., & Forster, C. (2007). BOLD fMRI deactivation of limbic and temporal brain structures and mood enhancing effect by transcutaneous vagus nerve stimulation. *Journal of Neural Transmission*, **114**(11), 1485–1493.

Legon, W., et al. (2014). Transcranial focused ultrasound modulates the activity of primary somatosensory cortex in humans. *Nature Neuroscience*, **17**(2), 322–329.

Leuchter, A. F., Cook, I. A., Jin, Y., & Phillips, B. (2013). The relationship between brain oscillatory activity and therapeutic effectiveness of transcranial magnetic stimulation in the treatment of major depressive disorder. *Frontiers in Human Neuroscience*, **7**, 37.

Leuchter, A. F., et al. (2015). Efficacy and safety of low-field synchronized transcranial magnetic stimulation (sTMS) for treatment of major depression. *Brain Stimulation*, **8**(4), 787–794.

Levkovitz, Y., et al. (2015). Efficacy and safety of deep transcranial magnetic stimulation for major depression: a prospective multicenter randomized controlled trial. *World Psychiatry*, **14**(1), 64–73.

Liu, J., et al. (2016). Transcutaneous vagus nerve stimulation modulates amygdala functional connectivity in patients with depression. *Journal of Affective Disorders*, **205**, 319–326.

Loo, C. K., et al. (2018). International randomized-controlled trial of transcranial direct current stimulation in depression. *Brain Stimulation*, **11**(1), 125–133.

Mantovani, A., et al. (2012). Long-term efficacy of repeated daily prefrontal transcranial magnetic stimulation (Tms) in treatment-resistant depression. *Depression and Anxiety*, **29**, 883–890.

Marangell, L. B., et al. (2002). Vagus nerve stimulation (VNS) for major depressive episodes: one year outcomes. *Biological Psychiatry*, **51**(4), 280–287.

Mayberg, H. S., et al. (1995). Induced sadness: a PET model of depression. *Human Brain Mapping*, Suppl 1, 396.

Mayberg, H. S., et al. (1997). Cingulate function in depression: a potential predictor of treatment response. *NeuroReport*, **8**, 1057–1061.

Mayberg, H. S., et al. (1999). Reciprocal limbic-cortical function and negative mood: converging PET findings in depression and normal sadness. *American Journal of Psychiatry*, **156**(5), 675–682.

McDonald, W. M., et al. (2011). Improving the antidepressant efficacy of transcranial magnetic stimulation: maximizing the number of stimulations and treatment location in treatment-resistant depression. *Depression and Anxiety*, **28**(11), 973–980.

Merton, P. A. & Morton, H. B. (1980). Stimulation of the cerebral cortex in the intact human subject. *Nature*, **285**, 227.

Merton, P. A., Hill, D. K., Morton, H. B., & Marsden. C. D. (1982). Scope of a technique for electrical stimulation of human brain, spinal cord, and muscle. *Lancet*, **2**(8298), 597–600.

Mervis, J. E., Capizzi, R. J., Boroda, E., & MacDonald III, A. W. (2017). Transcranial direct current stimulation over the dorsolateral prefrontal cortex in schizophrenia: a quantitative review of cognitive outcomes. *Frontiers in Human Neuroscience*, **11(44)**, 1–8.

Miranda, P. C, Lomarev, M., & Hallett, M. (2006). Modeling the current distribution during transcranial direct current stimulation. *Clinical Neurophysiology*, **117**(7), 1623–1629.

Miranda, P. C., Mekonnen, A., Salvador, R., & Ruffini, G. (2013). The electric field in the cortex during transcranial current stimulation. *Neuroimage*, **70**, 48–58.

Nahas, Z., et al. (2005). Two-year outcome of vagus nerve stimulation (VNS) for treatment of major depressive episodes. *Journal of Clinical Psychiatry*, **66**(9), 1097–1104.

Nobler, M. S., et al. (1994). Regional cerebral blood flow in mood disorders, III. Treatment and clinical response. *Archives of General Psychiatry*, **51**, 884–897.

Nobler, M. S., et al. (2000). Regional cerebral blood flow in mood disorders, V. Effects of antidepressant medication in late-life depression. *American Journal of Geriatric Psychiatry*, **8**(4), 289–296.

O'Reardon, J. P., et al. (2007). Efficacy and safety of transcranial magnetic stimulation in the acute treatment of major depression: a multisite randomized controlled trial. *Biological Psychiatry*, **62**(11), 1208–1216.

Pardo, J. V., Pardo, P. J., & Raichle, M. E. (1993). Neural correlates of self-induced dysphoria. *American Journal of Psychiatry*, **150**, 713–719.

Penry, J. K. & Dean, J. C. (1990). Prevention of intractable partial seizures by intermittent vagal stimulation in humans: preliminary results. *Epilepsia*, **31**(Suppl 2), S40–43

Petrides, G., et al. (2001). ECT remission rates in psychotic versus nonpsychotic depressed patients: a report from CORE. *Journal of ECT*, **17**(4), 244–253.

Polson, M. J., Barker, A., & Freeston, I. (1982). Stimulation of nerve trunks with time-varying magnetic fields. *Medical and Biological Engineering and Computing*, **20**(2), 243–244.

Robinson, R. G., Kubos, K. L., Starr, L. B., Rao, K., & Price, T. R. (1984). Mood disorders in stroke patients: importance of location of lesion. *Brain*, **107**, 81–93.

Rong, P., et al. (2016). Effect of transcutaneous auricular vagus nerve stimulation on major depressive disorder: a nonrandomized controlled pilot study. *Journal of Affective Disorders*, **195**, 172–179.

Roth, Y., Zangen, A., & Hallett, M. (2002). A coil design for transcranial magnetic stimulation of deep brain regions. *Journal of Clinical Neurophysiology*, **19**(4), 361–370.

Rush, A. J., et al. (2000). Vagus nerve stimulation (VNS) for treatment-resistant depressions: a multicenter study. *Biological Psychiatry*, **47**(4), 276–286.

Rush, A. J., et al. (2005). Vagus nerve stimulation for treatment-resistant depression: a randomized, controlled acute phase trial. *Biological Psychiatry*, **58**(5), 347–354.

Sackeim, H. A., et al. (2001). Vagus nerve stimulation (VNS™) for treatment-resistant depression: efficacy, side effects, and predictors of outcome. *Neuropsychopharmacology*, **25**(5), 713–728.

Sakel, M. (1937). A new treatment of schizophrenia. *American Journal of Psychiatry*, **93**(4), 829–841.

van Bockstaele, E. J., Peoples, J., & Telegan, P. (1999a). Efferent projections of the nucleus of the solitary tract to peri-locus coeruleus dendrites in rat brain: evidence for a monosynaptic pathway. *Journal of Comparative Neurology*, **412**(3), 410–428.

van Bockstaele, E. J., Peoples, J., & Valentino, R. J. (1999b). Anatomic basis for differential regulation of the rostrolateral peri-locus coeruleus region by limbic afferents. *Biological Psychiatry*, **46**(10), 1352–1363.

van Bockstaele, E. J., Pieribone, V. A., & Aston-Jones, G. (1989). Diverse afferents converge on the nucleus paragigantocellularis in the rat ventrolateral medulla: retrograde and anterograde tracing studies. *Journal of Comparative Neurology*, **290**(4), 561–584.

Williams, N. R., et al. (2018). High-dose spaced theta-burst TMS as a rapid-acting antidepressant in highly refractory depression. *Brain*, **141**, 1–5.

Zabara, J. (1985a). Peripheral control of hypersynchronous discharges in epilepsy. *Electroencephalography and Clinical Neurophysiology*, **61**, 5162.

Zabara, J. (1985b). Time course of seizure control to brief, repetitive stimuli. *Epilepsia*, **26**, 518.

Zabara, J. (1992). Inhibition of experimental seizures in canines by repetitive vagal stimulation. *Epilepsia*, **33**(6), 1005–1012.

Chapter 19

Subcallosal cingulate deep brain stimulation for treatment-resistant depression

Paul E. Holtzheimer and Helen Mayberg

Introduction

Major depressive disorder (MDD) is highly prevalent, disabling, costly, and lethal, thus making depression one of the most important medical problems in the United States and worldwide (Whiteford et al., 2013). Pharmacological and psychotherapeutic treatments can be effective in treating depression, but a substantial minority of patients remain treatment-resistant or relapse despite ongoing treatment. Electroconvulsive therapy (ECT) is one of the most effective treatments for depression, even showing efficacy in patients who have not responded to other standard interventions (UK ECT Review, 2003). However, 10% or more of patients with depression receiving ECT do not achieve meaningful therapeutic benefit, and at least half of those that do relapse within a few months. Thus, a conservative estimate places the prevalence of highly treatment-resistant depression (TRD) in the United States at approximately 1% (Holtzheimer & Mayberg, 2011), which rivals the all-case prevalence of other major neuropsychiatric disorders, such as schizophrenia (Kessler et al., 2005) and Alzheimer's dementia (Hebert et al., 2003). In the last 60 years, there has been no major advance in the treatment of MDD and there are essentially no evidence-based treatments for severe TRD.

For more than six decades, two predominant paradigms have guided treatment development for psychiatric disorders, including depression: a neurochemical paradigm that has led to the development of dozens of psychotropic medications, and a psychological/behavioural paradigm leading to the development of numerous psychotherapies. A third paradigm to guide treatment development is based on a neuroanatomical understanding of psychopathology. Within this paradigm, psychiatric disorders are posited to result from dysfunction within networks of brain regions that regulate mood, thought, behaviour, and related systems (e.g. sleep, appetite, libido, pain).

Treatments based in a neuroanatomical paradigm aim to directly target specific brain regions or networks of regions—via ablation or some form of non-ablative neurostimulation—to alter function of the system for therapeutic effect. Such interventions date back to the late nineteenth century, when cortical resection was tested as a treatment for aggressive psychosis (Hamani et al., 2011). This work culminated in the prefrontal leucotomy and was informed by elementary neural circuit models derived from animal studies and descriptions of patients following traumatic brain injury. Although these early neuroanatomical-based treatments appeared to have some efficacy, this was largely overshadowed by a high rate of significant adverse effects (developing seizure disorder and effects on cognition and personality). It should also be noted that even though these approaches were a mainstay of psychiatric treatments during the first half of the twentieth century—and critical in the history of psychiatry—none were ever subjected to rigorous testing as such, so there is essentially no scientific literature base to support these interventions.

As stereotactic neurosurgical techniques were introduced in the mid-twentieth century, more focused ablative lesions could be made within the brain. The hope was that smaller lesions could retain efficacy without the high rate of side-effects. This appeared to be the case, and stereotactic ablative procedures are still in use today for patients with severe, treatment-refractory psychiatric illness: anterior capsulotomy, anterior cingulotomy, subcaudate tractotomy, and limbic leucotomy (the combination of an anterior cingulotomy with a subcaudate tractotomy) (Hamani et al., 2011). Again, although these were and still are important treatment approaches for severe psychiatric illness, they were never subjected to careful scientific evaluation.

Over the past 20 years, non-ablative approaches to modulating neural function have developed, including transcranial magnetic stimulation (TMS, limited to surface cortical stimulation) and deep brain stimulation (DBS, used to target essentially any brain region). These approaches are often viewed as superior to ablation in that they are reversible and adjustable (i.e. stimulation parameters can be modified to optimize effect). Indeed, DBS of the anterior internal capsule has essentially replaced the anterior capsulotomy for the treatment of severe, treatment-refractory obsessive-compulsive disorder (OCD) (Greenberg et al., 2010). However, these approaches are still based on rather crude models of neural network function.

Neuroimaging methods have greatly improved over the past several decades, allowing the development of more sophisticated models of neural network function in neuropsychiatric disorders. Multiple strategies currently exist for examining the structure and function of the human brain *in vivo*. The most commonly used methods include single photon emission computed tomography (SPECT); positron emission tomography (PET); magnetic resonance imaging (MRI); and specific MRI-based approaches including functional MRI (fMRI, which can be performed during a task or at rest), diffusion weighted imaging (including diffusion tensor imaging which can be used to investigate the nature of white-matter tracts within the brain using an analytical approach called tractography), and magnetic resonance spectroscopy (which can analyse the metabolic nature of a specific brain region). Additional imaging methods include electroencephalography (EEG) and magnetoencephalography (MEG) which assess electrical activity within the brain with a very high level of temporal specificity.

This chapter presents six landmark papers that tell the developing story of one attempt to use a neural circuit-based approach to treat severe TRD. The first paper focuses on the development of the neural circuit model itself, based on converging data including those from numerous neuroimaging studies. From this work, a specific brain region, the subcallosal cingulate (SCC), was identified as being critically involved in the pathophysiology of TRD and potentially serving as a target for therapeutic neuromodulation. The remaining papers present the development of deep brain stimulation of the SCC as a treatment for TRD. As mentioned, this is an ongoing story, and this chapter concludes with a discussion of potential directions for future research, highlighting both the promises of this work and the challenges ahead.

Limbic-cortical dysregulation: a proposed model for depression

Main citation

Mayberg, H. S. (1997). Limbic-cortical dysregulation: a proposed model of depression. *Journal of Neuropsychiatry and Clinical Neurosciences*, 9, 471–481.

Background

Converging evidence dating back to the late nineteenth century implicated 'limbic' brain regions in the regulation of mood and affect. However, the potential role of these limbic structures in the pathophysiology of depression was not clear. As the number of structural and functional neuroimaging studies of depression increased, it became apparent that depression was unlikely to result from dysfunction of any specific brain region but, rather, from abnormalities within a distributed network of cortical and subcortical areas. In this paper, Mayberg proposes a working neural network model of depression based largely on neuroanatomical data.

Methods

Mayberg carefully reviews the literature on the structural and functional neuroimaging findings in depression, with particular emphasis on functional imaging studies published 10–15 years prior to this landmark paper. From this, a putative neural network model for depression is derived. The validity of this model is further supported by reference to complementary imaging data in non-depressed individuals as well as results from ablative surgical approaches to treating severe TRD.

Results

The model proposed consists of three primary components: a dorsal compartment, a ventral compartment, and the rostral anterior cingulate. The dorsal compartment consists of cortical brain regions, including the dorsolateral prefrontal cortex, inferior parietal cortex, and dorsal anterior and posterior cingulate cortices. This compartment is thought to be primarily involved in the cognitive aspects of the depressive syndrome, such as decreased attention, anhedonia, and psychomotor retardation. The ventral compartment is comprised of deeper cortical and subcortical brain regions, many of which had previously been included as part of the limbic system: subcallosal cingulate cortex, inferior lateral prefrontal cortex, anterior insula, hippocampus, and hypothalamus. This compartment is proposed to be involved in the neurovegetative aspects of depression, including disturbed sleep, appetite, and libido. The third component of the model includes only the rostral cingulate cortex (Brodmann Area 24a) which is presented as belonging to neither of the other systems, but serving rather to regulate interactions between these systems.

Depression is characterized by relatively decreased activity within the dorsal compartment and increased activity within the ventral compartment, potentially reflecting dysfunctional interaction between these systems. Remission of depression is characterized by increased dorsal compartment activity and decreased ventral compartment activity, presumed to be moderated in part by normal functioning of the rostral anterior cingulate. Therefore, a key role for the rostral anterior cingulate in treatment response, at least to antidepressant medications, is hypothesized.

Mayberg further highlights that though prior imaging studies are quite consistent in identification of which brain regions are involved in the depression network, there are inconsistences in the direction of involvement. For example, prefrontal cortical activity had been previously noted to be either increased or decreased in depression, depending on the study. Rather than attributing this to heterogeneity of symptoms or medication status between studies, Mayberg proposes that different brain-activity patterns may predict a patient's potential responsiveness to different antidepressant treatments. This is supported in part by a study showing that higher baseline rostral cingulate activity was associated with better response to antidepressant medication.

Conclusions and critique

The proposed model was arguably the most comprehensive to date and could be used to generate testable hypotheses regarding neural function in depression and in understanding response to various antidepressant treatments. The limitations were primarily based on the limited nature of the imaging and other data available. Mayberg proposed that the model was expected to evolve as new findings emerged. It was hoped that this process would eventually lead to the ability to identify which patients are more or less likely to respond to which antidepressant treatments and to provide direction for novel treatment development.

Subcallosal cingulate deep brain stimulation for treatment-resistant depression: proof of concept

Main citation

Mayberg, H. S., et al. (2005). Deep brain stimulation for treatment-resistant depression. *Neuron*, 45, 651–660.

Background

As the aforementioned model evolved, increased focus was placed on changes associated with response to different types of treatments, as well as brain-imaging findings associated with non-response that appeared similar despite the treatment modality. Converging data implicated the subcallosal or subgenual cingulate (SCC; Brodmann Area 25) in both the experience of depressed mood but also the antidepressant treatment response. Decreased SCC activity was seen following successful treatment with a diverse set of interventions, including antidepressant medications, placebo, transcranial magnetic stimulation, and electroconvulsive therapy. Further, the structural connectivity of the SCC with other brain regions implicated in the pathophysiology helped validate its role as a key node in the depression neural network. Direct connections with the prefrontal cortex, insula, hippocampus, hypothalamus, and brain stem supported the argument that SCC connectivity was involved in both the cognitive *and* neurovegetative symptoms of the depressive syndrome.

Guided by the success of deep brain stimulation of brain regions within the motor control network to treat medication-refractory Parkinson's disease, it was hypothesized that focal neuromodulation of the SCC and its connections to prefrontal and subcortical brain regions would have therapeutic benefit for patients with severe and highly treatment-resistant depression. A proof-of-concept trial was conducted to test the safety and efficacy of bilateral SCC DBS. Baseline and post-treatment resting-state PET scanning to measure regional cerebral blood flow was performed to assess for potential mechanisms of action.

Methods

As this study proposed to investigate one of the most invasive interventions for depression to date, eligibility criteria were extremely strict. To be included were adult patients, 18–60 years of age, who had been diagnosed with a major depressive episode that had not responded to at least four different classes of antidepressant medications. Patients with major psychiatric comorbidities (e.g. psychosis, substance use disorder) or contraindications to deep brain stimulation or PET scanning were excluded. Patients could remain on stable doses of their current psychiatric medications.

Bilateral implantation of electrodes into the SCC/SCC white matter was performed using stereotactic neurosurgical techniques. Each electrode array consisted of four individual contacts that could be used for monopolar or bipolar stimulation. Intraoperative testing of each electrode contact was performed with the patient awake and able to respond. Following surgery, open-label stimulation was initiated using parameters analogous to those used for DBS for movement disorders. Patients were evaluated clinically on a weekly basis for three months, then every other week until the six-month *a priori* endpoint. To evaluate safety, a comprehensive neuropsychological battery was performed at baseline, and at three and six months after the onset of stimulation. Blood-flow PET imaging was also performed after three and six months of active stimulation.

Results

Six patients were enrolled and received DBS system implantation. In addition to showing limited response to multiple antidepressant medications, all patients had received evidence-based psychotherapy for depression in the past, and all but one of the patients had previously received ECT. All were severely depressed as measured by the Hamilton Depression Rating Scale (HDRS). The average duration of current episode was 5.6 years. All but two patients met criteria for the melancholic subtype of depression and one patient was later reclassified as having a diagnosis of bipolar II disorder. Remission was defined as a HDRS score <8. At the six-month endpoint, two out of six patients were in remission, and one was near remission (HDRS = 9). With response defined as a ≥50% decrease in HDRS score from baseline to six months, four out of six patients were responders. Of note, the two non-responders included the one patient with bipolar II disorder, and neither patient met criteria for the melancholic subtype.

DBS was generally safe and well tolerated. Two patients developed persistent local infections post-operatively; these two patients showed limited benefit from long-term DBS, so the system was explanted in each case. A third patient developed a skin erosion over part of the system which resolved with antibiotic treatment. Importantly, there was no evidence of intracranial bleeding associated with the DBS surgery, and no patient showed a worsening of mood or increased suicidal ideation. There was no evidence of negative neuropsychological effects with short- or long-term DBS, and several patients showed cognitive improvements over time consistent with improvement in depression.

Compared to healthy controls, PET imaging at baseline showed increased blood flow in the SCC and decreased blood flow in the dorsal anterior cingulate, bilateral dorsolateral prefrontal cortices, and ventral striatum. After three months of SCC DBS, responders showed a reversal of these findings, with decreased blood flow in the SCC and increased blood flow in the dorsal anterior cingulate and bilateral dorsolateral prefrontal cortices, consistent with and extending the study hypotheses. Additionally, decreased blood flow was seen in the medial prefrontal cortex, insula, and orbitofrontal cortex (regions that had not appeared abnormal at baseline). After six months of SCC DBS, these findings persisted and were more pronounced.

Conclusions and critique

Although this was a small, open-label study, it provided the first proof-of-concept data suggesting that SCC DBS was a safe and effective treatment for patients with severe TRD. Additionally, PET imaging provided justification for the rationale that the effects of SCC DBS were not restricted to local changes in the area of stimulation but rather changes throughout a network of brain regions involved in the pathophysiology of depression. This study cohort was eventually expanded to a total of 20 patients, with long-term follow-up that further supported safety and efficacy (Lozano et al., 2008; Kennedy et al., 2011).

Subcallosal cingulate deep brain stimulation: replication and extension

Main citation

Holtzheimer, P. E., et al. (2012). Subcallosal cingulate deep brain stimulation for treatment-resistant unipolar and bipolar depression. *Archives of General Psychiatry*, 69, 150–158.

Background

Based on the initial proof-of-concept findings, a trial was designed to attempt to replicate but also extend the previous study. First, patients with bipolar II disorder were to be actively sought out for inclusion; although the one patient with bipolar II disorder was a non-responder in the previous study, there was no good scientific justification for the exclusion of bipolar II disorder patients based on the underlying depression model. Additionally, a blinded sham lead-in period was planned, to begin to better understand the potential for a placebo effect with this intervention.

Methods

Eligibility criteria were similar to the prior study. Adults aged 18–70 years with a diagnosis of major depressive episode were recruited. Duration of the current episode must have been at least 12 months, and patients must have failed at least four adequate trials of antidepressant medications in the current depressive episode. Additionally, patients must have failed or been intolerant to ECT at some point in their lifetime. Exclusion criteria included other major psychiatric comorbidity (e.g. obsessive-compulsive disorder, psychosis, post-traumatic stress disorder, substance use disorder), medical contraindication to DBS surgery, or having an implanted device. Patients were allowed to remain on stable doses of current psychotropic medications.

The baseline period was defined as the four weeks prior to surgery. Bilateral SCC DBS system implantation occurred using procedures similar to the initial proof-of-concept study. Following surgery, patients had a stimulation 'off' period lasting several days to several weeks, to allow for healing from the surgery. Patients were then told they would be randomized to four weeks of 'on' versus 'off' stimulation. However, stimulation remained off in all patients. Following this four-week period, all patients entered a six-month open-label stimulation phase. Stimulation parameters were similar to those used in the previous study. Initially, a blinded stimulation 'off' phase was planned, following the six-month open-label phase. This was eliminated from the protocol following the first three patients (as discussed in the 'Result' section). Patients were followed naturalistically for as long as they were willing to remain in the study.

Results

Seventeen patients were enrolled and received bilateral SCC DBS system implantation (ten patients with major depressive disorder and seven with bipolar II disorder). Duration of current episode averaged 5.5 years in this sample. Patients had failed an average of six adequate antidepressant medications in the current episode, and had an average of 24 lifetime medication trials. All patients completed the four-week sham lead-in phase, and 16 of 17 completed the six-month open-label phase. One patient had the system removed at 21 weeks due to infection; the system was reimplanted, and this patient contributed data to long-term naturalistic follow-up.

Following one month of sham stimulation, there was a modest but statistically significant within-group decrease in depression severity. However, no patient was an antidepressant responder following sham stimulation, and all but one patient continued to be moderately to severely depressed. At the six-month endpoint, 18% of the patients had achieved remission and 41% were responders. With long-term follow-up of up to two years, 58% of patients were in remission and 92% had achieved a response. Importantly, antidepressant efficacy appeared to be similar between patients with major depressive disorder and those with bipolar II disorder, and no patient experienced an episode of mania or hypomania during the study. Also, no patient achieving remission during the study had a depressive relapse during long-term follow-up.

As with the prior study, the DBS procedure was safe, with no intraoperative haemorrhages noted. The only serious adverse event associated with the DBS system was local skin infection occurring repeatedly in one patient. Overall, short- and long-term SCC DBS was well tolerated, with no negative effects of stimulation. Two patients attempted suicide during the study, though neither event was deemed to be related to DBS. There were no negative changes in neuropsychological function associated with long-term SCC DBS (results reported separately, see Moreines et al., 2014).

As previously described, a blinded stimulation 'off' phase was planned to follow the six-month open-label stimulation phase. The first three patients entered this phase, and all three showed a return of depressive symptoms (essentially returning to baseline severity) within 2–4 weeks. Stimulation was reinitiated in all three patients, and antidepressant efficacy returned, but at a much slower rate than seen during the six-month open-label phase. Once stimulation was reinitiated, but before antidepressant efficacy had returned, all three patients developed increased suicidal ideation requiring more intense outpatient monitoring. Due to ethical concerns, this phase of the study was removed from the protocol, and the remaining patients entered long-term naturalistic follow-up immediately after the six-month open-label stimulation phase.

Conclusions and critique

The results of this study continued to support the safety and potential efficacy of SCC DBS for severe TRD. Additionally, this study suggested that patients with bipolar II disorder could safely benefit from the intervention as well. A sham stimulation effect was identified, but this was seen to be quite modest. Blinded discontinuation was associated with a return in depressive symptoms in three out of three patients; although antidepressant efficacy could be regained with reinstatement of stimulation, it appeared to have a slower onset than when initially introduced. Finally, this study demonstrated that antidepressant efficacy of SCC DBS appeared to increase over time, a pattern also seen in the long-term follow-up of the initial proof-of-concept cohort (Lozano et al., 2008; Kennedy et al., 2011). This increase in antidepressant efficacy was often associated with a change of the stimulation contact from the one initially selected for chronic stimulation.

Although larger than the initial proof-of-concept study, this trial was still limited by small sample size. Additionally, for the six-month and long-term phases, open-label stimulation was provided, and there was no control group. Despite these limitations, this investigation provided a critically needed replication of the initial study and suggests further research was warranted.

Subcallosal cingulate deep brain stimulation for treatment-resistant depression: pivotal testing and negative findings

Main citation

Holtzheimer, P. E., et al. (2017). Subcallosal cingulate deep brain stimulation for treatment-resistant depression: a multisite, randomised, sham-controlled trial. *The Lancet Psychiatry*, 4, 839–849.

Background

In addition to the studies previously described, numerous reports from other independent research groups continued to support the safety and antidepressant efficacy of SCC DBS (Lozano et al., 2008, 2012; Kennedy et al., 2011; Puigdemont et al., 2012; Merkl et al., 2013). Among potential brain targets for DBS for TRD, the SCC region was by far the best studied, and all of the research was consistent in demonstrating impressive antidepressant effects in patients with severe and highly treatment-resistant depression. However, as with the initial studies, these additional studies all used open-label stimulation and no control group. Within this context, a large, multi-site, double-blind, randomized, sham-controlled study of SCC DBS was initiated. This study was sponsored by St Jude Medical (now a division of Abbott Labs).

Methods

A study enrolling up to 201 patients at up to 20 sites was planned. Adults aged 21–70 years with a moderate to severe major depressive episode were recruited; patients with bipolar disorder were excluded. Other eligibility criteria were very similar to prior studies: duration of the current episode of at least 12 months' duration, failure of at least four adequate antidepressant treatments, and no other major psychiatric or medical comorbidities, especially any condition that would be a contraindication for DBS surgery or having an implanted device. Patients could continue stable doses of current psychotropic medications.

Bilateral implantation of the DBS system into the SCC region was performed using stereotactic neurosurgical techniques, with targeting similar to that used in the studies previously described. Following surgery, there was a two-week pre-randomization period to allow patients to fully recover. Patients were then randomized to active (on) versus sham (off) stimulation using a 2:1 ratio, and entered a six-month double-blind, randomized, controlled phase. Following this, patients entered a six-month open-label extension phase, but investigators and patients remained blinded to treatment arm (active versus sham) during the initial six-month phase. Following this open-label phase, patients were invited to enrol in long-term naturalistic follow-up. Importantly, the Food and Drug Administration (FDA) in the United States mandated a futility analysis occur once about half of the planned enrolment and device implantation had been completed.

Results

Prior to the futility analysis, 128 patients enrolled in the study and 90 patients received DBS system implantation. Demographics and clinical characteristics were similar to those in prior SCC DBS studies with one notable exception: duration of current episode averaged 12.6 years in this cohort (compared to about 5.5 years in previous studies). When the futility analysis was performed, the results did not technically meet pre-established criteria for 'futility', but the sponsor chose to halt the study. All patients showed improvement in depression over the six-month double-blind phase and the six-month open-label phase, but there was no difference in efficacy between active and sham stimulation (both with a response rate of 17%, defined as a 50% or greater decrease in the Hamilton Depression Rating Scale). Further, patients receiving sham stimulation during the initial six-month phase showed no difference in trajectory of improvement during the open-label phase compared to patients who had been receiving active stimulation since randomization. However, with long-term (up to 24 months) open-label stimulation, approximately 40% of patients achieved an antidepressant response. No demographic or clinical characteristics were associated with shorter- or longer-term efficacy.

Overall, DBS was safe and well tolerated. Serious adverse events related to surgery or the DBS system included local skin infections, skin erosion over the system, and one post-operative seizure. Two patients died by suicide during the study. Both were initially randomized to sham stimulation and died during the open-label phase. However, these deaths were not attributed to active stimulation but, rather, worsening of the underlying depression despite ongoing stimulation.

Conclusions and critique

These findings were quite disappointing given the very positive results from earlier open-label studies. Of note, the study was not negative due to a greater than expected sham stimulation response rate: the study was powered based on a predicted sham response of 19% at six months, and the observed sham response was 17%. Instead, the response to active stimulation was much lower than that seen in prior open-label studies. On the one hand, these data might suggest that SCC DBS is not an effective treatment for severe

TRD. However, two important caveats must be considered. First, as already described, the duration of current episode for this patient sample was more than double that seen in prior studies. Although duration of current episode did not necessarily correlate with antidepressant response, this difference suggests that the patients recruited for this study represented a different population of TRD patients than those recruited for prior studies. Second, SCC targeting was performed using a similar anatomically-based algorithm as that used since the first SCC DBS study published in 2005. However, new data was emerging that suggested this approach to targeting was suboptimal and that connectivity-based targeting might be more precise.

Subcallosal cingulate deep brain stimulation for treatment-resistant depression: refining the target

Main citation

Riva-Posse, P., et al. (2014). Defining critical white matter pathways mediating successful subcallosal cingulate deep brain stimulation for treatment-resistant depression. *Biological Psychiatry*, 76, 963–969.

Background

The original rationale for targeting the SCC in patients with TRD was based on converging data implicating this region in depression and especially the antidepressant treatment response. However, as previously discussed, the rationale also included the structural connectivity of this region with other brain areas involved in depression: the hippocampus, prefrontal cortex, ventral striatum, and dorsal anterior cingulate. This was supported by PET findings in the initial proof-of-concept study showing blood-flow changes associated with response to SCC DBS in brain regions with established monosynaptic connections with the SCC. This implied that targeting the SCC for DBS must not only place the stimulation electrode in the SCC region but must also ensure that connections to other critical regions be targeted. To this point, an analysis of target location in a previous SCC DBS study showed that gross anatomical location did not differ between responders and non-responders (Hamani et al., 2009). However, given the significance of between-individual variability in the anatomy of this region, this approach does not consider whether there are differences in the SCC connections targeted in responders versus non-responders. To examine this, a diffusion tensor imaging (DTI)-based tractography analysis was performed on data collected in conjunction with the SCC DBS replication study described in the paper by Holtzheimer et al. (2012).

Methods

High-resolution structural MRI and DTI data were acquired prior to DBS surgery in 16 of the 17 TRD patients enrolled in Holtzheimer et al. (2012). A high-resolution computed tomography (CT) scan was acquired post-operatively to visualize the DBS electrodes. The post-operative CT scan was merged with the pre-operative MRI scan. The DBS contact used for chronic stimulation in each patient was identified on the merged scans. From this, a volume of tissue activation was modelled for each patient (Butson et al., 2011; Lujan et al., 2013). This volume of activation was then used as a seed for a probabilistic tractography analysis to show the projection of white-matter tracts presumed to be impacted by stimulation. The pattern of white-matter tracts impacted by stimulation was compared between responders and non-responders for six months of active SCC DBS stimulation; an additional analysis compared 24-month responders to six-month non-responders. To determine if the difference between DBS responders and non-responders could be explained by anatomical location of the SCC stimulation electrode alone, the average three-dimensional location of the stimulation contact in each group was compared.

Results

For the six-month comparison, data were from six responders versus ten non-responders. For the 24-month comparison, data from 12 responders were compared to the ten six-month non-responders. For the six-month comparison, findings showed that the stimulation contact impacted three main white-matter tracts in responders but not non-responders: forceps minor projecting bilaterally to the frontal pole (medial prefrontal cortex), cingulum bundle projecting to the rostral and dorsal anterior cingulate, and a white-matter tract projecting to the ventral striatum and anterior thalamus.

For the 24-month analysis, responders at 24 months showed the same pattern of white-matter tract impact as that seen in six-month responders. Importantly, there were six six-month non-responders who became 24-month responders. In these patients, the stimulation contact had been changed during long-term follow-up, suggesting that the revised contact location was better placed in white-matter tracts needing to be impacted for antidepressant efficacy.

Importantly, the structural anatomical location of the active stimulation contact did not significantly differ between responders and non-responders for either the six-month or 24-month analyses.

Conclusions and critique

These findings provided a critical insight into how targeting for SCC DBS might be optimized, while also validating that the mechanism of action of this intervention involved modulation of a complex network of brain regions involved in depression, with convergence at the SCC. Although somewhat limited by the qualitative nature of the primary analyses, this report suggested a new, more individualized and nuanced approach to DBS targeting—an approach that had not been used (or even known about) in the pivotal trial previously described.

Subcallosal cingulate deep brain stimulation for treatment-resistant depression: prospective testing using tract-based targeting

Main citation

Riva-Posse, P., et al. (2018). A connectomic approach for subcallosal cingulate deep brain stimulation surgery: prospective targeting in treatment-resistant depression. *Molecular Psychiatry*, 23, 843–849.

Background

Based on the analyses previously described, a study was initiated to test the efficacy of SCC DBS with targeting based on prospective DTI tractography, utilizing a connectomics approach.

Methods

Eligibility criteria for this study were virtually identical to those for the previous study at this site (Holtzheimer et al., 2012). MRI, including DTI and DTI-based tractography, were performed pre-operatively. Using an interactive process for the left and right hemisphere, a 3 mm seed (used to simulate the stimulation contact's volume of tissue activation) was placed in different regions within the SCC. The white-matter tracts impacted at each location were visually inspected. When the seed location that generated the tract pattern associated with antidepressant response to SCC DBS in the prior study was identified, the three-dimensional coordinates were noted, and this became the target for SCC electrode placement for that hemisphere. Patients then proceeded to bilateral DBS system implantation as in the prior study. Contact location was verified with a high-resolution post-operative CT scan, and the contact best approximating the pre-operatively determined target was chosen for chronic stimulation. Patients then received open-label SCC DBS.

Results

Eleven patients received DBS implantation and chronic stimulation. All had an SCC contact within each hemisphere that generated the tract pattern previously associated with a response. Following six months of active stimulation, eight of 11 patients (73%) were responders and six patients (55%) were in remission. As with prior studies, DBS was generally safe and well tolerated.

Conclusions and critique

Although small and open-label, this study provided support for the hypothesis that DTI-based targeting could help optimize target placement for SCC DBS. Response and remission rates at six months were notably higher in this study compared to prior trials (73% [with no need for contact change] versus 41%). These findings may help explain the negative results from the pivotal SCC DBS trials where non-DTI-based targeting was used.

Conclusion

The papers summarized in this chapter tell the ongoing story of the development of SCC DBS as a treatment for severe TRD. This represents one of the most comprehensive efforts to develop a novel intervention using a neuroanatomical paradigm of psychiatric illness. This story highlights the challenges involved and offers important insights into this process. First and foremost, this is a necessarily data-driven and iterative process. The model was largely based on neuroimaging data that identified brain regions and brain networks involved in the pathophysiology of depression and the antidepressant treatment response. This led to the initial hypothesis that modulation of the SCC would have antidepressant effects in patients with TRD. Subsequent investigation built upon lessons learned in prior studies. Second, these papers emphasize the importance of combining the clinical testing of such novel interventions with methods investigating mechanism of action. Only in this way can the models be refined to better inform future research. In the papers reviewed here, structural and functional neuroimaging were the primary techniques utilized. However, additionally useful approaches could include electrophysiological assays (e.g. assays of neural activity both local and remote to the area of stimulation).

The neuroanatomical paradigm for treatment development offers a promising alternative for patients who show inadequate response to pharmacological and psychotherapeutic approaches. Treatment development within this paradigm will be most successful if guided by a strong scientific rationale and carried out in a way that allows each clinical trial—whether successful or not—to optimally inform on the underlying neuroanatomical models.

References

Butson, C. R., Cooper, S. E., Henderson, J. M., Wolgamuth, B., & Mcintyre, C. C. (2011). Probabilistic analysis of activation volumes generated during deep brain stimulation. *Neuroimage*, **54**, 2096–2104.

Greenberg, B. D., Rauch, S. L., & Haber, S. N. (2010). Invasive circuitry-based neurotherapeutics: stereotactic ablation and deep brain stimulation for OCD. *Neuropsychopharmacology*, **35**, 317–336.

Hamani, C., Mayberg, H., Snyder, B., Giacobbe, P., Kennedy, S., & Lozano, A. M. (2009). Deep brain stimulation of the subcallosal cingulate gyrus for depression: anatomical location of active contacts in clinical responders and a suggested guideline for targeting. *Journal of Neurosurgery*, **111(6)**, 1209–1215.

Hamani, C., Snyder, B., Laxton, A. W., Holtzheimer, P. E., Mayberg, H. S., & Lozano, A. M. (2011). Surgical treatment of major depression. In: *Youmans Neurological Surgery*, 6th edn, ed. H. R. Winn. Philadelphia, PA: Elsevier Saunders.

Hebert, L. E., Scherr, P. A., Bienias, J. L., Bennett, D. A., & Evans, D. A. (2003). Alzheimer disease in the US population: prevalence estimates using the 2000 census. *Archives of Neurology*, **60**, 1119–1122.

Holtzheimer, P. E. & Mayberg, H. S. 2011. Stuck in a rut: rethinking depression and its treatment. *Trends in Neuroscience*, **34**, 1–9.

Holtzheimer, P. E., et al. (2017). Subcallosal cingulate deep brain stimulation for treatment-resistant depression: a multisite, randomised, sham-controlled trial. *The Lancet Psychiatry*, **4**, 839–849.

Holtzheimer, P. E., et al. (2012). Subcallosal cingulate deep brain stimulation for treatment-resistant unipolar and bipolar depression. *Archives of General Psychiatry*, **69**, 150–158.

Kennedy, S. H., et al. (2011). Deep brain stimulation for treatment-resistant depression: follow-up after 3 to 6 years. *American Journal of Psychiatry*, **168**(5), 502–510.

Kessler, R. C., et al. (2005). The prevalence and correlates of nonaffective psychosis in the National Comorbidity Survey Replication (NCS-R). *Biological Psychiatry*, **58**, 668–676.

Lozano, A. M., et al. (2012). A multicenter pilot study of subcallosal cingulate area deep brain stimulation for treatment-resistant depression. *Journal of Neurosurgery*, **116**, 315–322.

Lozano, A. M., Mayberg, H. S., Giacobbe, P., Hamani, C., Craddock, R. C., & Kennedy, S. H. (2008). Subcallosal cingulate gyrus deep brain stimulation for treatment-resistant depression. *Biological Psychiatry*, **64**, 461–467.

Lujan, J. L., et al. (2013). Tractography-activation models applied to subcallosal cingulate deep brain stimulation. *Brain Stimulation*, **6**(5), 737–739

Mayberg, H. S., et al. (2005). Deep brain stimulation for treatment-resistant depression. *Neuron*, **45**, 651–660.

Merkl, A., et al. (2013). Antidepressant effects after short-term and chronic stimulation of the subgenual cingulate gyrus in treatment-resistant depression. *Experimental Neurology*, **249**, 160–168.

Moreines, J. L., Mcclintock, S. M., Kelley, M. E., Holtzheimer, P. E., & Mayberg, H. S. (2014). Neuropsychological function before and after subcallosal cingulate deep brain stimulation in patients with treatment-resistant depression. *Depression and Anxiety*, **31**, 690–698.

Puigdemont, D., et al. (2012). Deep brain stimulation of the subcallosal cingulate gyrus: further evidence in treatment-resistant major depression. *International Journal of Neuropsychopharmacology*, **15**, 121–133.

Riva-Posse, P., et al. (2018). A connectomic approach for subcallosal cingulate deep brain stimulation surgery: prospective targeting in treatment-resistant depression. *Molecular Psychiatry*, **23**(4), 843–849.

Riva-Posse, P., et al. (2014). Defining critical white matter pathways mediating successful subcallosal cingulate deep brain stimulation for treatment-resistant depression. *Biological Psychiatry*, **76**, 963–969.

UK ECT Review. (2003). Efficacy and safety of electroconvulsive therapy in depressive disorders: a systematic review and meta-analysis. *Lancet*, **361**, 799–808.

Whiteford, H. A., et al. (2013). Global burden of disease attributable to mental and substance use disorders: findings from the Global Burden of Disease Study 2010. *Lancet*, **382**, 1575–1586.

Section VI

Special considerations

Chapter 20

Psychiatric ethics

Rachel E. Zettl and John Z. Sadler

Introduction

Anglo-American psychiatry, as a field, emerged from a nineteenth-century demand to address people who, for a variety of reasons, did not fit into the emerging social structures in the industrializing West. This lack of fit is recognized today as 'social deviance' (Porter, 2004). In the case of colonial Americans, beginning in their small communities and family farms, they tended the 'mad' through their own family and community connections. However, as America developed, with cities and industrialization, the family and community ties that made 'mad people' tolerable dissolved through migration to the emerging cities with their industrial jobs and fragmented social connections (Rothman, 2002a, 2002b; Scull, 1993). Increasingly, socially marginal groups were identified (lunatics, drunkards, widows, criminals, orphans, idiots) and came to be dehumanized as social problems which were a drain on personal, familial, and community resources. In eighteenth- and nineteenth-century America, various social institutions were invented, often, perhaps mostly, with humane good intentions, to aid these groups (or at least contain their threat to social stability). These institutions included the asylum, the jail, the hospital, the workhouse, the orphanage, and the special school. Borne from the stigma of their clients, these institutions were, from the beginning, at risk of losing public support and finances, as well as abusing the powers that the government had given them.

Like the medical and bioethics 'movement' that preceded it (Jonsen, 2000), contemporary psychiatric ethics emerged in large part as a social response to a series of abuses of medical privileges within the still-developing mental health system, as well as the self-conscious professionalizing of the field (Grob, 2015; Porter, 2004). Today, the challenges of industrialization and urbanization contribute to a similar demand for mental health ethics in the developing world: mentally ill people commonly experience the poverty, stigmatization, social isolation, and discrimination that accompany the fragmentation of family and community ties of industrial urbanization (Harpham, 1994; Srivastava, 2009; Turan & Besirli, 2008). With this background it should not be surprising that preoccupations with abuses, corruption, and professionalization occupy virtually all of our landmark paper selections—from professional policing of colleagues, to research abuses and exploitations, to contemporary conflict-of-interest concerns about influence peddling.

Identifying 'landmark papers' for a multifaceted topic like psychiatric ethics is a challenge. Unlike novel diseases or treatments, groundbreaking psychiatric ethics scholarship typically mirrors social changes and concerns which arise outside of the scientific and professional literature. For these reasons, simple citation analysis is inadequate. Moreover, citation analyses overlook cross- or interdisciplinary works. Identifying what counts as a landmark itself is puzzling. Is a landmark the first to address an idea? The most rigorous or persuasive presentation of an idea? The most influential in changing clinical practices? The most astute in anticipating the future? In making our selections for psychiatric ethics, we, in effect, mixed all of these values, and tried to identify papers that grasped as many of these considerations at once.

Moot points in psychiatry

Main citation

Little, R. B. & Strecker, E. A. (1956). Moot questions in psychiatric ethics. *American Journal of Psychiatry*, 113, 455–460.

Background

This paper from the 1956 *American Journal of Psychiatry* may be the first article in the English language to suggest 'psychiatric ethics' as a distinct variety of medical ethics. As a survey of practitioner views and behaviours, it also serves as an early example of what today we call 'empirical ethics' (i.e. social science studies involving themes relevant to clinical ethics). The second author, Edward Strecker, may be familiar to contemporary American psychiatrists as the namesake of the annual Strecker Award from the University of Pennsylvania, which since 1964 has recognized psychiatrists with outstanding career achievements.

The paper is a survey of psychiatrists in the Philadelphia area, and is crude in research design, data tabulation, and analysis by contemporary social science standards. What makes the paper important is the suggestion that the psychiatric field has unique ethical challenges which should be discussed openly. In their conclusions, the authors call for local chapters of the American Psychiatric Association (APA) to form ethics committees to assist members with these dilemmas, a suggestion which preceded the development of end-of-life related ethics committees in internal medicine by 20 years (Pontoppidan et al., 1976). Curiously, especially in the era of psychodynamic psychiatry and regarding slips of the tongue, the title of their paper characterizes the questions in psychiatric ethics as 'moot', which has a double meaning: in one sense, moot means 'open to discussion' or 'debatable', and in another, 'of little practical value or only academic interest'. The actual content of the paper supports the former meaning, but we wonder if then, as today, practicing clinicians had genuine ambivalence about the ethical challenges they faced (Geppert & Taylor, 2015).

Methods

This study was a survey questionnaire and content analysis, based on the presentation of nine questions which covered multiple ethical dilemmas experienced in psychiatry at that time, most still relevant today. The questionnaire was mailed to 67 male psychiatrists in the Philadelphia area, most of whom were affiliated with the Institute of Pennsylvania Hospital. Of the initial individuals contacted, 42 responded to the questions; however, only 38 were used due to the other four responses being 'too general'. Questions covered such topics as patient substance abuse, colleague substance abuse, and unethical behaviour, and various situations pitting a psychiatrist's duty to the patient's interest against social/collective interests, mostly involving confidentiality. The main goals were to identify the topics for which psychiatrists felt an ethical obligation to act. For many of the cases, respondents were asked to identify particular actions to be taken.

Results

In regard to the questions concerning physician ethics, danger to self or society, and a patient's spying against American interests, the majority of respondents answered consistently that they had an ethical responsibility to take some type of action. However, what those actions consisted of were often variable and inconsistent. In questions concerning patient's participation in criminal abortion and embezzlement, the majority of respondents stated they had no ethical responsibility to report the patient's actions. The physicians who indicated an ethical responsibility to act described multiple options for doing so. Generally, the majority of respondents were in agreement on the degree of ethical responsibility to act; however, the types of actions varied considerably from question to question.

Conclusions and critique

The respondents, by and large, took the study seriously and responded thoughtfully. As noted, the study by today's standards would be of limited generalizability because of the small sample size, selection biases of various kinds, the all-male participation (though this may have been representative of the field at the time), and a survey return rate that was less than ideal.

The study's importance derives from its groundbreaking discussion. The authors note that respondents were more confident in identifying ethical conflicts in practice than identifying how to resolve them. The authors' conclusions call for a broader professional context, a sounding board, and discussion for these matters, and specifically suggest ethics committees, set up under a professional/organizational umbrella. A more substantive historical study would be required to establish the role, if any, of this paper in provoking the APA and its district branches to form ethics committees, but the authors' foresight cannot be doubted.

A tale of two discernments about psychiatric standards of care

Main citations

Klerman, G. L. (1990). The psychiatric patient's right to effective treatment: implications of *Osheroff v. Chestnut Lodge*. *American Journal of Psychiatry*, 147, 409–418.
Stone, A. A. (1990). Law, science, and psychiatric malpractice: a response to Klerman's indictment of psychoanalytic psychiatry. *American Journal of Psychiatry*, 147, 419–427.

Background

Ten years after the tumultuous release of DSM-III and its signalling of biological/psychodynamic rivalries in psychiatry, this 1990 *American Journal of Psychiatry* exchange between two eminent psychiatrists was a signpost for several painful transitions in the field. These conflicts included rivalries between 'biological psychiatry' and 'psychodynamic psychiatry'; a movement toward evidence-based practice and formalizing standards of care; the rise of criterion-based diagnosis; and the enfeeblement, both clinical and economic, of long-term, intensive psychotherapy-oriented psychiatric hospitals. With our perspective from nearly three decades on, the core of the debate was clear, though the psychiatric field's response took decades to sort out in the midst of dramatic changes in psychiatric research, the funding of psychiatric care, and the diversification of the field (Frank & Glied, 2006). The debate at the time was whether psychodynamic treatment alone met standards of care, and whether patient Osheroff was negligently denied medications which could be, and appeared later to be, promptly effective. While the language of ethics is at most indirectly invoked in these two papers, the discussion is moral to the core.

Methods

The two essays, on casual examination, present an informal structure for the opening statements in a debate: for example, 'Resolved: the *Osheroff* case violated the psychiatric standard of care', with the 'for' statement by Gerald Klerman, and the 'against' by Alan Stone. We specify the 'informal' structure of a debate because the terms, and indeed the resolution proper, are not explicitly stated, such that the two authors are focusing on the same resolution. Rather, the authors voice strong disagreements about the significance of the *Osheroff* case for the field of psychiatry. Klerman considers the debates of the *Osheroff v Chestnut Lodge* trial and its lessons for the future of psychiatric practice, while Stone considers the ramifications of Klerman's claims about standards of care for legal and malpractice contexts. Both authors use the methods of rhetorical persuasion in order to sway readers to their position.

Summaries of the arguments

The gist of the public case involved the treatment of Dr Rafael Osheroff, a 42-year-old nephrologist from the Washington, DC area who had persistent depression after two years of outpatient treatment involving psychodynamic psychotherapy and antidepressants. His diagnoses at various facilities included depression with psychotic features; manic-depressive disorder, depressed phase; and narcissistic personality disorder. Admitted to Chestnut Lodge, Osheroff was treated in the hospital with psychodynamic therapy four times weekly, and the milieu for seven months, with no medications provided. His condition worsened, with a 40-pound weight loss, severe psychomotor agitation, and insomnia. The patient's requests for medications were denied. His family had him discharged and transferred to the Silver Hill Foundation, where he was treated with antipsychotic and antidepressant medications. At Silver Hill, Osheroff improved in three weeks and was discharged to outpatient care in three months, in the summer of 1979. He resumed his medical practice and maintained his improvement. In 1982, Osheroff filed a negligence lawsuit against Chestnut Lodge, claiming damages due to the withholding of medication. It was settled out of court later and a jury trial was avoided, with negotiations favouring Osheroff.

Klerman's argument

Klerman's argument had two major theses: (1) that patients have a right to effective treatment, and (2) that treatments with demonstrated scientific efficacy should be preferred over those without demonstrated efficacy. In this case, medications were the treatments of demonstrated efficacy. Acknowledging the rivalries in current American psychiatry between biological, psychodynamic, and behavioural treatments, Klerman emphasized the dispute over diagnosis and ensuing treatment between a biologically-driven depressive disorder and psychodynamically-driven narcissistic personality disorder. He reviewed the recent literature regarding these two conditions and found the treatment evidence for narcissistic personality disorder to be inferior. He found the persistence of the hospital in pursuing psychodynamic treatment in the face of the patient's deterioration problematic (e.g. ethically questionable). Klerman acknowledged that due to the social, economic, and practical barriers to conducting psychotherapy research, official guidelines for treatment were lacking (as compared to nowadays). However, he referred to an APA hospital utilization manual in claiming that psychotherapy for depression with psychotic features was not recommended, and medication or electroconvulsive therapy was indicated. He viewed the issue as not biological versus psychotherapeutic treatments, but 'opinion versus evidence' (Klerman, 1990, p. 415).

He concluded his discussion by addressing the larger issues for psychiatry as a field, recommending a responsibility to (1) make a thorough assessment and proper diagnosis, (2) communicate to the patient the results of the assessment and diagnosis, (3) disclose alternative treatments, (4) provide effective treatments, and (5) modify treatment plans and/or seek consultation if the patient fails to improve. With contemporary eyes, this discussion evokes various aspects of formal informed consent.

Stone's argument

In Stone's response, he shifts the main thrust of the argument away from standards of practice and, rather, to the legal procedures and implications of the *Osheroff* case.

He identifies his principal inquiry as how a malpractice attorney might use Klerman's paper in a case against a psychodynamically-oriented psychiatrist. Stone believes that Klerman's paper and position could be used by malpractice attorneys in the courts to penalize 'traditional' (e.g. psychodynamic) psychiatrists for practicing under this paradigm. In support of this claim, he accuses Klerman of making a tacit constitutional claim because of the latter's use of the phrase 'right to effective treatment'. Stone refutes any such constitutional claim. Stone also notes that Klerman's appeal to standard of care is not legitimate if based upon a single case (*Osheroff*). He warns that encouraging the courts to use the prevailing scientific evidence of the day in evaluating standards of care is a 'recipe for disaster'. Moreover, Stone resists the standard-of-care use of the DSM for diagnosis, worrying that this would lock the field into 'paradigm urged by Klerman' (Stone, 1990, p. 425). Invoking a legal precedent of a 'respectable minority' as justifiable clinical practice, Stone defends what he calls 'traditional' psychiatry from Klerman's biological-psychiatry colleagues.

Conclusions and critique

Over 25 years after the appearance of this discussion, much has changed in psychiatry—we have had the 'Decade of the Brain', the human genome has been mapped, the significance of epigenetics for gene expression and regulation has been explicated, psychotherapy efficacy research has proliferated, cost controls for care have become customary, references to evidence-based practice habitually issue from the mouths of medical students, informed consent is required, and the APA issues clinical care treatment guidelines for various DSM-defined conditions as a routine. It appears that history has favoured Klerman's position in that the changes to the field he envisioned (informed consent requirements, evidence-based practice, and DSM diagnosis) have prevailed, and Stone's fears about the courts dismembering psychiatry have not been realized. However, notably, the failure of long-term psychotherapy-only based hospitalizations did occur, as did, shortly after, managed-care imposed cost controls against exploitative for-profit psychiatric hospitals (Geyman, 2004).

We believe this exchange is of deep significance for psychiatric ethics in that it marked a turning-point in psychiatry. Today, not just biological treatments but all evidence-based treatments, leavened by clinical judgement and experience, along with patient values, provide the basis for standards of care (Sackett et al., 1996). That said, the value of evidence-based treatments in psychiatry remains debatable (Gupta, 2014).

Questions of competency

Main citation

Roth, L. H., Meisel, A., & Lidz, C. W. (1977). Tests of competency to consent to treatment. *American Journal of Psychiatry*, 134, 279–284.

Background

Today, psychiatrists are often called upon to render an opinion about whether a person is of 'sound mind' or mentally capable of making a deliberate choice in medical care (Leetjens et al., 2011). In 1977, the word 'competency' from law and today's notion of decision-making capacity were used interchangeably, though today we reserve 'competence' as the legal term and 'capacity' as a clinical term. The questions about decision-making capacity range from broad ones, such as the patient's ability to live independently, to managing financial affairs, to making a will, to consenting for medical treatment, or even to standing trial in a criminal court. Prior to the following paper, clinical practices for assessing decision-making capacity were not discussed, much less theorized, and were often haphazard. This paper initiated an ongoing and rich discussion about how psychiatrists are to make ethically justifiable decisions on behalf of patients who, for various reasons, may be compromised in their abilities to make decisions and conduct their affairs.

Methods

Loren Roth and colleagues review the law and medical literature to clarify how various tests of competency analyse a patient's decisions to accept or refuse treatment and to evaluate if they are applicable to clinical practice. The methodology goes beyond a literature review to critically engage with various methods used in assessing competency/capacity. Assessment methods ('tests') are evaluated based on their reliability; their acceptance by physicians, lawyers, and judges; and their balance of autonomy versus providing needed medical care (e.g. beneficence). Each approach to assessment is accompanied by a vivid case example. The authors employ the language of ethics in evaluating the relative value of these five forms of competency determination: evidence of choice, 'reasonable' outcome, rationality of the choice, the patient's ability to understand, and the patient's actual understanding.

Results

The sequence of the assessment techniques are presented in a rough order of complexity: the earliest one, 'evidence of choice', is fully observable but lacks nuance and easy applicability; the last, 'actual understanding', is precise in concept but difficult in execution, especially with patients who are uncooperative or have complex illnesses. The remaining three fall somewhere between these extremes of nuance and utility, implying a context-sensitive approach to assessment which was developed more explicitly by later authors, such as Drane (1984).

Conclusions and critique

The authors formulate five approaches to competency determination. The first, 'evidencing a choice', is crisply illustrated by the patient who blankly holds out an arm after a request for a blood draw. The authors find this one easy to determine, and protective against paternalism, but also find this method wanting in that it provides for little insight into the patient's understanding. The second, 'reasonable outcome of choice', depends upon the physician's assessment of reasonableness of the outcome based upon a patient's choice. Of the five, the authors seem most critical of this approach from the ethical standpoint, in that such an assessment defaults to the physician's judgement of rationality, not the patient's judgement or choices. The authors point out, presciently, that only patients who refuse physician treatments are likely to have their competency questioned, and that concern persists today. They are similarly critical of the third test, that of the patient providing 'rational reasons' for their choice, this time on the basis of the difficulty in ascertaining clinically whether the reason offered was determinative in the choice or simply a credible reason without any real potency for action. They note, as with the prior test, that irrationality is judged by the physician, and not the patient, thus potentially robbing the patient of autonomy otherwise warranted. They provide an example of a patient who refuses electroconvulsive therapy for a delusional reason, but the 'real' reason, undisclosed by the patient, is that she is afraid of the procedure. The former reason may be irrational, but the latter may well be rational, and indeed, a common concern. The fourth test, the 'ability to understand', is familiar today because it suggests that the patient's ability to understand risks, benefits, and alternatives to the proposed treatment is sufficient for competency. While the authors praise this test as closer to the intent of informed consent, they are troubled in the complexity of the determination, such as what to do if the patient's understandings of risks, benefits, and alternatives are mixed and/or incomplete. The last, 'actual understanding' involves an active dialogue between doctor and patient about the treatment options, with the patient demonstrating an ability to address the treatment stakes. This test, often favoured as the ideal today, is a tall order for significantly impaired or idiosyncratic patients, though it inspired practices involving the patient having to explain back, in their own terms, the treatment stakes.

This paper is still relevant today in mapping out the prevailing methods in assessing competence/capacity and is a landmark in exploring the ethical significance of these methods. Indeed, a recent review of instruments for measuring decision-making capacity acknowledges this paper as a major influence (Dunn et al., 2006).

Avoiding hubris: the ethical conduct and regulation of neuropsychiatric research

Main citation

Fins, J. J. (2003). From psychosurgery to neuromodulation and palliation: history's lessons for the ethical conduct and regulation of neuropsychiatric research. *Neurosurgery Clinics of North America*, 14, 303–319.

Background

Psychosurgery, the invasive destruction of brain tissue with therapeutic intent, was a dark chapter in twentieth-century American psychiatry, largely due to the use of prefrontal lobotomy on thousands of patients with scant evidence of safety or efficacy (Grob, 2015). Early in the twenty-first century, psychiatry and brain-related specialties were reopening the moral questions about physical manipulation of the brain. New neuromodulatory technologies, from transcranial magnetic stimulation to deep brain stimulation, were being explored for selected intractable neuropsychiatric conditions like obsessive-compulsive disorder, chronic depression, and Parkinson's disease. Some professional commentators (e.g. Ross et al., 2015) have dubbed the new century as bringing the birth of 'clinical neuroscience' with the distinctions between neurology, psychiatry, and even neurosurgery eroding. The new neuromodulatory therapies were due for an ethics assessment for the new century, and Joseph Fins' historical review was to clarify what has been learned from the past as well as what was yet to be.

Methods

Fins provides a historically informed literature review, drawing upon not just medical professional literature, but also legal, ethical, political, and public discourse about the use of psychosurgery in twentieth-century medicine and psychiatry. He summarizes his conclusions and provides a brief discussion and analysis of issues for the future of neuromodulation.

Results

The paper reviews the professional and public discourse about mid-twentieth-century uses of psychosurgery (the destruction of targeted brain tissue with therapeutic intent). He describes the peaks of the prefrontal leukotomy (lobotomy) for intractable psychopathology, exemplified by Egas Moniz's winning of the 1949 Nobel Prize in Medicine for the procedure, and the troughs of its use, through a discussion of Walter Freeman's hubris in using 'clinical experience' as the sole criterion for selecting suitable patients. Fins describes the heated public 'pros versus cons' discourse that lasted most of the mid-twentieth century, depicting the procedure as promising in some cases but mostly prone to abuse and misuse, and culminating in Congressional hearings in the 1970s about its proper use. Fins suggests that the psychosurgery debate was an important vector in the development of contemporary clinical research regulation via the National Commission for the Protection of Human Subjects in Biomedical and Behavioral Research in 1977. The National Commission later developed research ethics review boards, or Institutional Review Boards, partly in response to these and other research abuses.

The ethics core of the psychosurgery debate has several arms: (1) many of the conditions subject to the procedure were poorly defined, (2) the procedures were touted as specific treatments when, in retrospect, they were crudely non-specific, (3) the procedures were promulgated on tens of thousands of patients without adequate scientific evidence of safety and efficacy, and (4) the procedure was feared as not just a medical intervention but allegedly as also a social control intervention to neutralize disruptive citizens. Fins notes that contemporary research regulation and bioethical discourse will likely prohibit the excesses of the past; yet, he wonders how a proper balance between benefit and risk will be reached, even with better science and better oversight.

Conclusions and critique

Fins concludes with the recommendation to develop regulatory strategies that will balance benefits for those with intractable neuropsychiatric disorders against protections against wanton scientific progress and harms to human research subjects as well as patients. He offers an interesting analogy of intractable depression, obsessive-compulsive disorder, and Parkinson's disease as conditions worthy of palliation, not conventional 'therapy' as in a specific curative treatment for a specific condition. Such a palliative approach would shift to more patient-centred practice, where the terms of intervention are guided by patient values. He also situates his concerns about the use of neuromodulatory treatments in the context of social justice issues, so that 'physical' and 'mental' disorders can be treated equitably and available to all. Our reading of Fins' paper recalls Santayana's famous warning: 'Those who cannot remember the past are condemned to repeat it'.

Unwanted help: treatment of the homeless mentally ill

Main citation

Kahn, M. W. & Duckworth, K. S. (1998). Needing treatment, wanting nothing: ethical dilemmas in the treatment of the homeless mentally ill. *Harvard Review of Psychiatry*, 5, 274–80.

Background

By the turn of the twenty-first century, the problem of the homeless mentally ill was a familiar one and a result of 'deinstitutionalization' in the mid-twentieth century, an overconfidence in the new psychopharmacology, the sluggish development of community outpatient mental health, budget cutbacks, and a growing distrust in psychiatrists and involuntary hospitalization/treatment (Goldman & Morrissey, 1985). Today, encountering homeless mentally ill people is universal in our cities; however, our public policy still struggles with politically viable solutions. This paper addresses the problem on the ground, where the clinician and would-be patient meet.

Methods

This paper from the *Harvard Review of Psychiatry* provides a concise literature review, cast in the pedagogically attractive format of a case-discussion dialogue between the two authors.

Results

The authors discuss the ethics of the case of Ms A, who is a middle-aged mother of a young adult daughter. Ms A has some paranoid ideas, a 'subtle' thought disorder, and prefers to live, untreated, on the streets rather than in a home. Her daughter becomes aware of her condition and encourages a judge to sign an involuntary hospitalization order; the judge authorizes involuntary hospitalization and gives guardianship to her daughter. The authors present the case chronologically, presenting portions for discussion before moving on to the next development. In the midst of their discussion, the authors identify a large number of the ethical and socio-legal issues facing clinicians, families, and patients in seeking treatment for a patient who does not want mental healthcare.

Conclusions and critique

The 'landmark' properties of this paper do not reside in the novelty of the issues described, but rather in its identification of a contemporary ethics concern (the treatment-refusing homeless mentally ill) and the inventive collection of ethical issues associated with the resisting patient, presented in a format which captures the nitty gritty of actual clinical care. In the space of a relatively short review article, the authors explore a large range of ethical concerns in working with this population:

(1) The authors describe the historical transition of mental health law from a '*parens patriae*' (the state acts as a parent) approach to involuntary hospitalization and treatment, where the need for treatment was the justification for involuntary care, to the current approach, dominated by considerations of dangerousness to self or others (see also Goldman & Morrissey, 1985). They insightfully point out a 'malignant synergy' between two socio-political forces in making this change: a collision between liberal goals of boosting patient freedom and autonomy and a conservative desire to contain costs, with the two vectors converging to make access to treatment more difficult.

(2) They describe these dual legal justifications in ethical terms, where the need-for-treatment standard provides a low threshold for providing benefits to the patient, while undercutting their freedoms of choice. The inversion of these values characterizes the 'dangerousness' standard, identified as a 'libertarian' approach (Szasz, 1960), which strengthens individual freedom over patient benefit.

(3) They consider the trade-offs between *parens patriae* and libertarian approaches in terms of risk versus benefits for each. Insightfully, they note that risk is significant for both approaches—risks for unwanted treatments, as well as the risks of living on the streets with various impairments.

(4) They explore sensitivities to family members who have difficulty understanding either arm of the *parens patriae*/libertarian approach, as seen in the patient's daughter having trouble understanding why the mental health system seems so helpless.

(5) They also explore alternatives, such as guardianship, and the ethical pros and cons of this approach.

(6) Presciently, the authors explore the socioeconomics of the issue, reasoning that supported housing for the homeless might well be provided for years, compared to the costs of a single hospitalization. Here they anticipate the harm-reduction, 'housing-first' philosophy that has gained traction only in the past ten years.

The authors could not have anticipated all the responses to the refusing patient during the ensuing 20 years. These include the aforementioned harm-reduction, 'housing-first' approach (Tsemberis et al., 2004); much less, the vigorous 'recovery movement' focusing on housing, employment, and functioning over symptom control (Davidson et al., 2005); as well as the increasing role of peer support in recovery (Slade, 2009). This paper sets the stage for many of these changes which are still being played out in the twenty-first century.

Promoting accountability in leadership

Main citation

Cosgrove, L., Bursztajn, H., Krimsky, S., & McKivergan, M. A. (2009). Conflicts of interest and disclosure in the American Psychiatric Association's clinical practice guidelines. *Psychotherapy and Psychosomatics*, 78, 228–232.

Background

In the early years of the twenty-first century, longstanding concerns about conflicts of interest between clinicians and the pharmaceutical industry escalated as more and more facets of conflict-of-interest bias and frank research corruption appeared in the literature (Bekelman et al., 2003). In earlier years, the concern had been with industry's promotional efforts directed to individual physicians (e.g. dinners, tours, gadgets, samples) (Rodwin, 1993). However, over the years, new sources of conflict of interest were identified: consultation and advisory panel money for clinical trialists; industry sponsorship money for authors and committees of the recent *Diagnostic and Statistical Manual for Mental Disorders* (DSM); gag clauses for clinical trialists supported by industry who obtained results unfavourable to the sponsor's products; and, most egregiously, the withholding of publication of negative studies by industry sponsors. This latter effort seriously compromised the evidence and knowledge base for medications and devices that clinicians used with their patients. It also inspired an international movement to develop clinical trial registries to assure availability of all clinical trial data, with the American example being clinicaltrials.gov (De Angelis et al., 2004).

Lisa Cosgrove's group, in a series of studies over the past 20 years, began with examinations of DSM committee members' support by industry, and later turned to the financial ties with industry of the authors of the APA's treatment guidelines. A sample article from this latter effort is presented here, and illustrates the high-stakes impact of conflict of interest.

Methods

Using the method of 'multimodal screening', Cosgrove and colleagues searched for sources of industry support for members of the contemporary APA schizophrenia, bipolar disorder, and major depressive disorder clinical practice guidelines (CPG) committees. Each of the 20 committee members were investigated through online databases for disclosures in scientific publications and conferences, and American Patent and Trademark Office data. Financial support was counted for five years preceding the publication of the guideline. The authors defined financial support as including advisory or consulting committee membership, holding of patents or trademarks, collaborating on sponsored clinical trials involving company products, membership on a speaker's bureau, and various kinds of gifts. The authors had three investigators conduct independent searches, while a fourth member audited the other three searches and resolved questions about the coding.

Results

The results showed widespread financial support for the 20 CPG committee members among the three disorder groups: 90% of the members had at least one category of financial relationship, and 66.6% had three or more categories. All committee members of the schizophrenia and bipolar disorder CPGs had financial relationships, as did 60% of the major depressive disorder group. Of all the members who had financial relationships, over 70% had clinical research sponsorship or consultancies, 44% were on corporate advisory boards, 38% received honoraria, a third were on speaker's bureaus, and almost 17% held equity in one of the companies.

Conclusions and critique

The authors note that these three disorders groups are among the most commonly treated mental disorders. They describe the large economic impact of sales of medications for these disorders. They note that treatment guidelines affect all practicing clinicians who use them, and therefore reflect a powerful influence on everyday practice. They summarize the progress to date in efforts to minimize conflict-of-interest bias and corruption; and propose that an ad hoc committee should oversee the CPG committee members' financial relationships, and that amounts of support be disclosed, as currently few mechanisms exist in accounting for the magnitude of the financial influences identified in conflict-of-interest research. They recommend random audits to assure compliance with conflict-of-interest policies. Moreover, they recommend augmenting reporting requirements through '(1) an explicit statement listing all financial relationships (individual, family, or current research collaborators) regardless of whether or not an individual believes those relationships are relevant; ... (2) a disclosure of the total amount of money individuals received from each company; (3) an identification of the timing of the association; (4) no lower limit (e.g. USD 10,000) of disclosure ... because there is substantial evidence that even a small gift can influence behavior ...' (Cosgrove et al., 2009, p. 231).

We agree with the authors' concern for the limitations of their study, notably the potential to fail to detect financial relationships when they are, in fact, present. Moreover, the actual impact of financial interests on CPG decisions is very difficult to determine. Nevertheless, the significance of this study, as well as the Cosgrove et al. research group, has contributed to a growing awareness of conflict of interest in psychiatry, the impact of which, we think, will still be felt in years to come.

Conclusion

Psychiatry holds a unique social power in medicine, not shared by other specialties—the power to seclude, restrain, and treat patients without their consent. Such power has been long recognized and respected by the field, albeit also forgotten, as the history of psychiatry is too-often laden with episodes of patient abuses (Grob, 2015). The papers we have highlighted in this chapter express equally the noble intentions and the ethical lapses of the field, both of which have likely led to the seriousness of psychiatric ethics discussions over the past 60 years. We believe the foremost lesson from these papers is the need for constant vigilance about the use of psychiatric power, tempering it with the wisdom of balancing this power with caring and respect. Such ethical vigilance means that psychiatric ethics questions are rarely, if ever, 'resolved' but rather evolve and require new understandings, formulations, and responses.

Most of the papers discussed here are twentieth-century works addressing the moral challenges of twentieth-century psychiatry and mental health. But in addition to constant vigilance about abuses of psychiatric power, new challenges have emerged through social and scientific changes in the twenty-first century. In a 2015 overview of an extensive psychiatric ethics reference text, John Sadler and colleagues identify six areas posing relatively novel challenges for the field: (1) electronic communications, (2) multiculturalism, (3) new practice models, (4) new technologies, (5) scrutiny, and (6) clinical ethics informed by values.

The challenges of electronic communications are many; the concept of privacy is being rethought as trackable online behaviour creates 'digital phenotypes', the latter making the concept of consent for 'surveillance', commercial or otherwise, relevant. Already clinicians and organizations are developing guidance for use of social media and other digital communications. Finally, research has already begun on digital communications as a causative factor in psychopathology.

The potential for both virtual and literal migration has made late twentieth-century concerns about multiculturalism all the more relevant, as the values of tolerance of cultural difference prove insufficient to address issues of mental healthcare disparities and institutional discrimination against people of various identities—ethnic, gender, sexual, or otherwise.

The prevailing practice models of twentieth-century psychiatry—that of outpatient practice and hospital practice—have already been supplanted by team-based care, community outreach teams, patient-based self-help, and peer-support networks, as well as new partnerships between clinicians and patients in building collaborative networks ('co-production'). All of these are situated, in the USA, in various funding pathways—public, private, and governmental—rendering accountability even more complex than before.

Fins' paper introduced some of the many new technologies applicable to psychiatry—from therapeutic devices of varying degrees of invasiveness, to new drugs with new risks as well as benefits, as well as the ongoing problems with cost controls. If our colleagues in cancer treatment are signals, then psychiatry has its own looming crisis for extraordinarily expensive 'personalized medicine' interventions, further widening the disparities between 'haves' and 'have nots'.

As psychiatric practice becomes more embedded in social, cultural, and financial networks, it should not be too surprising that the scrutiny of psychiatrists by organizations and institutions grows almost daily. Clinicians are inundated with reporting requirements, billing justifications, patient volume and flow requirements, continuing education demands—the list goes on and on. From the ethics perspective, the care of the patient increasingly becomes marginalized as practice is increasingly driven by these non-personal and, indeed, dehumanizing bureaucratic demands. We would anticipate a tipping point in the near future where a backlash against such requirements is initiated by patients and their attorneys.

Psychiatric ethics itself is being transformed from an approach driven by rules of practice from law and guiding principles from organizations, into a practice which involves identifying guiding values and collaborating with stakeholders, negotiating mental healthcare at all levels of intervention, from access to care to diagnosis to treatment. These changes have already become imbricated in many of the aforementioned new models of practice. While adding complexity to practice, these models also provide for a habitual, communal vigilance about psychiatric power which we hope constitutes a more ethically conscientious future for psychiatry and its patients.

References

Bekelman, J. E., Li, Y., & Gros, C. P. (2003). Scope and impact of financial conflicts of interest in biomedical research: a systematic review. *Journal of the American Medical Association*, **289**(4), 454–465.

Cosgrove, L., Bursztajn, H., Krimsky, S., & McKivergan, M. A. (2009). Conflicts of interest and disclosure in the American Psychiatric Association's clinical practice guidelines. *Psychotherapy and Psychosomatics*, 78, 228–232.

Davidson, L., O'Connell, M. J., Tondora, J., Lawless, M., & Evans, A. C. (2005). Recovery in serious mental illness: a new wine or just a new bottle? *Professional Psychology: Research and Practice*, **36**(5), 480–487.

De Angelis, C., Drazen, J. M., Frizelle, F. A., et al. (2004). Clinical trial registration: a statement from the International Committee of Medical Journal Editors. *New England Journal of Medicine*, **351**, 1250–1251. doi:10.1056/NEJMe048225

Drane, J. F. (1984). Competency to give informed consent: a model for making clinical assessments. *Journal of the American Medical Association*, **252**(7), 925–927.

Dunn, L. B., Nowrangi, M. A., Palmer, B. W., Jeste, D. V., & Saks, J. D. (2006). Assessing decisional capacity for clinical research or treatment: a review of instruments. *American Journal of Psychiatry*, **163**, 1323–1334.

Frank, R. G. & Glied, S. A. (2006)/ *Better But Not Well: Mental Health Policy in The United States Since 1950.* Baltimore: Johns Hopkins University Press.

Geppert, C. M. A. & Taylor, P. (2015). What troubles psychiatrists: how psychiatrists view ethical dilemmas. In: *The Oxford Handbook of Psychiatric Ethics*, ed. S. Sadler, B. Fulford, & W. C. van Staden. Oxford: Oxford University Press; pp. 45–59.

Geyman, J. (2004). *The Corporate Transformation of Health Care: Can The Public Interest Still Be Served?* New York: Springer.

Goldman, H. H. & Morrissey, J. P. (1985). The alchemy of mental health policy: homelessness and the fourth cycle of reform. *American Journal of Public Health*, 75(7), 727–731.

Grob, G. N. (2015). A moral/ethical history of American psychiatry. In: *The Oxford Handbook of Psychiatric Ethics*, ed. S. Sadler, B. Fulford, & W. C. van Staden. Oxford: Oxford University Press; pp. 637–653.

Gupta, M. (2014). *Is Evidence-Based Psychiatry Ethical?* Oxford: Oxford University Press. Available from: http://dx.doi.org/10.1037/0735-7028.36.5.480 http://dx.doi.org/10.1037/h0046535

Harpham, T. (1994). Urbanization and mental health in developing countries: a research role for social scientists, public health professionals and social psychiatrists. *Social Science in Medicine*, **39**(2), 233–245.

Jonsen, A. R. (2000). *A Short History of Medical Ethics.* Oxford: Oxford University Press.

Klerman, G. L. (1990). The psychiatric patient's right to effective treatment: implications of Osheroff v. Chestnut Lodge. *American Journal of Psychiatry*, **147**, 409–418.

Leentjens, A. F. G., Rundell, J. R., Wolcott, D. L., Guthrie, E., Kathol, R., & Diefenbacher, A. (2011). Reprint of 'Psychosomatic medicine and consultation-liaison psychiatry: Scope of practice, process, and competencies for psychiatrists working in the field of CL psychiatry or psychosomatic. A consensus statement of the European Association of Consultation-Liaison Psychiatry and Psychosomatics (ECLPP) and the Academy of Psychosomatic Medicine (APM)'. *Journal of Psychosomatic Research*, **70**, 486–491.

Pontoppidan, H., et al. (1976). Optimum care for the hopelessly ill: a report of the clinical care committee of the Massachusetts General Hospital. *New England Journal of Medicine*, **295**, 362–364.

Porter, R. (2004). *Madmen: A Social History of Madhouses, Mad Doctors, and Lunatics.* Stroud, Gloucestershire, UK: Tempus Publishing.

Rodwin, M. A. (1993). *Medicine, Money, and Morals: Physicians' Conflicts of Interest.* New York: Oxford University Press.

Ross, D. A., Travis, M. J., & Arbuckle, M. R. (2015). The future of psychiatry as clinical neuroscience: why not now? *Journal of the American Medical Association: Psychiatry*, **72**(5), 413–414. doi:10.1001/jamapsychiatry.2014.3199

Rothman, D. J. (2002a). *Conscience and Convenience: The Asylum and Its Alternatives in Progressive America.* Hawthorne, NY: Aldine De Gruyter.

Rothman, D. J. (2002b). *Discovery of the Asylum: Social Order and Disorder in the New Republic.* Hawthorne, NY: Aldine De Gruyter.

Sackett, D. L., Rosenberg, W. M. C., Gray, J. A. M., Hyanes, R. B., & Richardson, W. S. (1996). Evidence-based medicine: what it is and what it isn't. *British Medical Journal*, **312**, 71.

Sadler, J. Z., van Staden, W. C., & Fulford, K. W. M. F. (2015). Introduction. In: *The Oxford Handbook of Psychiatric Ethics*, ed. S. Sadler, B. Fulford, & W. C. van Staden. Oxford: Oxford University Press; pp. 45–59.

Scull, A. (1993). *The Most Solitary of Afflictions. Madness and Society in Britain, 1700–1900.* New Haven and London: Yale University Press.

Slade, M. (2009). *Personal Recovery and Mental Illness: A Guide for Mental Health Professionals.* Cambridge: Cambridge University Press.

Srivastava, K. (2009). Urbanization and mental health. *Indian Journal of Psychiatry*, **18**(2), 75–76. doi: 10.4103/0972-6748.64028

Stone, A. A. (1990). Law, science, and psychiatric malpractice: a response to Klerman's indictment of psychoanalytic psychiatry. *American Journal of Psychiatry*, **147**, 419–427.

Szasz, T. S. (1960). The myth of mental illness. *American Psychologist*, **15**(2), 113–118.

Tsemberis, S., Gulcur, L., & Nakae, M. (2004). Housing first, consumer choice, and harm reduction for homeless individuals with a dual diagnosis. *American Journal of Public Health*, **94**(4), 651–656.

Turan, M. T. & Besirli, A. (2008). Impacts of urbanization process on mental health. *Anatolian Journal of Psychiatry*, **9**, 238–243.

Chapter 21

Forensic psychiatry

Stephen H. Dinwiddie

Introduction

Narrowly defined, forensic psychiatry can be considered as the practice of psychiatry within the social and conceptual space where issues of law and mental state meet—where society has concluded that resolution of legal issues can be more equitably achieved with the assistance of expert opinion. Though final determination of such questions lies within the province of the legal system, the forensic psychiatrist may be asked opinions as to insanity, competence to be tried or sentenced, ability to waive fundamental legal rights, and so on. But such questions, though of great intrinsic interest, are rarely posed to the general psychiatrist, and as a result forensic psychiatry, perhaps more than other psychiatric subspecialties, is often perceived as mysterious, baffling, and best avoided if at all possible.

A broader and more accurate definition of forensic psychiatry, however, would include within its ambit many aspects of everyday clinical practice as well—issues such as risk prediction, antisocial personality disorder, decisional capacity, and identifying and resolving ethical conflicts, not to mention treatment of mental illness afflicting individuals in custody (most of whom, eventually, will be released back into the community). Far from being an arcane area restricted to relatively few practitioners, forensic psychiatry is thus inextricably associated with routine practice. This chapter will discuss foundational papers in each of these aspects of forensic psychiatry.

Risk assessment and the prediction of dangerousness

Main citation

Steadman, H. J. & Keveles, G. (1972). The community adjustment and criminal activity of the Baxstrom patients: 1966–1970. *American Journal of Psychiatry*, 12, 80–86.

Background

Prior to the 1950s, great deference was accorded to psychiatric judgement by judicial and administrative authorities, and psychiatrists were quite confident in their abilities to predict long-term behaviour based on a combination of training, theory, and observation that was rarely (if ever) made explicit or assessed for accuracy. The legal system by and large deferred to this presumed expertise; in the absence of many effective treatments, individuals found to be in need of hospitalization because of risk of violence due to mental illness could look forward to lengthy inpatient stays. However, the introduction of antipsychotic medications caused dramatic changes in treatment—including a movement toward deinstitutionalization.

Johnnie Baxstrom, convicted on an assault charge in 1958, was nearing the end of his prison sentence. In 1961, he was determined to be mentally ill and transferred to Dannemora State Hospital, a facility operated by the New York Department of Corrections; even after his criminal sentence expired, facility psychiatrists considered him too dangerous to be released or even to be hospitalized in the civil system. Baxstrom's legal efforts to be released led to a 1966 American Supreme Court decision (*Baxstrom v Herold*, 1966) that found Baxstrom had been denied equal protection under the law: unlike the vast majority of civilly committed patients, Baxstrom (solely because of his criminal conviction years earlier) had not had the opportunity for judicial (as opposed to purely clinical) review of his supposed dangerousness. As a result of this decision, some 967 similarly situated patients housed at two hospitals for the 'criminally insane' were transferred to state psychiatric facilities and ultimately found clinically suitable for release, affording Henry Steadman and Gary Keveles an unparalleled opportunity to study the accuracy of psychiatrists' predictions of dangerousness. Their landmark study is described here.

Methods

Steadman and Keveles followed up all 47 women and a random sample of 199 of the 920 men to determine their outcomes and adjustments over a four-year period (1966–1970). Using State Department of Mental Hygiene records to identify those still in contact with the state system and a variety of methods (state record search, contact with family and friends, and death records), they were able to trace all but 14 of the patients.

Results

In an era of prolonged inpatient hospitalization, only about half (124 patients) of the sample were in state mental hospitals four and a half years after transfer. Some 27% were living in the community and another 14% had died in the interim. Of note, at the time of follow-up, only seven patients had returned to the correctional system or hospitals operated by the Department of Corrections—indeed, subsequent analyses found that only 26 of the total 967 patients released to other facilities were returned to either of the two hospitals for the criminally insane at any point during the four-and-a-half-year study period (Steadman, 1973). Of 121 patients who had been released into the community at some point, only 21 had been rearrested, leading to a total of 16 convictions.

Conclusions and critique

The authors concluded that, as far as predicting future 'dangerousness' accurately—even in a cohort of mentally ill criminal offenders—psychiatrists were extremely likely to overpredict. Contrary to expectation, reoffence was in fact quite rare, whether the outcome was a subsequent arrest (for a crime that either did or did not involve violence) or was simply some form of physical violence either in the hospital before release, which occurred in 15% of the patients, or subsequently in the community, which occurred in an additional 5%.

This study necessarily relied on official sources for information—arrest records, hospital notes, and the like—and thus was vulnerable to the usual associated methodological shortcomings. One (non-random follow-up of subjects) appears not to have been a significant flaw; they were able to obtain data on virtually all of the transferred patients, though it is likely a handful left the state.

Undoubtedly some of the released patients engaged in behaviours that might have been considered dangerous but did not result in police contact; moreover, as the authors noted, once known to law enforcement, individuals released from psychiatric facilities were (and still are) often transported for rehospitalization rather than arrest. Thus the 'true' rate of dangerous behaviour might have been substantially higher than what the authors were able to glean from records and perhaps the psychiatrists' predictions might not have been quite so inaccurate.

Conversely, many of the police contacts seem to have been for non-violent behaviours; some at least were arrested for minor crimes such as vagrancy or disorderly conduct. As the authors note, it seems likely that 'mental patients' might have been more likely to be brought to police attention and readmitted for such annoying but non-dangerous acts. Counting such contacts (as the authors did) as evidence of dangerousness would necessarily overestimate its base rate; and if such contacts were excluded, the psychiatrists' judgements would have been even worse.

An important caveat of this study is that 'dangerousness' was not clearly defined: psychiatrists and lawyers, apparently, were so familiar with a concept so obvious and so lacking in ambiguity that it needed no further thought—at the time. Even though the term was repeatedly used in the Supreme Court's decision on the original case, and even though a major purpose of the study was to determine the actual behaviour of inpatients at least implicitly identified by psychiatrists as posing significant social danger, Steadman and Keveles (quite properly) focused on clearer terms such as 'hospital readmission' or 'rearrest'. Elsewhere in discussing the study's results, Steadman (1973) emphasized the ambiguities involved in defining 'dangerousness'; and later studies would make it clear that prediction of violence (note here the shift in terminology) is highly nuanced.

This study prompted a 'second generation' of studies examining clinicians' ability to predict future violent behaviour in a much more rigorous way—using prospective research designs, carefully defined outcomes, strict determinations of which behaviours should count as 'dangerous' or 'violent', and study designs that account for a myriad of cognitive biases (Mossman, 1994). Much has been learned about historical and contextual factors associated with longer-term risk of violent behaviour, and the nebulous concept of 'dangerousness' has been substantially refined as researchers have realized that no one set of characteristics works for all.

Parallel investigations of suicidality have evolved as well (Hawton, 1987); and, mindful that accuracy of prediction remains low, over time clinicians have learned that rather than employing a dichotomous approach (e.g. violent versus non-violent, suicidal versus not), it is much more useful to focus on risk assessment and management rather than simple prediction of dangerous behaviour. A more nuanced approach based on identification of potentially modifiable factors and assessment of relative rather than absolute risk is now becoming the standard of care—an example of a 'forensic' skill that is increasingly being used in everyday practice.

The antisocial personality (part one)

Main citation

Cleckley, H. (1988). *The Mask of Sanity: An Attempt to Clarify Some Issues About the So Called Psychopathic Personality*. St Louis: C. V. Mosby.

Background

For most of Western history, individuals who were not overtly mentally ill but who seemed unable to comply with social norms were relegated to the criminal justice system—or perhaps to rough justice by fellow citizens. Their behaviour was attributed to a sinful nature, and (except for a few physicians such as Benjamin Rush) the problem of 'perversion of the moral faculties' excited little medical interest until the late nineteenth and early twentieth centuries. However, in the context of theories then current (such as Dr Cesare Lombroso's concept of the 'born criminal', Sir Francis Galton's espousal of eugenics, and studies of families such as the Jukes and Kallikaks), the concept of 'constitutional psychopathic inferiority' gained widespread acceptance in American psychiatry. The psychopathology of this group (which was applied to people with addictions, externalizing behaviours, homelessness, and even intractable epilepsy) was felt to occupy a middle ground somewhere between mental illness and unimpaired social function. From this inchoate concept, two lines of thought emerged that today define how we think of individuals now classified as 'psychopaths', 'sociopaths', or some cognate term. The first intellectual tradition can be traced primarily to Hervey Cleckley and *The Mask of Sanity*.

Cleckley published the first edition of his classic work, based on close clinical observation of a population of male inpatients, in 1941. Though his thinking evolved over time (the version printed in 1976 is generally considered the definitive statement of his ideas), Cleckley's desire was to better describe and characterize those puzzling individuals—whom he estimated (in 1941) accounted for perhaps a fifth of admissions to his hospital—whose rational and indeed often charming appearance belied an unstable, often predatory, and typically self-defeating lifestyle.

Methods

The Mask of Sanity is, par excellence, a work of clinical description rather than social science research. Cleckley vividly presents a number of cases histories that he considered to typify the psychopath, though not all would fit into today's conceptualization of the condition. An attempt is made to delineate the syndrome from other types of psychopathology, but it is done by gesturing at other conditions and highlighting differences rather than any empirical attempt to measure or even rigorously define the terms used.

Results

Cleckley identified some 16 characteristics that he felt defined the condition: superficial charm and good 'intelligence'; absence of delusions and other signs of irrational thinking; absence of 'nervousness' or psychoneurotic manifestations; unreliability; untruthfulness and insincerity; lack of remorse and shame; inadequately motivated antisocial behaviour; poor judgement and failure to learn by experience; pathological egocentricity and incapacity for love; general poverty in major affective reactions; specific loss of insight; unresponsiveness in general interpersonal relations; fantastic and uninviting behaviour with drink and sometimes without; suicide rarely carried out; sex life impersonal, trivial, and poorly integrated; and failure to follow any life plan.

Conclusions and critique

When Cleckley first published his description of these patients, the term 'psychopath' could refer to individuals who exhibited any of a wide variety of abnormal or unusual behaviours and lifestyles—indeed, in the view of Kurt Schneider, the term 'psychopathic personality' could fit anyone with an abnormal personality who suffered *or* caused society to suffer as a result of it (Mayer-Gross et al., 1956). Over time, the term 'psychopath' has become much more restricted and very closely associated with early-onset, persistent antisocial behaviour.

Cleckley believed that once the defining characteristics of the psychopath had been identified, the seasoned clinician would find little difficulty in recognizing and properly diagnosing the syndrome. Later study of the reliability of psychiatric diagnosis overall would undermine that belief. However, Cleckley's fundamental clinical insights *could* be more rigorously defined and studied; and the development of Robert Hare's original psychopathy checklist (Hare, 1980) and its subsequent versions—all based on characteristics identified by Cleckley—has allowed researchers (and clinicians) to reliably identify the syndrome and to study its causes and consequences.

The antisocial personality (part two)

Main citation

Robins, L. N. (1966). *Deviant Children Grown Up: A Sociological and Psychiatric Study of Sociopathic Personality*. Baltimore: Williams & Wilkins.

Background

At around the time that Cleckley was developing his ideas about psychopathy, Lee Robins was approaching the issue from a very different perspective. Trained as a sociologist,

Robins serendipitously gained access to some 22 years' worth of treatment records (which had been stored away, apparently forgotten) from a public-sector children's psychiatric clinic that closed at the end of the Second World War.

Methods

Many of the children treated at the clinic had been referred by the Juvenile Court, and the records allowed follow-up of these individuals (who had a high likelihood of being diagnosable with 'sociopathic personality' as adults) as well as of non-antisocial patients. The result was a sample of some 524 Caucasian patients (Robins concluded that the number of African-Americans in the sample was too small for meaningful study), of whom 406 had been referred for antisocial behaviour (typically theft or 'incorrigibility') and another 118 for other reasons. In addition, Robins identified 100 comparison subjects who had lived nearby but who had not been referred for evaluation or treatment. Remarkably, even after decades had elapsed, she was able to trace and interview over 80% of the patient group and over 90% of the comparison group. She used a structured interview format that included (among many other data points) inquiry about antisocial behaviours throughout childhood, adolescence, and adulthood.

Results

Nearly 75% of the men and some 40% of the women initially referred for antisocial behaviour had subsequently been arrested on a variety of charges ranging from drunkenness to murder. Early referral for antisocial behaviour seemed to strongly predict a pattern of dissocial behaviour that continued well into adulthood.

Overall, some 22% of the 'patient' sample could be reliably diagnosed with 'sociopathic personality' (the term used in the then-current diagnostic nomenclature), versus only 2% of the comparison sample. However, Robins went further: built into the interview were some 19 criteria (assessing areas of life function in which the individual might be considered to have failed to live up to social norms[1]) that could be used for diagnosis. She concluded that sociopathic individuals could be statistically (not just clinically) distinguished from those with 'hysteria', schizophrenia, anxiety neurosis, and alcoholism. By virtually every measure of function these individuals fared poorly in adulthood—with more instability in marriage, parenting, and employment; lower academic and occupational functioning; higher rates of problem drinking; and even indications of poorer health outcomes. Referral for antisocial behaviour as a youth predicted poor outcome

[1] Poor work history; receiving financial assistance from state, agencies, or relatives; repeated arrest; serious marital difficulties (if ever married); problematic alcohol use; drug use; truancy along with other school problems; impulsivity; belligerency; problematic sexual behaviour; suicide attempts; vagrancy; somatic complaints; pathological lying; poor ability to maintain social relationships; use of aliases; lack of guilt; poor performance when enlisted in the military; 'wild' behaviour in late adolescence.

over many domains in adulthood, with a high risk for continuing antisocial behaviour (Robins, 1978).

Conclusions and critique

Robins' study is remarkable in many ways. Not only did it provide an incredibly rich description of the life course of antisocial behaviour, but its methodology represented a tremendous scientific advance. Robins pioneered the use of structured interviews in psychiatric research, and rather than relying solely on 'clinical judgement' for diagnosis, she actually was able to quantify the level of diagnostic agreement. By using an explicit definition of sociopathy (as opposed to Cleckley's reliance on clinical judgement alone), her work presaged the development of truly operationalized diagnostic criteria to be used in the study of other illnesses, as well. Specifically in the case of antisocial personality disorder, her work profoundly influenced the Washington University and DSM-III (and later) diagnostic criteria for the disorder.

The sociological and scientific methods used by Robins in her study stand in sharp contrast to Cleckley's medical and naturalistic, even impressionistic, approach. How is it that two such disparate works can both be considered 'landmarks' in the field? Remarkably, despite profound differences in conceptualization and method, there is a striking degree of convergent validity. Both seem to have identified a very similar (and socially very problematic) group of individuals, with the psychopath representing a smaller, more extremely deviant group within the broader population of those meriting a modern diagnosis of antisocial personality disorder. Even so, organized psychiatry continues to struggle with reconciling two very different ways of identifying these individuals, and current (DSM-IV and later) diagnostic criteria represent something of a compromise.

Expert testimony

Strasburger, L. H., Gutheil, T. G., & Brodsky, A. (1997). On wearing two hats: role conflict in serving as both psychotherapist and expert witness. *American Journal of Psychiatry*, 154, 448–456.

Background

It would seem that serving as an expert witness is the very definition of the forensic psychiatrist. It possibly is—but in that case it is the rare psychiatrist indeed who will not, at least occasionally, serve in a forensic role. In the case of the treating psychiatrist being asked to opine on a variety of legal issues, whether criminal (such as fitness to stand trial or insanity) or civil (such as causation of psychological damages), a concern for dual agency immediately arises, setting up the potential for conflict between two ethical imperatives: the duty to act in the patient's best medical interest and the obligation in the courtroom for truth-telling. Before the issue was addressed by Larry Strasburger and collaborators, little attention was paid to this ethical pitfall.

Methods

The authors provide examples of role conflict for the simultaneously treating and testifying psychiatrist, and then discuss the differences between those two roles and the implications of those differences.

Results

The authors describe two scenarios in which the everyday clinician may leave the office to practice in the courtroom—and by doing so unknowingly commits an ethical breach. The first can occur when the treating psychiatrist determines that the patient requires civil commitment and/or enforced treatment. Taking such a step involves undermining the duty to maintain patient confidentiality in the service of protecting the well-being of the patient and perhaps of the community. In this situation, it is generally agreed that breach of confidentiality is justified (though the clinician should attempt to limit the information disclosed to the minimum necessary). Fortunately, the concern that taking such action inevitably undermines the treatment relationship seems not to be empirically justified (Katsakou & Priebe, 2006), though of course it would seem to be good practice to process the issue with the patient when appropriate.

The second scenario may occur when the clinician has established a treatment relationship with a patient who is involved in litigation of some sort. Probably the most commonplace situation involves allegation of personal injury (i.e. the patient has been exposed to a traumatic event of some sort and is pursuing legal remedy); less frequently, the issue may be a consequence of a contested divorce (e.g. involving child custody) or it may even arise in the context of criminal prosecution. Obviously, no conflict arises if there is no point of contact between treatment and the legal system. However, significant ethical conflicts arise once the clinician is asked to provide a professional opinion.

The authors first point out that there are fundamental differences between the nature of the treatment relationship (which involves empathy, an accepting stance toward the patient's narrative and hence openness to a certain kind of psychological rather than strictly factual 'truth' or causation, and allegiance toward the patient's best medical interests) and the role of the expert, which may not include any of these elements. It might seem that the roles can be seamlessly combined: the treater-expert should have a deeper and more accurate understanding of the patient, and hence a better understanding of the psychological effect of a putative trauma (or parenting ability, or degree of moral culpability in the case of criminal behaviour). In fact though, the methods of assessment and goals of evaluation can differ so greatly that one role or the other cannot survive. If nothing else, the naive clinician may go so far as to believe that emotional support of the patient should extend to actively advocating for his or her legal theory in the courtroom without reference to the legal fact base.

For the treating clinician, the goal is relief of symptoms; and when the modality of treatment is primarily psychotherapy, this may involve a deep and ongoing discussion about the meaning of the patient's experiences. Strict historical accuracy, in other words, is less important than the patient's perception of events (though a goal of treatment would be to assist the patient to re-evaluate life experiences in a more 'objective' way); and through this process the treater must be open to the deeper meaning of the patient's narrative, even if it seems inaccurate or even frankly implausible. This assumes, as it must, that both parties share a common goal—one of the healing of the patient—and thus the possibility of conflicting agendas is often disregarded. The requirement of some degree of 'belief' in the patient undercuts the treater's ability to properly consider other motives and the possibility of misattribution or outright malingering of symptoms.

This stance has clear implications for the conduct of evaluations. As opposed to the treater, the forensic clinician must take a more sceptical stance as to the accuracy of the individual's report of events and symptoms, and will generally rely more on collateral sources of information—not only prior treatment records but (depending on the nature of the medicolegal issue) police reports, arrest records, employee records, school records, or a variety of other sources. During the evaluation, confrontation may be used earlier and more frequently; and indeed it is an ethical requirement that the subject of the evaluation be explicitly informed that he or she is *not* a 'patient' and indeed that no therapeutic relationship at all is being established.

It may be that true objectivity in the case of the forensic clinician is an impossible goal (Diamond, 1959). Nonetheless, the purpose of the forensic evaluation and the reporting of findings is not to enhance the well-being of the patient but to assist the legal system (and therefore society) in fairly adjudicating disagreements. In carrying out this function, the forensic clinician's role cannot be conflated with that of a healer; if his or her opinions do not align with the plaintiff's legal agenda, their disclosure may well cause distress at a minimum. Combining the role of treater and expert risks betrayal of the supportive role of the clinician, to the patient's detriment, and can fatally undermine the objectivity needed to assist judicial decision-making.

Conclusions and critique

Prior to the publication of this paper, relatively little attention had been paid to the potential role conflicts the authors delineated. Since then, treatment guidelines promulgated by various professional societies have become much more attentive to such risks and have emphasized the need to separate roles whenever possible, while from the other side of the divide, ethics guidelines of the American Academy of Psychiatry and the Law explicitly address the potential for conflict in the ways identified in the paper. Any clinician facing the sort of role conflict identified by Strasburger and colleagues would be well advised to review the issues raised.

However, other, similar conflicts remain. The authors point out that there are circumstances under which both roles *must* be assumed—for example, in evaluations as to disability or in areas where there is a shortage of qualified professionals; and for such situations, the authors provide little guidance other than to advise awareness of the potential for conflict. Also unaddressed is the inherent conflict when a clinician chooses to work in a facility, such as a jail or forensic hospital, where one clinical responsibility is to restore capacity to participate in legal actions ranging from trial to determine guilt or innocence to execution. In such settings, part of the treating clinician's role may be to opine as to fitness to stand trial (so that successful treatment may eventuate in lengthy incarceration in the case of a finding of guilt) or even to restore the patient's ability to understand that he or she is facing the death penalty (and thus, at some level, arguably making the treater complicit in the process of legal execution).

Fortunately, the vast majority of psychiatrists will never have to deal with conflicts of that nature. However, as the authors note, even in everyday practice there is the potential for role conflict and hence ethical risk, and the clinician is well advised to be vigilant in identifying such conflicts and avoiding them to the degree possible.

Civil commitment and involuntary treatment

Main citation

Roth, L. H. (1979). A commitment law for patients, doctors, and lawyers. *American Journal of Psychiatry*, 136, 1121–1127.

Background

For centuries, physicians had the ability to admit and treat psychiatric patients against their will, based solely on clinical judgement and without legal oversight—a medically based and medically justified intervention to be employed on behalf of those too ill to understand their need for treatment. By the middle of the twentieth century, however (and in the context of growing public awareness of the abuses too often suffered by patients[2]), it became evident that the State's *parens patriae* obligation to care for individuals unable to properly care for themselves should be balanced against every citizen's right to autonomy—the freedom to conduct one's affairs as one sees fit unless one's behaviour impinges on the safety and well-being of others. This second justification for commitment, emphasizing the State's obligation to maintain an orderly society rather than its obligation to care for the incapacitated, implies that the State should exercise its 'police powers' to detain and medically incarcerate only those who are both significantly mentally ill and disruptive to society: only those, in other words, who by reason of mental illness present a pressing danger to themselves or others.

In the context of civil commitment, therefore, two models (or some mix thereof) contend to justify a social mechanism (i.e. preventive detention and imposed treatment) that is otherwise forbidden to the State and which can be triggered only by the presence of significant mental illness and (depending on the justification used) either inability to provide appropriate self-care or some significant degree of dangerousness.

[2] Admittedly a very slowly growing and intermittent awareness—as exemplified in the USA from the time of Dorothea Dix's work in the mid-1800s to the publication of Albert Deutsch's *The Shame of the States* in 1948 and, ultimately, to a number of legal actions (e.g. *Wyatt v Stickney*, 1972).

Methods

Loren Roth reviewed existing ethical justifications for commitment laws, identified problems with the existing criteria, and proposed an alternate approach.

Results

Building on ethical principles earlier proposed by Alan Stone (1975), Roth suggested that a relatively brief period of civil commitment in order to pursue treatment, over the individual's objection, could be justified if several conditions were met: that the individual suffered from a reliably diagnosed mental illness[3]; that in the absence of treatment, the immediate prognosis was one of major distress; that treatment was available; that the illness substantially impaired the person's ability to understand or communicate about the possibility of treatment; and the risks and benefits associated with treatment were such that the reasonable person would consent to treatment.

These Stone–Roth criteria are explicitly based on a *parens patriae* rather than dangerousness justification and are geared to the relief of suffering. For this reason, they do not distinguish between two very different legal processes—limiting the individual's physical freedom (i.e. civil commitment to an inpatient setting) and limiting the individual's freedom to refuse unwanted care (i.e. judicially enforced treatment). However, if a distinction is made between commitment and treatment, this can lead to the odd situation wherein a patient can be civilly committed, yet can refuse treatment for the condition that led to his or her hospitalization in the first place—a circumstance perhaps more easily accepted by lawyers than by doctors (Appelbaum & Gutheil, 1979).

Roth recognized this problem and so proposed a second test for civil commitment, requiring presence of mental illness plus recent evidence of dangerous behaviour such as an act of violence or credible threat thereof. He suggested that, since many such individuals would in fact have the ability to competently accept (or refuse) treatment, treatment should be offered but not compelled—the burden then swinging to the patient to balance the desires of freedom to accept or decline treatment against the presumed desire to regain physical freedom. Commitment, under this proposal, would be time-limited and judicially reviewed and extended if necessary. In this way, not only could two differing justifications for involuntary detention be harmonized, but treatment for 'dangerousness' rather than severe mental illness could be distinguished and appropriate safeguards put in place.

Conclusions and critique

For the most part, civil commitment and involuntary treatment are controlled by state statutes and so vary depending on location. To the extent that a trend can be identified, laws have generally tended to favour a 'police power' or 'dangerousness' approach rather than a *parens patriae* or 'need of treatment' justification, though often elements of both

---

[3] Implied, but not specifically stated in this criterion, was that the illness was non-trivial: Roth specifically noted presence of psychosis in this regard.

are present. Not all have explicitly separated the legal questions of commitment and treatment, and less attention has been paid to processing treatment refusal differently based on suffering versus dangerousness—though fortunately, in practice, there appears to be substantial overlap in the patients identified under either schema (Monahan et al., 1982).

It can be argued that regardless of the justification presented in a given case, the clinician's duty to his or her patient should include taking steps to ensure the patient's safety (and at times that of others) and relieve suffering when possible. However, Roth's attempt to simultaneously distinguish between justifications for these different kinds of actions and to balance competing ethical interests should remind us that, even under circumstances of extreme illness, the ability to enforce limits on physical freedom and to impose treatment (over the patient's objections) does not relieve the clinician of the responsibility of balancing conflicting responsibilities to relieve suffering as well as to safeguard patient autonomy.

Decisional capacity

Main citation

Appelbaum, P. S. & Grisso, T. (1988). Assessing patients' capacities to consent to treatment. *New England Journal of Medicine*, 319, 1635–1638.

Background

The concept of informed consent came rather late to medicine. In the USA, a strongly paternalistic view that justified physicians withholding information or even (if believed to be necessary) lying to patients held sway well into the nineteenth century; and it was not until 1914 (in a case dealing with an unwanted operation) that Justice Benjamin Cardozo wrote:

> Every human being of adult years and sound mind has a right to determine what shall be done with his own body; and a surgeon who performs an operation without his patient's consent commits an assault for which he is liable in damages. This is true except in cases of emergency where the patient is unconscious and where it is necessary to operate before consent can be obtained.(*Schloendorff v Society of New York Hospital*, 1914, p. 92)

This holding indicates that if an individual is both legally ('of adult years') and clinically (of 'sound mind') able to comprehend the proposed treatment, the decision as to accept or decline it should be made by the patient rather than the treater. However, what does being 'of sound mind' mean in this context? This paper is selected as an example of a number of studies the authors have carried out by which a fundamentally *legal* concept can be subjected to empirical study.

Methods

This paper draws on earlier empirical work by the authors and provides a systematic review of what functions might be considered to be part of the legal and ethical construct of decisional capacity.

Results

Paul Appelbaum and Thomas Grisso identified four different components contributing to decisional capacity. One (arguably the most basic) is the simple ability to communicate a choice at all. However, even this has its complications. Is a simple, one-time indication sufficient? What if the individual cannot stably choose—or cannot recall having done so a few minutes later, or repeatedly and rapidly changes the decision? The authors argue that conditions such as extreme ambivalence, impairment in level of consciousness, severe thought disorder, or short-term memory disruption could undermine even this fundamental component of decision-making.

A second construct emphasizes the patient's ability to incorporate and understand information relevant to the decision at hand—such as the nature of the proposed procedure and its potential risks and benefits. This implies a certain level of cognitive function including the ability to recall relevant information and to weigh the probabilities of various possible outcomes; and thus this level of capacity could be undermined by deficits in memory, basic intellectual function, or attention span.

However, focusing on the purely cognitive component of the choice risks scant assessment of true appreciation—which requires not simply a recitation of facts but the patient's ability to emotionally grasp the import of the information. As the authors note, this is no warrant of the reasonableness of the decision itself. The issue is one of determining what weight the patient him or herself places on specific risks and benefits, rather than whether the ultimate decision would be one that most people would endorse.

A final level of decisional capacity assesses the process by which a decision is reached, rather than on the weight accorded the information: the ability to rationally manipulate relevant information in a way logically consistent with the weight assigned to it. Although in this article the authors do not specifically mention this, this level of 'rational manipulation of information' is now generally thought to imply that the individual can appropriately understand the necessary information, assign it proper importance relevant to the specific clinical circumstances, and use it to reach a decision that is congruent with stably held values and beliefs.

Conclusions and critique

In earlier works (Appelbaum & Grisso, 1995; Grisso et al., 1995), Appelbaum and Grisso had empirically assessed patients' decisional capacities and, in doing so, had undermined the commonly held, prejudiced belief that severe psychiatric illness must inherently undermine decisional capacity—or that lack of such illness could be taken to assure presence of such ability. This article is not 'foundational' in the sense that it represents even the earliest of the authors' thoughts on the topic. Though the article provides the clinician with excellent practical advice as to how to go about assessing decisional capacity and how to think through the various models of capacity as the courts might, perhaps its most important message is that rather than thinking of decisional capacity in binary terms, it behooves the treating physician to consider it as a point along a spectrum. Of course, the ultimate determination of a legal capacity (such as the ability to make a sufficiently informed choice) is made by the legal system, but, in practice, clinicians must frequently weigh in on such matters and make recommendations in a manner timelier than courts may be able to routinely do.

In this regard, the authors do not explicitly suggest here that the four views of decisional capacity discussed are intrinsically hierarchical, though that conceptualization has since become commonplace. Over time, there seems to have been a movement toward attempting to balance risk of erroneous assessment of capacity against potential harm to the patient—that is, deferring more to the patient's stated desires when risk associated with accepting an 'incompetent' decision is low, but requiring a greater degree of confidence that the individual has sufficient decisional capacity when the stakes are higher.

Rigorous analysis of the components of decisional capacity has had fundamental influence on issues relating to research (e.g. how to assess and quantify ability to consent to clinical studies) as well as on the day-to-day clinical assessment of ability to consent to a wide variety of treatments. Breaking down a global, often impressionistic and imprecise binary judgement ('has capacity/lacks capacity') into well-defined parts allows the clinician to assess decision-making in a more systematic way, and perhaps more importantly, provides a means by which the clinician can identify specific barriers to true capacity and address deficits, so as to restore or enhance patient autonomy.

Conclusion

The evolution of forensic psychiatry depends heavily on advances in psychiatry and in many basic sciences. What impact will new knowledge about (for example) behavioural genetics or behavioural neuroscience have on violence prediction, or on how psychopathic or otherwise antisocial individuals should be dealt with by the criminal justice system? How should functional neuroimaging studies of lying be incorporated into the legal system?

At the same time, the field is shaped by social changes that, eventually, are incorporated into the law. It may seem that some ethical questions can be regarded as settled—but new variations constantly arise. What degree of decisional capacity should be demonstrated if an individual requests physician-assisted suicide? As treatment methods improve and risks decrease, should barriers against civil commitment and involuntary treatment be lowered? Or consider the psychiatrist treating patients accused of criminal behaviour—how should the testifying expert deal with not just dual loyalties, but multiple and conflicting duties to the patient, the legal and correctional systems, and society at large?

The forensic psychiatrist therefore practices within the ever-changing social and conceptual space where issues of law and mental state meet—where society has concluded that resolution of legal issues can be more equitably achieved with the assistance of expert opinion. However, as this chapter demonstrates, forensic psychiatry is far from being an arcane area of psychiatry best left to a relatively few practitioners with a puzzling fondness for the law. One way or another, forensic issues permeate the everyday practice of psychiatry, and in that sense, every psychiatrist must at times be a forensic psychiatrist.

References

Appelbaum, P. & Grisso, T. (1995). The MacArthur Treatment Competence Study I: mental illness and competence to consent to treatment. *Law and Human Behavior*, **19**(2), 105–126.

Appelbaum, P. & Gutheil, T. (1979). 'Rotting with their rights on': constitutional theory and clinical reality in drug refusal by psychiatric patients. *Bulletin of the American Academy of Psychiatry and the Law*, 7(3), 306–315.

Baxstrom v Herold [1966] 383 US 197.

Diamond, B. L. (1959). The fallacy of the impartial expert. *Archives of Criminal Psychodynamics*, **3**(2), 2221–2236.

Grisso, T., Appelbaum, P., Mulvey, E. P., & Fletcher, K. (1995). The MacArthur Treatment Competence Study II: measures of abilities related to competence to consent to treatment. *Law and Human Behavior*, **19**(2), 127–148.

Hare, R. D. (1980). A research scale for the assessment of psychopathy in criminal populations. *Personality and Individual Differences*, **1**, 111–119.

Hawton, K. (1987). Assessment of suicide risk. *British Journal of Psychiatry*, **150**, 145–153.

Katsakou, C. & Priebe, S. (2006). Outcomes of involuntary psychiatric admission—a review. *Acta Psychiatrica Scandinavica*, **114**, 232–241.

Mayer-Gross, W., Slater, E., & Roth, M. (1956). Psychopathic personality and neurotic reactions. In: *Clinical Psychiatry*, ed. W. Mayer-Gross, E. Slater, & M. Roth. Baltimore: Williams and Wilkins; pp. 91–186.

Monahan, J., Ruggiero, M., & Friedlander, H. D. (1982). Stone–Roth midel of civil commitment and the California dangerousness standard. *Archives of General Psychiatry*, **39**(11), 1267–1271.

Mossman, D. (1994). Assessing predictions of violence: being accurate about accuracy. *Journal of Consulting and Clinical Psychology*, **62**(4), 783–792.

Robins, L. N. (1978). Sturdy childhood predictors of adult antisocial behaviour: replications from longitudinal studies. *Psychological Medicine*, **8**(4), 611–622.

Schloendorff v Society of New York Hospital [1914] 105 N.E.

Steadman, H. J. (1973). Implications from the Baxstrom experience. *Bulletin of the American Academy of Psychiatry and the Law*, **1**, 189–196.

Stone, A. A. (1975). *Mental Health and Law: A System in Transition*. DHEW Publication ADM 75–176. Washington, DC: US Government Printing Office.

Wyatt v Stickney [1972] 344 F. Supp. 373.

Chapter 22

Suicide

Danuta Wasserman, Marcus Sokolowski, and Vladimir Carli

Introduction

Suicide is a leading cause of death, particularly among young and middle-aged men. According to the World Health Organization (WHO), over 800,000 people take their own lives each year worldwide, while attempted suicide is about 20 times more frequent than completed suicide. Moreover, as reported by the WHO, suicide accounts for just over half of the violent deaths in the world (WHO, 2014).

Throughout the nineteenth century, the notion of suicide as a complex social and medical phenomenon became more prevalent. Preceding Emile Durkheim (1897/2005), Henry Morselli's work on many aspects of suicide is arguably the most significant contribution during that time (Morselli, 1882; Goldney & Schioldann, 2000). Emile Durkheim's theory was very influential by highlighting the critical role social factors have on suicidal behaviours. Edwin Shneidman's theory of psychache introduced the idea that suicide is a result of overwhelming and intolerable psychological pain (Shneidman, 1993). Norman Farberow and Edwin Shneidman further expanded their theory of suicide, focusing on the communicative aspects, and saw suicide as a cry for help (Farberow & Shneidman, 1961). Suicidal people communicate their pain and cries for help in many different ways, which evokes many different responses, from empathy to ambivalence to aggression (Maltsberger & Buie, 1974; Wolk-Wasserman, 1986; Wasserman & Wasserman, 1994). Erwin Stengel's theory of suicide comprises both individual and interpersonal aspects; he understood suicide as an extremely personal act, greatly influenced by social relationships with a serious social impact (Stengel, 1964). Since then, a lot of research has been done on the determinants of suicide that can be associated with risk and protective factors, providing the foundation upon which prevention strategies and national suicide plans have been built (Wasserman & Wasserman, 2009).

The causes of suicidal behaviour are complex, and many different and interacting contributing factors have been described. According to the stress-vulnerability model, many factors can lead towards a predisposition for suicide diathesis: genetic make-up, exposure to psychological stress, and adverse environmental conditions, especially in the developmental stages of childhood and adolescence (Wasserman et al., 2007). There are strong associations between suicide and inequity, social exclusion, and socioeconomic deprivation (Li et al., 2011; Maris, 1997; Stack, 2001).

The process of suicidal behaviours is also complex; it can range from suicidal ideation (communicated through verbal or non-verbal means), to planning of suicide, attempting suicide, and, in the worst case scenario, completed suicide. Once again, these behaviours are influenced by interacting biological, psychological, social, environmental, and situational factors (Wasserman & Sokolowski, 2016). Suicide is a global problem taking the lives of too many, yet it is preventable.

We have selected three areas within the field of suicide prevention that we believe to be important and to help us to appreciate the complexity of the field. Firstly, information about effective preventive strategies is needed to develop and implement successful national suicide prevention programmes. Secondly, talking about suicide is of the utmost importance to reduce the stigma surrounding the topic and to increase suicide research. Lastly, the genetics of suicidal behaviour is a widely studied topic that is important as it provides an understanding of the diathesis of suicide.

Effective suicide prevention strategies

Main citations

Mann, J. J., et al. (2005). Suicide prevention strategies: a systematic review. *Journal of the American Medical Association*, 294, 2064–2074.

Zalsman, G., et al. (2016). Suicide prevention strategies revisited: 10-year systematic review. *Lancet Psychiatry*, 3, 646–659.

Related reference

Wasserman, D., et al. (2015). School-based suicide prevention programmes: the SEYLE cluster-randomised, controlled trial. *Lancet*, 385, 1536–1544.

Background

Suicide prevention efforts have been occurring for decades (Lester, 2001). As early as 1906, suicide prevention programmes were being initiated—in London by the Suicide Prevention Department of the Salvation Army, and in New York by the National Save-A-Life League (Mishara, 2001). Around the 1950s, many more programmes were established, by the Suicide Prevention Agency in Vienna (1948) (Ringel, 1988), the Suicide Prevention Service in Berlin (1956) (Bezencon, 2001), and the Los Angeles Suicide Prevention Centre (1958) (Litman et al., 1961). In 1956, a crisis line initiative was launched in London by the Samaritans, founded by Edward Chad Varah (Varah, 1962), which was taken up by numerous countries, using the concept of 'befriending' (Jennings et al., 1978). Now, there are an incalculable number of suicide prevention services operating in many countries all over the world (Bertolote, 2004). In 1960, the International Association for Suicide Prevention (IASP) was founded in Vienna by Erwin Ringel (along with the support of Norman Farberow, Walter Pöldinger, and Vera Aigner), with the purpose of preventing suicidal behaviour, mitigating its effects, and providing support to those involved (Ringel 1988, 1997). The Finnish Suicide Prevention Project (1986–1996) was the first-ever national research-oriented suicide prevention programme to be thoroughly implemented and evaluated, providing a base of knowledge of how to use these research results in practical preventive activities (Lönnqvist, 1988). These efforts, and many others, have been very important for suicide prevention.

Knowledge about which are the effective evidence-based suicide prevention strategies is critically required to support the development of national suicide prevention programmes and to reduce suicide rates worldwide. In particular, evidence-based strategies are needed for young people, as suicidal behaviours amongst adolescents are a global problem that needs critical attention. In several countries, suicide rates have been decreasing in the general population but have been stable or increasing among the younger population.

To date, the evidence around suicide prevention is currently provided by a multitude of papers and about several different strategies. These strategies can be categorized as either public health strategies (targeting entire populations or groups at increased risk) or healthcare strategies (targeting patients with mental disorders). Although there are many published papers, the overall quality of evidence is relatively low, most studies have a quasi-experimental design, and insufficient numbers of randomized controlled trials (RCTs) are available.

Describing the evidence for each strategy goes beyond the scope of this chapter. For this reason, we present two systematic reviews as main papers: the first one published in 2005 (Mann et al., 2005) and an update published 10 years later (Zalsman et al., 2016). These reviews can be considered the most important evidence in the field. Additionally, we selected one RCT evaluating different school-based suicide prevention strategies targeting adolescents (Wasserman et al., 2015).

Methods

To examine the evidence in regard to the effectiveness of specific suicide prevention interventions and to create a guide for subsequent prevention programmes and research, a group of international experts completed a systematic review (Mann et al., 2005). Relevant RCTs, cohort studies, systematic reviews, meta-analyses, population studies, and ecological studies published between 1966 and June 2005 were identified and then analysed. Ten years later, suicide prevention strategies were revisited by European experts to re-examine the evidence of the effectiveness of such interventions (Zalsman et al., 2016). A systematic review identified all papers published between 1 January 2005 and 31 December 2014, covering the same areas for suicide prevention as in the Mann et al. review; interventions including public education, physician education, screening, treatments, internet or hotline support, media strategies, and restricting access to suicide means were highlighted (Mann et al., 2005). A narrative synthesis was given as neither of these systematic reviews allowed for a formal meta-analysis because of the heterogeneity of populations and methodology.

The Saving and Empowering Young Lives in Europe (SEYLE) study was a multi-centre, cluster-randomized controlled trial that measured the efficacy of school-based preventive interventions throughout 168 schools in ten European countries. Each school partaking in the study was randomly allocated to one of three interventions or a control group (Wasserman et al., 2015). The interventions included: Question, Persuade, and Refer (QPR) (Tompkins et al., 2010)—a gatekeeper training module to help school staff members identify suicidal behaviours and direct at-risk individuals to the appropriate care; the Youth Aware of Mental health programme (YAM) (Wasserman et al., 2018)—a universal intervention in which students were educated about mental health awareness and provided with the skills to manage negative life events and suicidal behaviours; and a selective and indicated screening intervention by professionals (ProfScreen) (Kaess et al., 2014), that provided referral for treatment based on the participants' responses to a questionnaire. The effectiveness of the interventions was measured by the number of incident suicide attempts and severe suicidal ideation in comparison with the control group during the follow-up period.

Results

In the reviews by Mann et al. (2005) and Zalsman et al. (2016), physician education, means of suicide restriction, treatment of suicidal patients, and school-based prevention programmes showed to be the most promising methods for reducing suicide rates.

Physician education

Studies from Japan, Hungary, and Sweden showed that education of physicians—to ensure that they correctly screen, diagnose, and treat depressed patients—is an important component of suicide prevention (Takahashi, 1998; Rihmer et al., 2001; Rutz, 2001; Rutz et al., 1997). These studies also showed that a considerable decline in suicide rates was often associated with increased prescription rates for treatment of depression.

Treatment

In several countries, a correlation between higher rates of antidepressant prescriptions and a reduction in suicide rates was found (Carlsten et al., 2001; Hall, 2003; Gibbons et al., 2005; Olfson et al., 2003). It was also noted that RCTs are required to provide further evidence that selective serotonin reuptake inhibitors, which are effective for treatment of major depression, reduce suicide rates. Evidence was found for the use of lithium as an effective method in reducing suicidal behaviours among individuals with mood disorders (Cipriani et al., 2013; Baldessarini et al., 2006; Kessing et al., 2005). Anticonvulsant mood stabilizers were also suggested to have protective effects against suicidal behaviours (Gibbons et al., 2009). A meta-analysis found that clozapine reduced the risk of suicide in psychosis as compared with other dopamine and serotonin-receptor antagonists (Asenjo Lobos, 2010).

Psychological treatments (including cognitive therapy, problem-solving therapy, interpersonal therapy, and outreach) showed encouraging results for reducing repeated suicidal behaviours in comparison to standard aftercare (Brown et al., 2005; Hawton et al., 2000; Guthrie et al., 2001; Beautrais et al., 2010; Dieserud et al., 2000). Notably, compared to the recipients of standard care, cognitive therapy reduced the rate of repeated suicide attempts by half (Brown et al., 2005). Furthermore, amongst adolescents and adults, as well as individuals with schizophrenia and borderline personality disorder, cognitive behaviour therapy (CBT) was identified as an effective treatment to reduce suicidal ideation and behaviours (Taylor et al., 2011; Bateman et al., 2007; Marshall & Rathbone, 2011; Weinberg et al., 2006). Correspondingly, dialectical behaviour therapy (DBT) was a particularly effective treatment for adolescents (Linehan, 2006).

Means of suicide

Suicide rates were lowered by restricting access to common lethal methods. Restricting access to firearms (Loftin et al., 1991; Lester & Leenaars, 1993; Ludwig & Cook, 2000), pesticides (Gunnell et al., 2007), and barbiturates (Nielsen & Nielsen, 1992; Oliver & Hetzel, 1973; Carlsten et al., 1996; Retterstøl, 1989) resulted in decreased suicide rates in countries where those methods were common. Adding barriers at popular suicide sites (Beautrais, 2001; Law et al., 2014), changing the packages of analgesics (Hawton, 2002), making the use of catalytic converters in vehicles compulsory (McClure, 2000; Kelly & Bunting, 1998; Shelef, 1994; Mott et al., 2002), and introducing antidepressants with a lower toxicity, additionally contributed to a reduction in suicides. Studies showed that the risk of suicide by firearms is significantly increased by being available in the household (Anglemyer et al., 2014). Thus, restriction of means of suicide is a primary strategy to be considered and included in nationwide suicide prevention plans (Pirkis et al., 2013).

The media has been suggested to help suicide prevention efforts. One study showed that subway suicides drastically reduced by 80% after the media decreased the coverage of subway suicides in Vienna, Austria in 1987 (Etzersdorfer & Sonneck, 1998). How the media reports suicide is of particular importance to avoid cluster suicidal acts (Schmidtke & Häfner, 1988). Therefore, guidelines have been put in place by the WHO to ensure media outlets do not sensationalize suicide. For example, the media should not give detailed explanations of suicide methods or show any pictures of the act (WHO, 2008, 2017).

School-based prevention programmes

Evidence was found to support the efficacy of universal school-based programmes in preventing suicidal behaviours. In the SEYLE study (Wasserman et al., 2015), the YAM intervention was significantly effective in reducing suicidal ideation and suicide attempts compared to the control group, thus showing significant preventive effects. In fact, incident suicide attempts reduced by more than 50% as a result of the YAM intervention.

Conclusions and critique

The first review completed by Mann et al. (2005) concluded that physician education and restriction of means of suicide appeared to be the most promising methods for reducing suicide rates. Other preventive methods showed encouraging developments at the time, including public screening, media education, and screening programmes, although they required further investigation of efficacy. Future research was needed to address the knowledge deficits, issues faced in under-resourced developing countries, and longer-term trends in suicide rates.

Ten years later, Zalsman et al. (2016) examined the updated evidence and identified significant signs of progress, advances, and findings for suicide prevention strategies. Data further supported the efficacy of several suicide prevention strategies as indicated in the Mann et al. review (2005); the evidence strengthened restricting access to lethal means and providing pharmacological and psychotherapy treatments as effective suicide prevention strategies. The quality of studies involving school-based prevention programmes had improved and was found to be an effective strategy in reducing suicide attempts. Education of primary care physicians in depression recognition and treatment was previously identified as a promising suicide preventive strategy, but unfortunately no new studies had been performed to further determine the efficacy of the intervention. Several strategies, while promising, remained inconclusive in terms of their effectiveness and require further research; these include general public awareness campaigns, gatekeeper education, telephone and internet interventions, follow-up, and chain of care.

The systematic reviews concluded that future research needs to target specific population samples when assessing the efficacy of evidence-based suicide interventions: for example, different age and gender groups, different patient types, and different ethnicities.

Talking about suicide does not increase suicide

Main citation

Gould, M., et al. (2005). Evaluating iatrogenic risk of youth suicide screening programs. *Journal of the American Medical Association*, 293, 1635–1643.

Related references

Dazzi, T., Gribble, R., Wessely, S., & Fear, N. T. (2014). Does asking about suicide and related behaviours induce suicidal ideation? What is the evidence? *Psychological Medicine*, 44, 3361–3363.

Blades, C. A., Stritzke, W. G. K., Page, A. C., & Brown, J. D. (2018). The benefits and risks of asking research participants about suicide: a meta-analysis of the impact of exposure to suicide-related content. *Clinical Psychology Review*, 64, 1–12.

Background

Throughout history, suicide has commonly been understood as a forbidden topic. For many, suicide was seen as a crime or a sin (Alvarez, 1990). Whereas now, much has been done to shift this perspective and create a scientific understanding of suicide (Wasserman & Wasserman, 2009).

There is still much debate about whether or not being exposed to suicide-related content increases the risk of suicidal behaviours. Some health professionals, researchers, and ethics committees are wary and behave reluctantly in exposing individuals to suicide-related content in fear of increasing suicidal behaviours in vulnerable people. Consequently, it is becoming increasingly important that these concerns are addressed, as they pose a significant obstacle for suicide prevention at all levels of influence. To reduce suicide attempts and suicidal behaviours, it is imperative to develop effective suicide prevention strategies. However, the fear and stigma associated with discussing suicide has created an enormous barrier in suicide research and suicide prevention. Thus, it is vital that we address the notion that talking about suicide does not increase the risk of suicide.

While there remains a need for further investigation, several studies have provided evidence to support the idea that talking about suicide does not cause iatrogenic effects of suicide. In fact, discussing suicide-related content has resulted in a reduction of suicidal ideation and behaviours.

Methods

Madelyn Gould and colleagues (2005) performed a RCT to examine whether or not youth suicide screening programmes created an iatrogenic effect of distress or suicidal ideation. The aim was to identify whether a screening programme that questioned youth about suicidal behaviours resulted in increased levels of suicidal ideation or distress among high-school students. The study, which comprised a two-day screening strategy, involved 2,342 participants who were students from six different high schools in the New York State region. Classes were randomly allocated to either the experimental group or the control group. The experimental group received two surveys that both included suicide-related questions, while the control group only received suicide-related questions in the second survey, not the first. Levels of distress were measured after the first survey, and before completing the second survey two days later; the results between the two groups were then compared.

Results

The results found that neither levels of distress nor depressive feelings differed between the experimental group and control group instantly after the first survey. Moreover, being exposed to suicide-related questions did not increase the likelihood of reporting suicidal ideation between the experimental and the control group. Among the participants classified as high risk, there was no difference in the increase of distress or suicidal ideation between the experimental and control group following the first survey. In fact, among the high-risk participants who had attempted suicide, were depressed, or both, the experimental group participants showed lower levels of distress or suicidal ideation than the same high-risk participants in the control group.

Overall, there was no evidence that suicide screening created iatrogenic effects of suicide. Thus, the study concluded that it is safe to complete screening in high schools as part of preventing suicidal behaviours.

Conclusions and critique

The study by Gould et al. (2005) focused on adolescents and was one of the first studies to provide much needed information about the safety of screening young people for suicide risk. More recently, Dazzi et al. completed a review of published articles between 2001 and 2013 that have investigated whether discussing suicide leads to an increase of suicide-related behaviours (Dazzi et al., 2018). The literature review included studies comprising various population groups: adults, adolescents, at-risk populations, and the general population. No evidence was found to suggest that being asked suicide-related questions increased suicidal behaviours.

Finally, a meta-analysis of 18 studies conducted between 2000 and 2017 was performed by Blades et al. (2018), with the aim to identify whether levels of distress, suicidal ideation, or suicide attempts increased as a result of either being exposed to suicide-related content or discussing suicide. The results revealed that compared to pre-exposure, there was a significant, although small, reduction in suicidal ideation after being exposed to suicide-related content. In fact, compared to the control group, those who participated in the experimental suicide-related exposure conditions were less likely to report a suicide attempt afterwards, suggesting that some small benefits to participants may be associated with suicide-related research.

These studies are considered landmark papers showing that talking about suicide does not increase suicide.

The advent of molecular and population genetic studies to suicide research

Main citation

Nielsen, D. A., Goldman, D., Virkkunen, M., Tokola, R., Rawlings, R., & Linnoila, M. (1994). Suicidality and 5-hydroxyindoleacetic acid concentration associated with a tryptophan hydroxylase polymorphism. *Archives of General Psychiatry*, 51, 34–38.

Background

By the early 1990s, it was clear that suicide involved both biological alterations and some form of a heritable, genetic component. The biological aspects were being investigated at relatively detailed levels of serotonin (5-HT) receptor/transporter binding and 5-HT metabolic enzymes. Initial observations of serotonin and 5-hydroxyindoleacetic acid in discrete areas of the brain of suicide victims (Lloyd et al., 1974; Beskow et al., 1976) and reduced 5-HT metabolite 5-hydroxyindoleacetic acid (5-HIAA) levels in cerebrospinal fluid (CSF) (Asberg et al., 1976) suggested a 5-HT deficiency in suicide in line with the monoamine hypothesis of depression. Meanwhile, a number of family, adoption, and twin studies had shown that there is an overall genetic component involved in suicide (Roy, 1993). There were, however, no actual genomic loci being studied in suicide genetics, except in one isolated and largely neglected study from the late 1970s (Comings,

1979). David E. Comings reported a yet to be replicated polymorphism in a brain protein he named Pc-1, which was more frequent in suicides of various psychiatric disorders. However, it remains unknown to this day which gene or genetic variant was behind these early observations. There was a wide gap between the more detailed biochemical understandings of serotonergic deficiencies versus its genetics.

For other psychiatric disorders such as schizophrenia, manic depression, autism, alcoholism, and Alzheimer's disease, the interest in specific 'candidate' genes was advancing steadily throughout the 1980s. David Goldman was a researcher and proponent of genetic approaches in psychiatry during this period, as gene-cloning technologies started to become more widely used. During his research of other psychiatric disorders (e.g. alcoholism), Goldman had cited Comings' paper from 1979 several times. A study by David Nielsen, Goldman, and colleagues subsequently introduced this rapidly evolving era of modern genetics to suicide research (Nielsen et al., 1994). They reported about a newly discovered genetic variant (today called single-nucleotide polymorphism, or SNP) in a candidate gene that is important for serotonin metabolism—tryptophan hydroxylase (TPH)—and also observed association with both CSF 5-HIAA and suicidal behaviour.

Subsequently, this new area of genetic research was starting to be used by other investigators, in parallel with the technological progress in genetics, bringing us to the current-day situation of having well over one hundred candidate genes in different neurosystems (Sokolowski et al., 2015), studies of gene-environment (GxE) interactions (Caspi et al., 2003) and epigenetic mechanisms (McGowan et al., 2009), as well as testing the association of millions of non-hypothesized SNPs by genome-wide methods (Perlis et al., 2010). This paper by Nielsen, Goldman, and colleagues can be said to have initiated the use of modern molecular and population genetic study approaches in suicide genetics research (Nielsen et al., 1994).

Methods

The design was a basic case-control study. Cases were criminal offenders and arsonists, who were mainly divided into impulsive ($n = 56$) or non-impulsive ($n = 14$) groups depending on the premeditation of their crime, whereas controls ($n = 20$) were healthy volunteers without psychiatric disorders. Cases were diagnosed with mainly antisocial personality disorder (APD) or intermittent explosive disorder (IED). Both cases and controls were from the same ethnic population (Finnish), which is important to reduce biases from genetic population stratification. Crucially, all subjects were also evaluated for a history of suicide attempts (confirmed by medical records, third party, or scars), and there were some instances of completed suicide.

The genotype of subjects was determined by so-called single-strand conformation polymorphism (SSCP) analysis, first presented in 1990, which can detect variation in DNA composition without sequencing. A polymerase chain reaction was performed on a part of the TPH gene to obtain sufficient DNA for analysis, followed by *Hae*III enzymatic digestions of the amplified DNA fragments to obtain smaller-size fragments for SSCP analysis. The digested and denatured single-strand DNA was evaluated for its migration in a native gel, and the genotype was inferred by observing different fragments, named as either homozygous 'UU' or 'LL' genotypes (or when observing both, heterozogotic 'U/L'). The development of the method used to identify this first-known genetic variant in TPH intron 7 had been published in a separate paper by Nielsen, Dean and Goldman (1992), two years prior to the current association study—a method made possible only due to the cloning and sequencing of TPH cDNA in 1990. The genetic association analyses were performed by comparing the frequency of U/L alleles or UU/UL/LL genotype counts between different groups by using Pearson χ^2-tests. In addition, allele frequencies and genotype counts were also compared to a sampling of CSF levels of 5-HIAA by liquid chromatography.

Results

Among all subjects (cases and controls), the frequency of the rarer U allele was 0.41, something which today is called a 'common' (>0.01) SNP frequency. This allele frequency did not differ significantly across cases (0.44 for impulsive and 0.39 for non-impulsive) or controls (0.35).

There were several notable findings in this study. First, in impulsive cases there was a significant correlation between the genotype and CSF 5-HIAA, with UU cases having higher 5-HIAA than the impulsive UL/LL cases. Such correlation was not found among non-impulsive cases of controls. Second, suicidal *cases* had significantly lower frequency of the U allele (0.32) than did non-suicidal *cases* (0.54), no matter if the cases were impulsive or non-impulsive (thus analysed in a pool of all cases, without using the controls). Third, there were significantly less UU-carrier *cases* that had performed multiple (two or three) lifetime suicide attempts, compared to UL/LL-carrier *cases*. Fourth and finally, there was no significant difference in genotype when comparing the impulsive cases having different psychiatric diagnoses (APD /IED), non-impulsive cases, and controls.

Conclusions and critique

The main point of interest for the field of suicide genetics is that a newly identified genetic variant (the TPH L allele) was associated for the first time ever with suicidality. This genetic variant was later also sequenced by the authors and then renamed A779C, whereby the reported L allele corresponded to a C allele in the DNA (Nielsen et al., 1997), and clearly motivated different researchers to try and replicate these initial TPH observations of Nielsen et al. Today, this SNP is also named rs1799913, being in linkage disequilibrium with another nearby SNP rs1800532 (or A218C) (Nielsen et al., 1997), often studied interchangeably with A779C.

The association was performed as a set of within comparisons in three subgroups (impulsive or non-impulsive cases, or controls). To be statistically conservative, it should have employed a multiple comparison correction accounting for the number of independent tests made, likely rendering the association with suicidality non-significant (given the nominal $P = 0.016$). It is also noteworthy that if one were to instead compare suicidal *cases* with *controls* (pooled or not with the non-suicidal cases), the observed association would also be rendered non-significant (an analysis not presented in the results). However, both these issues were addressed in a follow-up replication study by the authors published a few years later (Nielsen et al., 1998).

Curiously, Nielsen et al. observed the more common C allele as being the risk allele which was over-represented in relation to suicidality, while many others subsequently observed association of the A allele (González-Castro et al., 2014). This type of problem with consistent allele direction has turned out to be very usual in the studies of single, common SNPs which are correlated with causal genetic variants. Such so-called 'flip-flop' phenomena have been explained by the fact that both sampling and ethnic differences can lead to different linkage disequilibrium (LD) patterns, and that single SNP associations may be complicated by other risk factors (SNPs or environmental factors) (Lin et al., 2007). This may happen if, for example, the originally studied population is of a particular ancestry, as was the case with the Nielsen et al. studies (1994). Another explanation, expressed by Comings (who had published the observation of the (yet unreplicated) Pc-1A polymorphisms in suicides), was that the problems of replicating single genetic loci should actually be expected rather than surprising, if suicidality is a polygenic disorder (Comings, 2003). Comings further suggested that it makes more sense to study the 'additive and epistatic effects of multiple genes', which is today acknowledged and beginning to be applied in suicide genetics (Mullins et al., 2014; Sokolowski et al., 2016; Schild et al., 2013), after the first genome-wide study published in suicide genetics (Perlis et al., 2010).

While neither Nielsen, Goldman, nor Comings retained any particular focus on suicide genetics later on, but rather continued with investigations of other disorders, they made the initial contributions that moved the suicide research field from being all about twin and family studies, to investigating the molecular genetics of nature and nurture (Wasserman et al., 2007; Caspi et al., 2003) and their (often epigenetic) interactions.

Conclusion

Suicide is a global problem. Therefore, suicide prevention strategies—both universal (targeting the general public and population), selective (targeting vulnerable groups), and indicated (targeting individuals with diagnosed psychiatric disorders)—that are effective and supported by evidence-based research should be considered and implemented by public health policymakers and healthcare providers.

At the moment, quantitative methods of research dominate the field of suicidology. While quantitative methods are important, they are unable to provide a deeper understanding beyond simple linear cause and effect thinking. Therefore, moving forward, more qualitative research is needed to fill some of the knowledge gaps and to acquire a complete understanding of suicidal behaviours and barriers to the implementation of evidence-based methods (Wasserman et al., 2018; Rogers & Apel, 2010; Hjelmeland & Knizek, 2010).

The study from Gould et al. (2005) has been one of the most notable efforts to provide evidence that suicide risk is not increased by asking questions about suicide. Since that study, a significant amount of evidence has been accumulated showing that the concerns regarding the increased risk for individuals participating in suicide-related research are unsubstantiated. Instead, participation in suicide-related research may even be associated with small benefits. Therefore, as previously suggested by Dazzi and colleagues, ethical concerns about future research should be relaxed and more of a focus ought to be placed upon a risk–benefit analysis of evidence-based research (Dazzi et al., 2014). Otherwise, future research that is necessary may be hindered.

Developments and knowledge about the genetics of suicide and their interaction with the environment are continually evolving, enabling the creation of improved means for diagnosis, prevention, and treatment of suicidal behaviours in the future.

In this chapter, the described studies are considered landmark papers in the field of suicidology, showing the effectiveness of many suicide prevention methods, that talking about suicide does not increase suicide, and the genetics of suicidal behaviour.

References

Alvarez, A. (1990). *The Savage God: A Study of Suicide*. New York: W. W. Norton.

Anglemyer, A., Horvath, T., & Rutherford, G. (2014). The accessibility of firearms and risk for suicide and homicide victimization among household members: a systematic review and meta-analysis. *Annals of Internal Medicine*, **160**(2), 101–110.

Asberg, M., Träskman, L., & Thorén, P. (1976). 5-HIAA in the cerebrospinal fluid. A biochemical suicide predictor? *Archives of General Psychiatry*, **33**(10), 1193–1197.

Asenjo Lobos. C., et al. (2010). Clozapine versus other atypical antipsychotics for schizophrenia. *Cochrane Database of Systematic Reviews*, 11, CD006633.

Baldessarini, R. J., Tondo, L., Davis, P., Pompili, M., Goodwin, F. K., & Hennen, J. (2006). Decreased risk of suicides and attempts during long-term lithium treatment: a meta-analytic review. *Bipolar Disorder*, **8**(5p2), 625–639.

Bateman, K., Hansen, L., Turkington, D., & Kingdon, D. (2007). Cognitive behavioral therapy reduces suicidal ideation in schizophrenia: results from a randomized controlled trial. *Suicide and Life-Threatening Behavior*, **37**(3), 284–290.

Beautrais, A. L. (2001). Effectiveness of barriers at suicide jumping sites: a case study. *Australian and New Zealand Journal of Psychiatry*, **35**(5), 557–562.

Beautrais, A. L., Gibb, S. J., Faulkner, A., Fergusson, D. M., & Mulder, R. T. (2010). Postcard intervention for repeat self-harm: randomised controlled trial. *British Journal of Psychiatry*, **197**(1), 55–60.

Bertolote, J. M. (2004). Suicide prevention: at what level does it work? *World Psychiatry*, **3**(3),147–151.

Beskow, J., Gottfries, C. G., Roos, B. E., & Winblad, B. (1976). Determination of monoamine and monoamine metabolites in the human brain: post mortem studies in a group of suicides and in a control group. *Acta Psychiatrica Scandinavica*, **53**(1), 7–20.

Bezencon, E. (2001). The international federation of telephonic emergency services. In: *Suicide Prevention: Resources for the Millennium*, ed. D. Lester. New York: Routledge; pp. 274–282.

Blades, C. A., Stritzke, W. G. K., Page, A. C., & Brown, J. D. (2018). The benefits and risks of asking research participants about suicide: a meta-analysis of the impact of exposure to suicide-related content. *Clinical Psychology Review*, **64**, 1–12.

Brown, G. K., Have, T. T., Henriques, G. R., Xie, S. X., Hollander, J. E., & Beck, A. T. (2005). Cognitive therapy for the prevention of suicide attempts: a randomized controlled trial. *Journal of the American Medical Association*, **294**(5), 563–570.

Carlsten, A., Allebeck, P., & Brandt, L. (1996). Are suicide rates in Sweden associated with changes in the prescribing of medicines? *Acta Psychiatrica Scandinavica*, **94**(2), 94–100.

Carlsten, A., Waern, M., Ekedahl, A., & Ranstam, J. (2001). Antidepressant medication and suicide in Sweden. *Pharmacoepidemiology and Drug Safety*, **10**(6), 525–530.

Caspi, A., et al. (2003). Influence of life stress on depression: moderation by a polymorphism in the 5-HTT gene. *Science*, **301**(5631), 386–389.

Cipriani, A., Hawton, K., Stockton, S., & Geddes, J. R. (2013). Lithium in the prevention of suicide in mood disorders: updated systematic review and meta-analysis. *British Medical Journal*, **346**, f3646.

Comings, D. E. (1979). Pc 1 Duarte, a common polymorphism of a human brain protein, and its relationship to depressive disease and multiple sclerosis. *Nature*, **277**(5691), 28–32.

Comings, D. E. (2003). The real problem in association studies. *American Journal of Medical Genetics Part B: Neuropsychiatric Genetics*, **116B**(1), 102.

Dazzi, T., Gribble, R., Wessely, S., & Fear, N. T. (2014). Does asking about suicide and related behaviours induce suicidal ideation? What is the evidence? *Psychological Medicine*, **44**(16), 3361–3363.

Dieserud, G., Loeb, M., & Ekeberg, Ø. (2000). Suicidal behavior in the municipality of Bærum, Norway: a 12-year prospective study of parasuicide and suicide. *Suicide and Life-Threatening Behavior*, **30**(1), 61–73.

Durkheim, E. (2005). *Suicide: A Study in Sociology*. London: Routledge.

Etzersdorfer, E. & Sonneck, G. (1998). Preventing suicide by influencing mass-media reporting. The viennese experience 1980–1996. *Archives of Suicide Research*, **4**(1), 67–74.

Farberow, N. L. & Shneidman, E. S. (1961). *The Cry For Help*. New York: McGraw-Hill.

Gibbons, R. D., Hur, K., Bhaumik, D. K., & Mann, J. J. (2005). The relationship between antidepressant medication use and rate of suicide. *Archives of General Psychiatry*, **62**(2), 165–172.

Gibbons, R. D., Hur, K., Brown, C. H., & Mann, J. J. (2009). Relationship between antiepileptic drugs and suicide attempts in patients with bipolar disorder. *Archives of General Psychiatry*, **66**(12), 1354–1360.

Goldney, R. D. & Schioldann, J. A. (2000). Pre-Durkheim suicidology. *Crisis*, **21**(4), 181–186.

González-Castro, T. B., Juárez-Rojop, I., López-Narváez, M. L., & Tovilla-Zárate, C. A. (2014). Association of TPH-1 and TPH-2 gene polymorphisms with suicidal behavior: a systematic review and meta-analysis. *BMC Psychiatry*, **14**(1), 196.

Gould, M. S., et al. (2005). Evaluating iatrogenic risk of youth suicide screening programs: a randomized controlled trial. *Journal of the American Medical Association*, **293**(13), 1635–1643.

Gunnell, D., Fernando, R., Hewagama, M., Priyangika, W., Konradsen, F., & Eddleston, M. (2007). The impact of pesticide regulations on suicide in Sri Lanka. *International Journal of Epidemiology*, **36**(6), 1235–1242.

Guthrie, E., et al. (2001). Randomised controlled trial of brief psychological intervention after deliberate self poisoning. Commentary: another kind of talk that works? *British Medical Journal*, **323**(7305), 135.

Hall, W. D. (2003). Association between antidepressant prescribing and suicide in Australia, 1991–2000: trend analysis. *British Medical Journal*, **326**(7397), 1008.

Hawton, K. (2002). United Kingdom legislation on pack sizes of analgesics: background, rationale, and effects on suicide and deliberate self-harm. *Suicide and Life-Threatening Behavior*, **32**(3), 223–229.

Hawton, K., et al. (2000). Psychosocial versus pharmacological treatments for deliberate self harm. *Cochrane Database of Systematic Reviews*, 2, CD001764.

Hjelmeland, H. & Knizek, B. L. (2010). Why we need qualitative research in suicidology. *Suicide and Life-Threatening Behavior*, **40**(1), 74–80.

Jennings, C., Barraclough, B. M., & Moss, J. R. (1978). Have the Samaritans lowered the suicide rate? A controlled study. *Psychological Medicine*, **8**(3), 413–422.

Kaess, M., et al. (2014). Risk-behaviour screening for identifying adolescents with mental health problems in Europe. *European Child and Adolescent Psychiatry*, **23**(7), 611–620.

Kelly, S. & Bunting, J. (1998). Trends in suicide in England and Wales, 1982–96. *Population Trends*,92, 29–41.

Kessing, L. V., Søndergård, L., Kvist, K., & Andersen, P. K. (2005). Suicide risk in patients treated with lithium. *Archives of General Psychiatry*, **62**(8), 860–866.

Law, C., Sveticic, J., & Leo, D. D. (2014). Restricting access to a suicide hotspot does not shift the problem to another location. An experiment of two river bridges in Brisbane, Australia. *Australian and New Zealand Journal of Public Health*, **38**(2), 134–138.

Lester, D. (2001). *Suicide Prevention: Resources for the Millennium*. New York: Routledge.

Lester, D. & Leenaars, A. (1993). Suicide rates in Canada before and after tightening firearm control laws. *Psychological Reports*, 72(3), 787–790.

Li, Z., Page, A., Martin, G., & Taylor, R. (2011). Attributable risk of psychiatric and socio-economic factors for suicide from individual-level, population-based studies: a systematic review. *Social Science & Medicine*, **72**(4), 608–616.

Lin, P-I., Vance, J. M., Pericak-Vance, M. A., & Martin, E. R. (2007). No gene is an island: the flip-flop phenomenon. *American Journal of Human Genetics*, **80**(3), 531–538.

Linehan, M. M. (2006). Two-year randomized controlled trial and follow-up of dialectical behavior therapy vs therapy by experts for suicidal behaviors and borderline personality disorder. *Archives of General Psychiatry*, **63**(7), 757.

Litman, R. E., Shneidman, E. S., & Farberow, N. L. (1961). Los Angeles suicide prevention center. *American Journal of Psychiatry*, **117**, 1084–1087.

Lloyd, K. G., Farley, I. J., Deck, J. H., & Hornykiewicz, O. (1974). Serotonin and 5-hydroxyindoleacetic acid in discrete areas of the brainstem of suicide victims and control patients. *Advances in Biochemical Psychopharmacology*, **11**(0), 387–397.

Loftin, C., McDowall, D., Wiersema, B., & Cottey, T. J. (1991). Effects of restrictive licensing of handguns on homicide and suicide in the district of Columbia. *New England Journal of Medicine*, **325**(23), 1615-1620.

Lönnqvist, J. (1988). National suicide prevention project in Finland: a research phase of the project. *Psychiatria Fennica*, **19**, 125–132.

Ludwig, J. & Cook, P. J. (2000). Homicide and suicide rates associated with implementation of the Brady Handgun Violence Prevention Act. *Journal of the American Medical Association*, **284**(5), 585–591.

Maltsberger, J. T. & Buie, D. H. (1974). Countertransference hate in the treatment of suicidal patients. *Archives of General Psychiatry*, **30**(5), 625–633.

Mann, J. J., et al. (2005). Suicide prevention strategies: a systematic review. *Journal of the American Medical Association*, **294**(16), 2064–2074.

Maris, R. W. (1997). Social and familial risk factors in suicidal behavior. *Psychiatric Clinics of North America*, **20**(3), 519–550.

Marshall, M. & Rathbone, J. (2011). Early intervention for psychosis. *Schizophrenia Bulletin*, **37**(6), 1111–1114.

McClure, G. M. G. (2000). Changes in suicide in England and Wales, 1960–1997. *British Journal of Psychiatry*, **176**(1), 64–67.

McGowan, P. O., et al. (2009). Epigenetic regulation of the glucocorticoid receptor in human brain associates with childhood abuse. *Nature Neuroscience*, **12**(3), 342–348.

Mishara, B. L. (2001). Helplines and crisis intervention services: challenges for the future. In: *Suicide Prevention: Resources for the Millennium*. New York: Routledge; pp. 153–172.

Morselli, E. A. (1882). *Suicide: An Essay on Comparative Moral Statistics*. New York: Appleton.

Mott. J. A., et al. (2002). National vehicle emissions policies and practices and declining US carbon monoxide-related mortality. *Journal uf the American Medical Association*, **288**(8), 988–995.

Mullins, N., et al. (2014). Genetic relationships between suicide attempts, suicidal ideation and major psychiatric disorders: a genome-wide association and polygenic scoring study. *American Journal of Medical Genetics Part B: Neuropsychiatric Genetics*, **165**(5), 428–437.

Nielsen, A. S. & Nielsen, B. (1992). [Pattern of choice in preparation of attempted suicide by poisoning—with particular reference to changes in the pattern of prescriptions]. *Ugeskr Laeger*, **154**(28), 1972–1976.

Nielsen, D. A., Dean, M., & Goldman, D. (1992). Genetic mapping of the human tryptophan hydroxylase gene on chromosome 11, using an iatronic conformational polymorphism. *American Journal of Human Genetics*, **51**(6), 1366–1371.

Nielsen, D. A., Goldman, D., Virkkunen, M., Tokola, R., Rawlings, R., & Linnoila, M. (1994). Suicidality and 5-hydroxyindoleacetic acid concentration associated with a tryptophan hydroxylase polymorphism. *Archives of General Psychiatry*, **51**(1), 34–38.

Nielsen, D. A., Jenkins, G. L., Stefanisko, K. M., Jefferson, K. K., & Goldman, D. (1997). Sequence, splice site and population frequency distribution analyses of the polymorphic human tryptophan hydroxylase intron 7. *Brain Research Molecular Brain Research*, **45**(1), 145–148.

Nielsen, D. A., et al. (1998). A tryptophan hydroxylase gene marker for suicidality and alcoholism. *Archives of General Psychiatry*, **55**(7), 593–602.

Olfson, M., Shaffer, D., Marcus, S. C., & Greenberg, T. (2003). Relationship between antidepressant medication treatment and suicide in adolescents. *Archives of General Psychiatry*, **60**(10), 978–982.

Oliver, R. G. & Hetzel, B. S. (1973). An analysis of recent trends in suicide rates in Australia. *International Journal of Epidemiology*, **2**(1), 91–101.

Perlis, R. H., et al. (2010). Genome-wide association study of suicide attempts in mood disorder patients. *American Journal of Psychiatry*, **167**(12), 1499–1507.

Pirkis, J., Spittal, M. J., Cox, G., Robinson, J., Cheung, Y. T. D., & Studdert, D. (2013). The effectiveness of structural interventions at suicide hotspots: a meta-analysis. *International Journal of Epidemiology*, **42**(2), 541–548.

Retterstøl, P. N. (1989). Norwegian data on death due to overdose of antidepressants. *Acta Psychiatrica Scandinavica*, **80**(S354), 61–68.

Rihmer, Z., Belsö, N., & Kalmár, S. (2001). Antidepressants and suicide prevention in Hungary. *Acta Psychiatrica Scandinavica*, **103**(3), 238–239.

Ringel, E. (1988). Founder's perspectives—then and now. *Suicide andLife Threatening Behavior*, **18**(1), 13–19.

Ringel, E. (1997). *Der Selbstmord: Abschluss Einer Krankhaften Psychischen Entwicklung; Eine Untersuchung an 745 Geretteten Selbstmördern*. Eschborn, Germany: Klotz.

Rogers, J. R. & Apel, S. (2010). Revitalizing suicidology: a call for mixed methods designs. *Suicidology Online*, **1**, 92–94.

Roy, A. (1993). Genetic and biologic risk factors for suicide in depressive disorders. *Psychiatric Quarterly*, **64**(4), 345–358.

Rutz, W. (2001). Preventing suicide and premature death by education and treatment. *Journal of Affective Disorders*, **62**(1), 123–129.

Rutz, W., Wålinder, J., Von Knorring, L., Rihmer, Z., & Pihlgren, H. (1997). Prevention of depression and suicide by education and medication: impact on male suicidality. An update from the Gotland study. *International Journal of Psychiatry in Clinical Practice*, **1**(1), 39–46.

Schild, A. H. E., Pietschnig, J., Tran, U. S., & Voracek, M. (2013). Genetic association studies between SNPs and suicidal behavior: a meta-analytical field synopsis. *Progress in Neuro-Psychopharmacology and Biological Psychiatry*, **46**, 36–42.

Schmidtke, A. & Häfner, H. (1988). The Werther effect after television films: new evidence for an old hypothesis. *Psychological Medicine*, **18**(3), 665–676.

Shelef, M. (1994). Unanticipated benefits of automotive emission control: reduction in fatalities by motor vehicle exhaust gas. *Science of the Total Environment*, 146–147, 93–101.

Shneidman, E. S. (1993). *Suicide as Psychache: A Clinical Approach to Self-Destructive Behavior*. Lanham, MD, USA: Jason Aronson.

Sokolowski, M., Wasserman, J., & Wasserman, D. (2015). An overview of the neurobiology of suicidal behaviors as one meta-system. *Molecular Psychiatry*, **20**(1), 56–71.

Sokolowski, M., Wasserman, J., & Wasserman, D. (2016). Polygenic associations of neurodevelopmental genes in suicide attempt. *Molecular Psychiatry*, **21**(10), 1381–1390.

Stack, S. (2001). Sociological research into suicide. In: *Suicide Prevention: Resources for the Millennium*. New York: Routledge; pp. 17–29.

Stengel, E. (1964). *Suicide and Attempted Suicide*. Baltimore, MD.: Penguin Books.

Takahashi, K. (1998). Suicide prevention for the elderly in Matsunoyama Town, Higashikubiki County Niigata Prefecture: psychiatric care for elderly depression in the community. *Folia Psychiatrica et Neurologica Japonica*, **100**, 469–485.

Taylor, L. M. W., Oldershaw, A., Richards, C., Davidson, K., Schmidt, U., & Simic, M. (2011). Development and pilot evaluation of a manualized cognitive-behavioural treatment package for adolescent self-harm. *Behavioural and Cognitive Psychotherapy*, **39**(5), 619–625.

Tompkins, T. L., Witt, J., & Abraibesh, N. (2010). Does a gatekeeper suicide prevention program work in a school setting? Evaluating training outcome and moderators of effectiveness. *Suicide and Life-Threatening Behavior*, **40**(5), 506–515.

Varah, C. (1962). How 'the Samaritans' combat suicide. *Mental Health (London)*, **21**(4), 132–134.

Wasserman, C., Postuvan, V., Herta, D., Iosue, M., Värnik, P., & Carli, V. (2018). Interactions between youth and mental health professionals: the Youth Aware of Mental health (YAM) program experience. *PLOS One*, **13**(2), e0191843.

Wasserman, D., Geijer, T., Sokolowski, M., Rozanov, V., & Wasserman, J. (2007). Nature and nurture in suicidal behavior, the role of genetics: some novel findings concerning personality traits and neural conduction. *Physiology & Behavior*, **92**(1–2), 245–249.

Wasserman, D., et al. (2015). School-based suicide prevention programmes: the SEYLE cluster-randomised, controlled trial. *Lancet*, **385**(9977), 1536–1544.

Wasserman, D. & Sokolowski, M. (2016). Stress-vulnerability model of suicidal behaviours. In: *Suicide: An Unnecessary Death*, 2nd edn. Oxford/New York: Oxford University Press; pp. 21–37.

Wasserman, D. & Wasserman, C. (eds). (2009).*Oxford Textbook of Suicidology and Suicide Prevention: A Global Perspective*. Oxford/New York: Oxford University Press.

Wasserman, D. & Wasserman, J. (1994). Danger of assisted suicide for patients with mental suffering. *Lancet*, **344**(8925), 822–823.

Weinberg, I., Gunderson, J. G., Hennen, J., & Cutter, C. J. (2006). Manual assisted cognitive treatment for deliberate self-harm in borderline personality disorder patients. *Journal of Personality Disorders*, **20**(5), 482–492.

Wolk-Wasserman, D. (1986). Suicidal communication of persons attempting suicide and responses of significant others. *Acta Psychiatrica Scandinavica*, **73**(5), 481–499.

World Health Organization. (2008). *Preventing Suicide: A Resource For Media Professionals.* Geneva: World Health Organization.

World Health Organization. (2014). *Preventing Suicide: A Global Imperative*, ed. S. Saxena, E. G. Krug, & O. Chestnov. Geneva: World Health Organization.

World Health Organization. (2017). *Preventing Suicide: A Resource For Media Professionals, Update 2017.* Geneva: World Health Organization.

Zalsman, G., et al. (2016). Suicide prevention strategies revisited: 10-year systematic review. *Lancet Psychiatry*, **3**(7), 646–659.

Chapter 23

Research methodology

Robert D. Gibbons

Introduction

Psychiatry has long been a very fertile area for methodological and statistical research. One reason is that psychiatric research is a microcosm of scientific work in general, with diverse subfields in particular. These psychiatric subfields include imaging, genetics, molecular biology, mental health services research, psychiatric epidemiology, and research related to the development of taxonomies based on clinical symptomatology (e.g. diagnosis) and biology (biological subtyping), to name a few. Each of these important areas has methodological features of interest related to experimental design, statistical modelling, and techniques for measurement.

While there have been many important contributions in mental health statistics and related quantitative research methodology, the chapter focuses on those areas that were motivated by problems considered in psychiatry and psychology, yet have spilled over to many other fields in the biological, social, and physical sciences. Notably, these areas include the analysis of longitudinal data, inter-rater agreement, and measurement. With respect to longitudinal data analysis (LDA), the chapter focuses on the paper by Robert Gibbons and colleagues (1993), since it led to the widespread adoption of mixed-effects regression models in the medical sciences, and the paper by Donald Hedeker and colleagues (2008), since it introduced the location-scale model for analysis of intensive longitudinal data. With respect to item response theory (IRT) and computerized adaptive testing (CAT), the chapter focuses on the paper by Gibbons et al. (2012), since it generalized the field of IRT-based CAT to the measurement of multidimensional constructs (e.g. depression). Finally, in the area of inter-rater agreement, the chapter focuses on the pioneering paper by Jacob Cohen (1960) which developed the kappa statistic—the most widely used measure of inter-rater agreement in psychiatric research and many other areas of medicine and beyond.

While there are many notable examples of papers from each of these areas in the psychiatric literature, the chapter focuses on four foundational sets of papers. The interested reader is referred to the landmark papers on mixed-effects regression models by Laird (1982), and multidimensional IRT by Bock and Aitkin (1981), which present critical contributions to LDA and IRT from the fields of biostatistics and psychometrics respectively.

Some conceptual and statistical issues in analysis of longitudinal data

Main citation

Gibbons, R. D., et al. (1993). Some conceptual and statistical issues in analysis of longitudinal psychiatric data. *Archives of General Psychiatry*, 50, 739–750.

Background

At the time that this paper was written, longitudinal studies were the exception rather than the rule as they are today. As the authors note, 'statistical methods for analysing these data are rarely commensurate with the effort involved in their acquisition' (Gibbons et al., 1993, p. 739). The traditional approach to analysis of longitudinal data often relied upon simple endpoint analyses, restricted to only those subjects who completed the study, or imputing the last available observation as though it were the final observation. This latter approach, known as last observation carried forward (LOCF), was a favourite of the American Food and Drug Administration (FDA). The FDA viewed the approach of imputing the last available observation as what would have been observed at the end of the study as a conservative approach, and therefore preferred it to the more statistically sophisticated and more complete analysis of all of the available data under more general assumptions for the missing data. There are those in the FDA who continue to be under the misconception that imputing the last available observation is a more ideal approach. It was not until 2009, when FDA statisticians conducted an extensive simulation study and performed reanalysis of 25 new drug application (NDA) datasets, that this misconception was clarified (Siddiqui et al., 2009). These authors discovered that analyses based on LOCF can yield 'substantial biases in estimators of treatment effects and can greatly inflate Type I error rates of statistical tests', whereas the methods described in this 1993 landmark paper show mixed-effects regression models 'lead[s] to estimators with comparatively small bias, and controls Type I error rates at a nominal level in the presence of missing completely at random (MCAR) or missing at random (MAR) and some possibility of missing not at random (MNAR) data' (Siddiqui et al., 2009, p. 227).

There are several interesting backstories regarding this paper. The National Institute of Mental Health (NIMH) had recently completed its Treatment of Depression Collaborative Research Program (TDCRP) study (Elkin et al., 1989). The study was originally designed as a comparison of two psychotherapies—interpersonal psychotherapy (IPT) and cognitive behaviour therapy (CBT); however, objections from outspoken members of the psychiatric community led to the addition of a pharmacotherapy treatment arm—imipramine plus clinical management (IMI-CM) and, of course, placebo plus clinical management (PLA-CM). The original analysis of these data were conducted using LOCF and the following predefined contrasts stated in their null form as (1) no difference between the two psychotherapies, (2) no difference between pharmacotherapy and placebo, and (3) no difference between pharmacotherapy and the two combined psychotherapies. These pre-specified analyses failed to identify a statistically significant difference between pharmacotherapy and psychotherapy, and ultimately led to insurance reimbursement for psychologists and social workers performing psychotherapy (following several lawsuits).

A meeting was held at the University of Pittsburgh between several leading figures in psychiatry at the time and two of the statisticians who ultimately authored this landmark paper. The question was whether the analysis of the TDCRP data was appropriate and whether newer approaches to the more complete analysis of longitudinal data would lead to the same or different conclusions. The statistical authors obtained the NIMH TDCRP dataset, reanalysed them using linear mixed-effects regression models, and took the opportunity to publish the results of their analysis along with a very detailed discussion of statistical issues in longitudinal data analysis. As a side note, the authors decided to submit the paper to the leading substantive journal in psychiatry at the time, the *Archives of General Psychiatry*, where they thought it would have the greatest impact on statistical practice. The editor, Dr Daniel X. Freedman, complained that 'his readers barely understood the biology published in the journal, how would they possibly be able to understand complex statistical issues' (personal communication). However, he agreed to send it out for review. The statistical reviewer, Professor Joe Fleiss of Columbia University's Department of Biostatistics, explained that this was the most clearly written description of this new area of statistics that he had ever seen, that it could not be made clearer, and that Freedman had to publish it, which he did.

Methodology

The paper makes several important points about the analysis of longitudinal data in general and the usefulness of mixed-effects regression models (which the authors called 'random regression models'—RRM) in particular. They begin by describing the various approaches to longitudinal data analysis at the time that included endpoint analyses, repeated-measures analysis of variance (ANOVA), and multivariate repeated measures analyses. The strengths and weaknesses of these methods are compared, and then the more general approach based on RRM is described. The key features highlighted in the paper include (1) the treatment of missing data, (2) borrowing strength across individuals, (3) the use of all available data to estimate the person-specific time trends which form the basis for the analysis, (4) inclusion of time-varying and time-invariant covariates, and (5) various forms of correlated errors of measurement. The authors also provide a non-technical description of the statistical theory of estimation, which is a mixture of marginal maximum likelihood and empirical Bayes for the person-specific trends. The authors then illustrate the analytical approach in a reanalysis of the TDCRP data.

Results

Results of the reanalysis of the TDCRP data were informative. The two psychotherapies were not statistically differentiable; however, imipramine had a significantly faster rate of improvement relative to placebo. When data through 12 weeks of treatment were analysed, a significant improvement in patients treated with pharmacotherapy over psychotherapy was found. None of the analyses showed a difference between the two psychotherapies relative to each other or relative to placebo. This was a markedly different result than originally found using LOCF.

Conclusions and critique

Regardless of which horse you bet on, this paper laid the foundation for the use of generalized mixed-effects regression models for analysis of longitudinal psychiatric data. Surprisingly, based on its citations, this paper also led to widespread use of modern statistical methods for longitudinal data analysis throughout most areas in medical research, as well as many areas in the behavioural and social sciences. At the time of publication of this book, this paper has been cited over 825 times. Although it presents advanced statistical concepts, it does so without a single equation. Perhaps this accounts for its large impact on statistical practice among non-statisticians.

Computerized adaptive testing of mental health disorders

Main citations

Gibbons R. D., et al. (2012). Development of a computerized adaptive test for depression. *Journal of the American Medical Association Psychiatry*, 69, 1104–1112.

Gibbons R. D., et al. (2013). The CAD-MDD: a computerized adaptive diagnostic screening tool for depression. *Journal of Clinical Psychiatry*, 74, 669–674.

Gibbons R. D., et al. (2014). Development of the CAT-ANX: a computerized adaptive test for anxiety. *American Journal of Psychiatry*, 171, 187–194.

Gibbons R. D. (2016). Computerized adaptive diagnosis and testing of mental health disorders. *Annual Review of Clinical Psychology*, 12, 83–104.

Gibbons R. D., Kupfer, D., Frank, E., Moore, T., Beiser, D., & Boudreaux, E. (2017). Development of a computerized adaptive suicide scale. *Journal of Clinical Psychiatry*, 78, 1376–1382.

Background

Traditional mental health screening and measurement have been based largely on classical test theory. Fixed-length scales are developed based on clinical judgement and are scored by a counting operation, the sum of the individual item ratings. Typically, short-form versions of these scales are developed to minimize patient and clinician burden. In some cases, ratings are based on clinician judgement (e.g. the Hamilton Rating Scale for Depression—HAM-D) and in other cases, ratings are based on self-report (e.g. Patient Health Questionnaire (PHQ)-9). An alternative to full-scale administration is to develop a very large bank of symptom items and adaptively administer a much smaller set of these that are targeted to the severity of each individual. The paradigm shift is from fixed-length tests with varying precision across individuals or within the same individual over time, to adaptive tests which fix the precision of measurement and allow the items to vary both in number and in content from subject to subject. The net result is that we can increase the precision of measurement, by extracting the information from hundreds and possibly thousands of symptom items that would take hours to administer, and decrease the burden of measurement for the clinician to a minute or two.

Unlike educational measurement in which computerized adaptive testing (CAT) is based on unidimensional item response theory (IRT), in mental health measurement, the constructs are inherently multidimensional and CAT must incorporate this multidimensionality in order to obtain accurate measurements. Multidimensional IRT (MIRT)-based CAT was initially introduced in the first of these landmark papers, in 2012 (Gibbons et al., 2012). The specific MIRT model used is the bifactor model (Gibbons & Hedeker, 1992) which was the first confirmatory item-factor analysis model, appropriate for binary and/or ordinal (Gibbons et al., 2007) item responses. The collection of landmark papers identified here illustrates the use of this technology for the measurement of depression, anxiety, mania, hypomania, and suicidality. These landmark papers also describe the first computerized adaptive diagnostic (CAD) screener for major depressive disorder (MDD).

Methodology

While the development of a traditional psychiatric measurement instrument is relatively straightforward, the development of CAT is far more complex, as illustrated in these papers. First, we begin by using clinical judgement and existing measurement instruments to create a large bank of hundreds, and possibly thousands, of symptom items. Second, we administer either the entire bank of items or subsets of the bank to a large number of individuals (e.g. 1,000 or more) and obtain the item responses. The critical goal is that the patients represent the full range of symptomatology, and therefore patients with and without the mental health disorder of interest are included in the calibration sample. Third, the calibration data are analysed using a bifactor IRT model which assumes that all items are dependent on the primary dimension of interest (e.g. depression) and a subdomain from which the items are drawn (e.g. mood disorder, cognitive impairment, somatization, suicidality). Our interest is typically in the primary dimension; however, the presence of the subdomains incorporates residual dependence among the items based on the subdomain from which they were drawn. From this statistical analysis phase, we can identify a subset of the total item bank that fully characterizes the primary dimension of interest and provides information throughout the entire severity range, from feelings of sadness through suicidality. Fourth, from a subset of subjects that took the entire bank of items, we can simulate the adaptive testing and optimize a series of CAT-tuning parameters. Examples of possible parameters include the uncertainty at termination, secondary termination criteria based on remaining item information, and parameters that select the next maximally informative item or the second most informative item conditional on the current estimated severity score. Fifth, the live CAT is then administered to a new sample of patients, which controls and validates against existing scales or gold-standard structured clinical interviews such as the Structured Clinical Interview for the DSM (SCID) for DSM-5 diagnoses. The development of CAT is far more time and resource intensive than the development of a traditional mental health measurement tool based on classical test theory; however, once developed it is much easier to use and has numerous advantages over traditional instruments.

It should be noted that diagnosis and measurement are fundamentally different things. For diagnosis, or diagnostic screening, we require items at the threshold or tipping point between a negative and a positive diagnostic classification; whereas for measurement, we want to centre the items at the severity level of the individual. While MIRT-based CAT is used for measurement, these authors use machine learning (Random Forests) for diagnostic screening. The difference is that for diagnosis there is an external criterion (i.e. DSM-5 diagnosis), where for measurement, the CAT is criterion-free.

Results

In their 2012 paper, Gibbons et al. showed that for the measurement of depression, using an average of 12 adaptively administered items, they were able to extract information from a 389-item bank, yet maintain a correlation of $r = 0.95$ with the 389-item bank score. Test–retest reliability was $r = 0.92$, which is substantially higher than test–retest reliability for the PHQ-9 ($r = 0.8$), despite repeat assessment using different items (Beiser et al., 2016). Similar results were obtained for anxiety, mania, hypomania, and suicidality. For diagnostic screening, they were able to reproduce an hour-long SCID DSM-5 clinician diagnosis with sensitivity of 0.95 and specificity of 0.87 using an average of four items in 36 seconds. In the same subjects, the PHQ-9 had sensitivity of only 0.7.

Conclusions and critique

Adaptive testing of mental health disorders opens up new opportunities for increasing the precision of mental health diagnostic screening and measurement, and in tandem decreasing patient burden and eliminating clinician burden. Using cloud-based administration, screening and measurement is no longer limited to the clinic or clinician's office. Indeed, these authors have illustrated daily depression measurement in a patient's home over a six-month period (Sani et al., 2017). Since different items are presented on repeated assessments, the response bias associated with repeated administration of traditional fixed-length tests is eliminated.

Applications of this emerging technology are being used to screen and measure mental health constructs in primary care, emergency medicine, obstetrics and gynaecology, as well as to perform large-scale detection and monitoring in jails, bond courts, juvenile justice, detention, and foster-care systems. A prime example of the robust application of this tool is at UCLA, where they recently screened their entire freshman class for depression, anxiety, and suicidality using these methods. They immediately triaged those with significant pathology to internet cognitive therapy, face-to-face psychotherapy, and/or pharmacotherapy based on their CAT-based estimated severity of illness. New tests for substance abuse, psychosis, post-traumatic stress disorder, functional impairment, and well-being in cancer survivors are either currently available or being developed and/or validated, as are detailed self-rated and parent-rated assessments of children as young as seven.

Inter-rater agreement

Main citations

Cohen, J. (1960). A coefficient of agreement for nominal scales. *Educational and Psychological Measurement*, 20, 37–46.
Fleiss, J. L., Cohen, J., & Everitt, B. S. (1969). Large sample standard errors of kappa and weighted kappa. *Psychological Bulletin*, 72, 323-327.
Fleiss, J. L. (1971). Measuring nominal scale agreement among many raters. *Psychological Bulletin*, 76, 378–382.
Kraemer, H. C. (1980). Extension of the kappa coefficient. *Biometrics*, 36, 207–216.

Background

The coefficient kappa has a long and rich history in psychiatric research. Kappa is a chance-corrected measure of nominal-scale agreement among raters that has widespread application to the problem of establishing inter-rater agreement. The problem is of particular importance in psychiatric research because it provides an index of the degree to which two or more clinicians will agree on a potentially fallible diagnostic classification. The original contribution by Cohen, in 1960, considered the case of two raters making a binary diagnostic classification. Kappa has been extended in several ways to include (1) weighted kappa which differentially weights different misclassifications, (2) multiple response categories, (3) more than two raters, (4) unequal number of ratings per subject, and (5) multiple choices in which a subject may be simultaneously classified in two or more categories. Kappa has been used extensively to establish the inter-rater reliability of DSM classifications. Most recently, the DSM-5 has been shown to have unacceptably low inter-rater agreement for several common disorders, including major depressive disorder (Regier et al., 2013). Discussion of a kappa-like statistic can be found as early as Galton (1892).

Methodology

In the most general case, kappa measures the agreement between two or more raters who classify each of 'N' individuals into 'C' mutually exclusive categories. It is essentially the difference between observed and expected chance agreement divided by the expected chance disagreement. If the raters are in complete agreement, then kappa = 1. To measure the probability of chance agreement, kappa uses the marginal observed proportions for each category and rater. If, for example, one rater rated the diagnosis present 40% of the time and the other rated it present 50% of the time, then the probability that they would both rate a patient positive is $0.4 \times 0.5 = 0.2$, and the probability of both rating a patient negative is $0.6 \times 0.5 = 0.3$. The probability of chance agreement is therefore $0.2 + 0.3 = 0.5$. Although a relatively simple idea, it has played a major role in psychiatric research methodology because of the general uncertainty in diagnostic classifications and their importance in understanding the biology, genetics, and epidemiology of psychiatric disorders.

Results

As previously noted, Cohen, Joseph Fleiss, and Helena Kraemer have extended kappa in numerous ways that are highly relevant to psychiatric research. Kappa is quite conservative in its magnitude and becomes even more conservative as the rate of the underlying disorder becomes small. The most recent high-profile use of kappa is in connection with the DSM-5 field trials. Estimates of kappa were quite low for common disorders such as major depressive disorder (kappa = 0.28). Overall, three diagnoses (post-traumatic stress disorder, complex somatic symptom disorder, and major neurocognitive disorder) were in the very good range (kappa = 0.60–0.79), seven (schizophrenia, schizoaffective disorder, bipolar I disorder, binge eating disorder, alcohol use disorder, mild neurocognitive disorder, and borderline personality disorder) were in the good range (kappa = 0.40–0.59), four (major depressive disorder, generalized anxiety disorder, mild traumatic brain injury, antisocial personality disorder) were in the questionable range (kappa = 0.20–0.39), and one (mixed anxiety-depressive disorder) was in the unacceptable range (kappa < 0.20). Differences in inter-rater reliability between previous iterations of the DSM criteria and the current criteria have been attributed to differences in the experimental protocols, where the current field trials have been argued to be more representative of routine practice (Kraemer, 2012).

Conclusions and critique

Inter-rater reliability or agreement has played an important role in psychiatric research, and the development of kappa as a more rigorous way of statistically describing the degree of agreement grew out of the need to measure agreement in psychiatric research studies. Unlike other areas of medicine in which diagnosis is aided by often reliable laboratory tests, including results of imaging and molecular genetic tests, psychiatric research has made limited progress in the identification of such diagnostic aids. Instead, careful description of the manifestation of these disorders, in terms of psychopathological symptoms and behaviour, forms the foundation of psychiatric diagnostic classifications and sets an upper limit on the degree to which different raters agree on the diagnostic classification of a given patient. The development of kappa has been an important addition to the psychiatric research methodology literature because it provides an improved index of agreement that is adjusted for chance.

Location-scale models

Main citations

Hedeker, D., Mermelstein, R. J., & Demirtas, H. (2008). An application of a mixed-effects location scale model for analysis of Ecological Momentary Assessment (EMA) data. *Biometrics*, 64, 627–634.

Hedeker, D., Mermelstein, R. J., & Demirtas, H. (2012). Modeling between- and within-subject variance in Ecological Momentary Assessment (EMA) data using mixed-effects location scale models. *Statistics in Medicine*, 31, 3328–3336.

Background

The majority of statistical theory and practice concerns the mean function. For example, in a randomized clinical trial of a new medical treatment, we are interested in whether the treatment decreases the severity of the illness as measured by a quantitative score on a psychological or behavioural trait. When the data are longitudinal, generalized mixed-effects regression models (see the section 'Some conceptual and statistical issues in analysis of longitudinal data') can be used to estimate the difference in average rate of change between treated and control subjects over the course of the study. The treatment that produces the largest average change in rate of improvement is generally selected as the best treatment for that indication. Two different treatments with similar rates of improvement are often considered exchangeable, assuming that their side-effect profiles are comparable.

With advances in measurement (see the section 'Computerized adaptive testing of mental health disorders') and as 'high-frequency' and 'intensive' longitudinal datasets become available, new and highly innovative approaches to the analysis of these data can involve not only the mean function, but the variability as well. Working in the area of smoking-cessation research, these authors have developed 'location-scale' mixed-effects models that can simultaneously model both the mean and variance of a data-intensive longitudinal study. This model allows us to identify treatments and interventions which not only maximize the average clinical response, but do so in a way that minimizes variability. Two treatments that are equivalent in terms of their reduction in average symptomatology may be quite different in terms of the variability in that symptomatology as measured over time. Covariates including, but not limited to, treatment alone may also be important predictors of the variability in the responses from the overall mean trend line. We seek the treatment that produces a large and statistically significant reduction in average severity over time, while at the same time a treatment that minimizes both within-subject and between-subject variability in the longitudinal response process.

Methodology

The location-scale model is a generalized mixed-effects regression model that includes a linear model for the mean function and a log-linear model for the variance function. In terms of the variance function, we can estimate the effects of covariates (including treatment) on both between-subject (BS) and within-subject (WS) variance components. For BS, we can only examine the effects of individual-level (time-invariant) covariates, whereas for the WS variance component, both individual-level and time-specific covariate effects are estimatable. In addition, the WS variance can itself vary between individuals, above and beyond the effects accounted for by the covariates. In this way, individual units or subjects are allowed to deviate in their own specific way from the overall mean trend line, but they are also allowed to vary in terms of the variability of their deviations from the overall trend line over time. Here, the mean refers to the location of the measurement and the scale refers to its variance; hence, the term mixed-effects location-scale model. These authors have developed estimation procedures for these models and developed software that can be used by investigators to fit these models within intensive longitudinal data.

Results

The landmark papers listed here present applications of this new statistical methodology to mood-regulation problems in adolescent smoking studies. They found that in terms of negative affect (NA) and positive affect (PA), there is considerable BS variability in both. In addition, the mean and variance are positively correlated for NA (higher scores show more variability) and negatively correlated for PA (higher scores show less variance). Greater negative affect leads to more variable responses over time, and the reverse is true for greater positive affect. Smoking increases the mean negative affect and the within-subject variability, but not the between-subject variability. By contrast, smoking had no effect on positive affect.

Conclusions and critique

The development of the mixed-effects location-scale model is a major advance for psychiatric research methodology. It exposes a completely new dimension of the longitudinal treatment-response process that has, for the most part, been previously unexplored. As intensive longitudinal data become more available in psychiatric research, through the use of ecological momentary assessments, daily diaries, experience sampling, and high-frequency administration of computerized adaptive tests, these new statistical models will help us answer even more penetrating questions regarding the nature of the longitudinal response process and our ability to identify differential treatment effects.

Conclusion

This chapter highlights only a handful of important statistical contributions to psychiatric research methodology. The chapter leaves out far more than has been included. Statistical contributions to causal inference, imaging, and molecular genetics are some areas not highlighted. However, the chapter attempts to highlight those statistical advances, such as the mixed-effects location-scale model, that were directly motivated by problems in psychiatric research or problems that are particularly relevant to the psychiatric research community. As technology increases our access to various forms of high-dimensional data, the need for relevant statistical methods will continue to grow. An important cautionary note regarding the availability of 'big data' in psychiatric research is that 'big data' are invariably observational data, and observational data are highly prone to bias. A randomized clinical trial with a few hundred participants may well have the same or even more information than a slightly biased observational dataset that includes half the American population (Meng, 2014).

References

Beiser, D., Vu, M., & Gibbons, R. (2016). Test-retest reliability of a computerized adaptive depression test. *Psychiatric Services*, **67**, 1039–1041.

Bock, R. D. & Aitkin, M. (1981). Marginal maximum likelihood estimation of item parameters: application of an EM algorithm. *Psychometrika*, **46**, 443–459.

Cohen, J. (1960). A coefficient of agreement for nominal scales. *Educational and Psychological Measurement*, **20**(1), 37–46.

Elkin, I., et al. (1989). National Institute of Mental Health Treatment of Depression Collaborative Research Program: general effectiveness of treatments. *Archives of General Psychiatry*, **46**, 971–982.

Galton, F. (1892). *Finger Prints*. London: Macmillan.

Gibbons, R. & Hedeker, D. (1992). Full-information item bi-factor analysis. *Psychometrika*, **57**, 423–436.

Gibbons, R. D., et al. (1993). Some conceptual and statistical issues in analysis of longitudinal psychiatric data. *Archives of General Psychiatry*, **50**, 739–750.

Gibbons, R., et al. (2007). Full-information item bi-factor analysis of graded response data. *Applied Psychological Measurement*, **31**, 4–19.

Gibbons R. D., et al. (2012). Development of a computerized adaptive test for depression. *Journal of the American Medical Association Psychiatry*, **69**, 1104–1112.

Hedeker, D., Mermelstein, R. J., & Demirtas, H. (2008). An application of a mixed-effects location scale model for analysis of Ecological Momentary Assessment (EMA) data. *Biometrics*, **64**, 627–634.

Kraemer, H., Kupfer, D., Clarke, D., Narrow, W., & Regier, D. (2012). DSM-5: how reliable is reliable enough? *American Journal of Psychiatry*, **169**(1), 13–15.

Laird, N. M. & Ware, J. H. (1982). Random-effects models for longitudinal data. *Biometrics*, **38**, 963–974.

Meng, X-L. (2014). A trio of inference problems that could win you a Nobel Prize in statistics (if you help fund it). In: *Past, Present, and Future of Statistical Science*, ed. X. Lin, C. Genest, D. L. Banks, G. Molenberghs, D. W. Scott, & J-L. Wang. Boca Raton, FL: CRC Press; pp. 537–562.

Regier, D., et al. (2013). DSM-5 field trials in the Unites States and Canada. Part II: Test-retest reliability of selected categorical diagnoses. *American Journal of Psychiatry*, **170**(1), 59–70.

Sani, S., Busnello, J., Kochanski, R., Cohen, Y., & Gibbons, R. (2017). High frequency measurement of depressive severity in a patient treated for severe treatment resistant depression with deep brain stimulation. *Translational Psychiatry*, 7, e1207.

Siddique, O., Hung, J., & O'Neill, R. (2009). MMRM vs. LOCF: a comprehensive comparison based on simulation study and 25 NDA datasets. *Journal of Biopharmaceutical Statistics*, **19**, 227–246.

Index

Tables and figures are indicated by *t* and *f* following the page number

For the benefit of digital users, indexed terms that span two pages (e.g., 52–53) may, on occasion, appear on only one of those pages.

Note: The only names included in the index are those of cited authors of each landmark paper.

B

E

O

Q

T